Behavioral Neurology

Third Edition

JONATHAN H. PINCUS, M.D.
Professor of Neurology
Yale University School of Medicine

GARY J. TUCKER, M.D.
Professor and Chairman
Department of Psychiatry and Behavioral Sciences
University of Washington School of Medicine

New York   Oxford
OXFORD UNIVERSITY PRESS
1985

OXFORD UNIVERSTIY PRESS

Oxford   London   New York   Toronto
Delhi   Bombay   Calcutta   Madras   Karachi
Kuala Lumpur   Singapore   Hong Kong   Tokyo
Nairobi   Dar es Salaam   Cape Town
Melbourne   Auckland

and associated companies in
Beirut   Berlin   Ibadan   Mexico City   Nicosia

Published by Oxford University Press, Inc., 200 Madison Avenue
New York, New York 10016

Library of Congress Cataloging in Publication Data
Pincus, Johathan H., 1935-
Behavioral neurology.
Includes bibliographies and index.
1. Neuropsychiatry.   2. Neurology.   3. Human
behavior.   I. Tucker, Gary J., 1934-   . II. Title.
[DNLM: 1. Mental Disorders.   2. Nervous System
Diseases. WL 100 P649b]
RC341.P56   1985   616.89   84-29579
ISBN 0-19-503554-2
ISBN 0-19-503555-0 (pbk.)

Printing (last digit): 9   8   7   6   5   4   3   2   1

Printed in the United States of America

Behavioral Neurology

This book is dedicated to our teachers, Gilbert H. Glaser and Thomas P. Detre, whose interests have stimulated our own.

"It ought to be generally known that the source of our pleasure, merriment, laughter, and amusement, as of our grief, pain, anxiety, and tears, is none other than the brain. It is specially the organ which enables us to think, see, and hear, and to distinguish the ugly and the beautiful, the bad and the good, pleasant and unpleasant. Sometimes we judge according to the perceptions of expediency. It is the brain too which is the seat of madness and delirium, of the fears and frights which assail us, often by night, but sometimes even by day; it is there where lies the cause of insomnia and sleep-walking, of thoughts that will not come, forgotten duties, and eccentricities. All such things result from an unhealthy condition of the brain."

Hippocrates

CONTENTS

INTRODUCTION

It is a truism that the mind does not exist apart from the brain, yet the practice of categorizing diseases as "neurological" and "psychiatric" suggests otherwise. According to convention, neurology deals with "organic disease," that is, disease of the brain, in which symptoms can be closely correlated with specific alterations of brain structure or a disorder of physiological or biochemical function. Psychiatry is designated as the province of "functional disturbances," which are defined as thought and behavior disorders that cannot be correlated with alterations of brain structure or biological function. The primary cause of functional disorders is traditionally related to stressful environmental influences. Hence, the term "functional" carries the implication of reversibility. This division, however practical with reference to the proper referral of patients, obscures important aspects of behavioral disorders. It is incorrect to conceive of any disturbance of behavior or thought as "functional" because thoughts, feelings, and memories are as much the result of brain activity as movement, sensation, and speech. In addition, "functional" disturbances of intellect and behavior that result from environmental influences are often irreversible.

There is strong evidence that environmental influences at certain stages of life can produce permanent changes within the nervous system. One such change is amblyopia ex anopsia, a form of acquired blindness that affects infants and children who have uncorrected strabismus. Strabismus makes normal binocular vision impossible. To avoid double vision the child "suppresses" visual impulses arising from the weak eye by means of a cortical process that is not well understood. If the condition is not treated, and if the child is not forced to use the weak eye, permanent blindness in that eye develops. This form of blindness occurs commonly only in childhood, rarely if ever beginning in adulthood, despite the fact that adults with acquired weakness of extraocular muscles also frequently "suppress" the image from the weak eye.

A similar condition has been reproduced in kittens. If the eyelid of the neonatal kitten is sewn shut for three months and then opened, vision is permanently lost in that eye. The same is not true for the adult cat. The cells of the visual cortex of the neonatal kitten are, like those of the adult cat, endowed with the ability to respond to patterns of light (angles or forms). Eyelid closure in the first three months of life results in the permanent loss of this cortical reaction, though normal retinal and geniculate responses to visual stimuli are retained.

Histological changes accompany this alteration in ocular physiology. When radioactive proline fucose is injected into one eye, the material is carried along the visual pathways transsynaptically to the occipital cortex. Ordinarily, the fourth layer of occipital cortical cells is labelled in columns that are equal in width to unlabelled interspersed parallel columns that represent connections from the uninjected eye. Following the closure of one eye early in life, there is a marked reduction in the size of the field from the closed eye in layer IV of the occipital cortex and a corresponding increase in the field from the normal eye. A similar change in morphology has been described in the somatosensory area of the mouse after removing vibrissae (whiskers) on one side early in life (Woolsey and VanDerLoos, 1970). This demonstrates in a different sensory system the flexibility of neuronal architecture in response to an environmental manipulation.

Loss of activity in the visual and somatosensory pathways (disuse atrophy) is probably not the main factor that disrupts the normal response of developing sensory cortex when subjected to prolonged sensory deprivation. This is suggested by the finding that after both eyes of the newborn monkey are closed at birth for 17 days or more, most occipital cortical cells can be activated by the usual visual stimuli. The receptive fields and columnar organization are normal histologically. Thus, one could speculate that pathways from the two eyes are competing for cortical representation and, with one eye closed, the contest is unequal and the dendritic connections from the closed eye are taken over by neuron terminals from the open eye and the connections from the closed eye are rendered ineffective (Kuffler and Nichols, 1976).

Profound differences in cortical responsivity can also result from the loss of conjugate vision produced by cutting a peripheral nerve to one of the extraocular muscles. The effect on cortical physiology is permanent only when the operation is performed early in life. Though both eyes receive visual stimulation, almost all of the cells in the occipital cortex are driven by one or the other eye, while virtually none are driven by both. This is the reverse of the normal situation, and binocular representation largely disappears. In these experiments it is clear that binocular vision depends on binocular conjugate stimulation and that cortical connections, present at birth, can be rendered permanently ineffective by environmental manipulations (Weisel and Hubel, 1965).

A possible analogy to these experiments may be seen in behavioral imprinting studies carried out by ethologists. Artificially hatched goslings must not be allowed full sight of a human being between hatching and transmission to the mother because their following drive is likely to become immediately and permanently attached to human beings. Young goslings who have been exposed to human beings stare calmly at humans without any display of fear and do not resist handling. They pipe piteously if left without human contact and soon follow humans reliably, never again regarding an adult goose as parent. This is a classic example of the manner in which a single experience can permanently imprint behavior in animals, though only during a definite early period of life (Lorenz, 1970).

Similar results have been obtained in experiments with mammals. If dogs are handled by humans between four and eight weeks of age, they are more tractable and tame than animals that have not had human contact in the early weeks of life (Fuller, 1967).

Another possible analogy to these experiments may be seen in the work of Harlow et al. (1971). Infant monkeys were taken away from their mothers and "raised" by surrogate mothers (rag dolls). Though they were healthy and well developed, and showed no sign of abnormality in solving problems, these monkeys were unable to establish normal heterosexual relations even after transfer to a colony of normal monkeys. Partial and total social isolation during the first six months of life also led to severe, irreversible abnormalities in the adult monkey's behavior. The actual neurophysiological and neurochemical correlates of this state are not known. Isolation does not produce such abnormalities in older monkeys raised by a normal mother.

An extensive literature has documented parallel structural, biochemical, and electrophysiological abnormalities of sensory systems when these systems are deprived of appropriate sensory input during early life (Blakemore and Cooper, 1978; Valverde, 1970; Riesen, 1975). Conversely, an enriched and stimulating environment enhances the branching of cortical dendrites and the development of dendritic spines (Valverde, 1971; Volkmar and Greenough, 1972; Bennett, Diamond, and Rosenzweig, 1964). Similarly, the histological development of the motor system is accelerated by use and retarded by nonuse (Sammeck, 1976; Schapiro and Vukovich, 1970). Studies in which rodents, dogs, and monkeys were isolated from mother and peers in early life have demonstrated later neurochemical, histological, and electrophysiological defects (Prescott, 1971).

These findings provide an experimental context in which the effects of early environment upon human development may be understood. Delay of motor and social development has been described in institutionalized infants who have suffered maternal deprivation in the first year of life. Though these children made dramatic gains when given the benefit of good maternal care, starting in the second year, residual impairments that persisted at least through the preschool years were noted. Deficits were seen in their capacity for forming emotional relationships, in impulse control, and in areas of thinking and learning that reflect adaptive capacities and imagination (Provence and Lipton, 1962). Though the permanence of such deficits has not been fully demonstrated in humans, and genetic influences on the thought processes of previously institutionalized children have not been completely ruled out, it would appear that the human nervous system also has a potential for development that is largely determined by genetic factors but may be changed permanently by experience and is particularly susceptible to irreversible change during the first months and years of life.

Why is the immature nervous system so susceptible? In a consideration of this question, a brief account of the normal alterations in the brain that are known to occur early in postpartum life may be useful. The number of nerve cells does not substantially change after birth, yet the brain increases in size tremendously during the first year of life and does not fully complete its growth until adolesence. Two factors are primarily responsible for the enlargement of the brain during this period. One is the formation of myelin sheaths, which facilitate axonal conducting, and the other is the development of dendritic connections between nerve cells. The temporal association of myelin and dendritic development with the period of susceptibility of the immature brain to environmental influences suggests that these factors may be related. If so, axonal conducting and myelin formation are likely to be less important than dendrite development in determining susceptibility to the environment, since axons have a more limited functional capacity and respond in an all-or-none fashion. Dendrites are capable of more prolonged and graduated electrical responses. Also, there is evidence that functional dendritic connections are developed in response to environmental influences during the period of rapid brain growth.

Axonal impulses are indistinguishable from animal to animal. Even the most sophisticated neurophysiologist would be hard pressed to tell if a propagated action potential came from the axon of a worm, a frog, or a human being. The major neurophysiological difference between species is not in the nature of nerve impulses but rather in the number of nerve cells and the type and number of dendritic connections between them. Similarly, the real difference between such sensations as pain, smell, and sight is not primarily determined by the pattern of axonal impulses.

The dendritic connections made by afferent nerves subserving the sensory organs, rather than axonal patterns, are what endow electrical messages with individual sensory significance, even though intensity is a function of the frequency of axonal impulses. Yet the mechanism(s) by which nerves make contact with each other is (are) still not clear. We do know that this is not a random process, but quite specific. Thus, a sensory nerve carrying information from a stretch receptor in the quadriceps muscle has a synaptic contact with a motor nerve—not any motor nerve but the nerve that supplies that very same muscle. Though the factors involved in the organization of these connections are not fully known, they are clearly under some kind of genetic control.

A persuasive hypothesis has been advanced that individual neurons take up different positions and reach different, specific targets because they have different underlying substrates to grow on. These newly formed neurons then become a part of the substrate for their neighbors, which differentiate later. Such a mechanism would allow a small number of genes to control the detailed architecture of a large number of neurons (Levinthal, 1980).

Since dendrites are a major determinant of the number and kind of contacts between nerve cells, and consequently in the passage of neural information (impulses) from one cell to another, it is surprising that so little is known about alterations of these structures in disease states. By means of a variety of standard histological techniques it is possible to stain cell bodies, axons, myelin, and glia, but it has been difficult for the pathologist to discern alterations in dendrites by light or electron microscopy.

Many disorders of nervous system function are so incapacitating that one would expect to find histopathological changes with standard techniques; yet in such disorders as idiopathic epilepsy, mental retardation, infantile autism, learning disorders, dystonia musculorum deformans, schizophrenia, and affective psychosis, no consistent histopathological changes have been described that would indicate the etiology. The failure to find such changes with hematoxolin and eosin stains has contributed to the development of the concept of "functional" or "idiopathic" disease. The absence of lesions demonstrable by standard histological techniques has too often led to the assumption that no abnormality exists. Yet, in "idiopathic" epilepsy, electroencephalographic spikes, which are mainly dendritic in origin, are the laboratory findings that most consistently reflect abnormality (Brazier, 1958); and in Golgi-stained preparations from animals with experimentally induced epilepsy, neurons in the region of the epileptic focus (induced by alumina gel) have shown a striking loss of dendritic spines and other changes in dendritic structure (Westrum et al., 1965). There is also some evidence that a diminution in the number of dendrites may be correlated with severe mental retardation even in the absence of other changes (Huttenlocher, 1974). Similarly, Alzheimer's dementia, ganglioside storage disorders, Down's syndrome, and Menke's disease are associated with profound structural alterations of dendrites (Purpura, 1979; Scheibel, 1979), and it is not unrealistic to hope that increased understanding of these and other genetic-chromosomal illnesses will lead to effective treatment in future.

Many recent advances have been made toward elucidating the nature of certain genetic disorders by the use of high resolution techniques and recombinant DNA methodology. Cytogenetic abnormalities, for example, constitute the largest group of clearly defined causes of mental retardation. The most frequent of these is Down's syndrome (Mongolism, Trisomy 21). The second most common disorder of this type is the Fragile X syndrome in which a piece of one X chromosome "hangs loosely" and sometimes breaks off (Sutherland, 1979). Symptomatic mental retardation in this syndrome is most marked in males but many female heterozygotes may be mildly retarded (Turner et al., 1980). Conceivably a similar, as yet undiscovered, X-linked chromosomal abnormality could be involved in learning disorders such as congenital dyslexia that would explain their increased prevalence among males. Since the Fragile X syndrome affects a specific, limited region of the X chromosome, it is likely that the clinical consequences are the result of the loss of a very few genes. These, hopefully, will soon be identified by recombinant DNA methodology that is now being used to construct a genetic map of the X chromosome, which should make it possible to locate the defective genes in X-linked diseases.

Microdeletions of material from the 15th chromosome are now generally recognized to be responsible for a neurologic syndrome associated with mental retardation and a peculiar behavioral trait, insatiable appetite (the Prader-Willi syndrome). Other deletions are associated with retardation, Wilms tumor, aniridia and genito-urinary abnormalities. Retinoblastoma has been associated with a microdeletion of chromosomal material. Microdeletions, identified by linkage techniques, may explain Huntington's chorea and be involved in affective disorders, alcoholism, and other neurologic and psychiatric disorders (Gerald and Bruns, 1980; Housman and Gusella, 1980; Gusella et al., 1983; Ledbetter et al., 1981).

While the genetic basis of behavioral syndromes is being investigated by linkage and other techniques, the study of their morphological concomitants will of necessity depend on the development of quantitative methods to measure changes in dendritic arborization and synaptic contacts. Several promising initiatives have already been published. Measuring the angle between bifurcating branches and planar angles of computerized reconstructions of Golgi stains, Matthysse (1980) is studying changes in Purkinje cell structure in a variety of genetic diseases. Buell and Coleman (1979) have used a computer-microscope system to compare the size of dendritic trees in the brains of aged individuals who are nondemented and demented. They found that neurons die as aging proceeds but that dendritic trees in the surviving cells in the nondemented aged become more extensive. Perhaps this increase in branching represents plasticity in response to the loss of cells. In the demented aged brain, however, such neuronal plasticity does not seem to exist.

These morphologic studies have underscored the importance of dendritic alterations and focused attention on dendritic functioning. Dendrites are activated in several different ways. One way is through the release, by a presynaptic cell, of transmitter chemicals that act at the postsynaptic receptor site and are then rapidly inactivated or removed. Another is by hormonal secretion into the extracellular fluid of substances that affect general neuronal excitability by altering cellular metabolism and the membrane environment for longer periods of time than transmitters. Several chemicals are probable transmitters in the central nervous system—acetylcholine, norepinephrine, dopamine, serotonin, and certain amino acids as well (e.g., gamma-aminobutyric acid and glycine). Particular transmitter substances do not always have either an excitatory or an inhibitory effect; rather it is the nature of the interaction of the transmitter with postsynaptic (dendritic) membrane that determines its action. Each nerve cell in the human brain receives messages from many other cells—some inhibitory and some excitatory. Each cell averages the sum of these effects in making the "decision" to fire.

There is growing evidence that disturbances in the synthesis, release, storage, and inactivation of transmitter substances and changes in the dendritic receptor sites at which they work may lead to profound neurological and behavioral changes. Although there are many more questions than answers, recent progress in this area has suggested that certain amino acids, which probably act as transmitters, play an important role in movement disorders, sleep disturbances, and psychotic states.

These advances have created more common ground for psychiatrists and neurologists. Interest in the biochemical basis of Parkinson's disease and chorea leads to an interest in the chemical basis of depression, mania, and thought disorders, and vice versa, because disturbances in the metabolism of the same catecholamines have been demonstrated, or are suspected, to exist in all these disorders. The widespread use of phenothiazines has unfortunately led to many cases of tardive dyskinesia, a movement disorder which psychiatrists are obliged to recognize and to understand to the degree that current knowledge allows. Similarly, the student of schizophrenia must learn about the schizophrenialike psychosis of epilepsy, drug-induced psychosis, and the many neurological conditions that are often mistaken for schizophrenia.

In this book we attempt to explore the traditional border zone between neurology and psychiatry. In large part, this will be a discussion of "clinical synaptology" and will require the grouping of disorders that seldom are discussed in the same book, let alone the same chapter. Seizure disorders are presented with special emphasis on complex partial seizures and the cognitive and behavioral disturbances with which they may be associated. The role of the limbic system in the production of psychosis and episodic violence is explored. The symptoms of dementia are discussed in terms of anatomical locus and etiological considerations. The evidence that schizophrenia is an organic disorder of brain function is presented along with criteria by which it can be distinguished from diseases that can cause similar symptoms. Affective psychoses, movement disorders, and sleep disorders are described, with emphasis on their treatment. On the basis of what is known about the mechanism of action of drugs that affect these conditions, tentative hypotheses concerning their etiology are proposed. Elements in the medical history and examination that are important in differentiating these conditions are stressed. Also included is a discussion of commonly misdiagnosed conditions with hints as to how they may be differentiated. These include hysteria, hyperventilation syndrome, and headache.

REFERENCES

Bennett, E., M. C. Diamond, D. Krech and M. R. Rosenzweig.   Chemical and anatomic plasticity of the brain. *Science* 146:610, 1964.

Blakemore, C. and G. F. Cooper.   Development of the brain depends on the visual environment. *Nature* 228:477, 1978.

Brazier, M. A. B.   The development of concepts relating to the electrical activity of the brain. *J. Nerv. Ment. Dis.* 126:303, 1958.

Buell, S. J. and P. D. Coleman.   Dendritic growth in the aged human brain and failure of growth in senile dementia. *Science* 206:854, 1979.

Fuller, J. L. Experiential deprivation and later behavior. *Science* 158:1645, 1967.

Gerald, P. S. and G. A. P. Bruns. Recombinant DNA and the analysis of cytogenetic disorders associated with mental retardation. *Arch. Neurol.* 37: 734, 1980.

Gusella, J. F., N. S. Wexler, P. M. Conneally, et al. A polymorphic DNA marker genetically linked to Huntington's disease. *Nature* 306:234, 1983.

Harlow, H. F., M. K. Harlow, and S. J. Suomi. From thought to therapy: Lessons from a primate laboratory. How investigation of the learning capability of rhesus monkeys has led to the study of their behavioral abnormalities and rehabilitation. *Am. Scien.* 59:538, 1971.

Housman, D. and J. Gusella. DNA polymorphism-potential for neurological diagnosis. *Arch. Neurol.* 37:734, 1980.

Huttenlocher, P. R. Dendritic development in neocortex of children with mental defect and infantile spasms. *Neurology* 24:203, 1974.

Kuffler, S. W. and J. G. Nicholls. From Neuron to Brain. A Cellular Approach to the Function of the Nervous System. Sinauer Associates Inc. Sunderland, Massachusetts, 1976.

Ledbetter, D. H., V. M. Riccardi, S. D. Airhart et al. Deletions of chromosome 15 as a cause of the Prader-Willi syndrome. *New Engl. J. Med.* 304: 325, 1981.

Levinthal, C. Genetic and environmental control of neural development. *Arch. Neurol.* 37:732, 1980.

Lorenz, K. Studies in Animal and Human Behavior, Vol. I. translated by Robert Martin. Methuen & Co. Ltd. London, 1970.

Matthysse, S. Genetics of neuronal form. *Arch. Neurol.* 37:732, 1980.

Prescott, J. W. Early somatosensory deprivation as an ontogenetic process in the abnormal development of the brain and behavior. In Medical Primatology pp. 356-375. Karger Co., Basel, 1971.

Provence, S. and R. Lipton. Infants in Institutions. International University Press, New York, 1962.

Purpura, D. P. Pathobiology of cortical neurons in metabolic and unclassified amentias. Research Publications: Association for Research in Nervous and Mental Disease 57:43, 1979. Raven Press, New York. Ed. Robert Katzman.

Riesen, A. H. The Developmental Neuropsychology of Sensory Deprivation. Academic Press, New York, 1975.

Sammeck, R. Myelin changes induced by detraining. *J. Physiol.* 266:16P, 1976.

Schapiro, S. and K. R. Vukovich. Early experience: Effects upon cortical dendrites. *Science* 167:292, 1970.

Scheibel, A. Dendritic changes in senile and presenile dementias. Research Publications: Association for Research in Nervous and Mental Disease 57: 107, 1979. Raven Press, New York. Ed. Robert Katzman.

Sutherland, G. R. Hereditable fragile sites on human chromosomes. II. Distribution, phenotypic effects and cytogenetics. *Am. J. Hum. Genet.* 31:136, 1979.

Turner, G., R. Brookwell, A. Daniel et al. Heterozygous expression of

X-linked mental retardation and X chromosome marker Fra(X) (q27) *New Eng. J. Med.* 303:662, 1980.

Valverde, F. Rate and extent of recovery from dark rearing in the visual cortex of the mouse. *Brain Res.* 33:1, 1971.

Volkmar, F. R. and W. J. Greenough. Rearing complexity affects branching of dendrites in visual cortex of rats. *Science* 176:1445, 1972.

Weisel, T. V. and D. H. Hubel. Extent of recovery from the effects of visual deprivation in kittens. *J. Neurophysiol.* 28:1060, 1965.

Westrum, C. E., L. E. White, and A. A. Ward, Jr. Morphology of the experimental epileptic focus. *J. Neurosurg.* 21:1033, 1965.

Woolsey, T. A., H. VanDerLoos. The structural organization of layer IV in the somatosensory region (SI) of mouse cerebral cortex. The description of a cortical field composed of discrete cytoarchitectonic units. *Brain Res* 17:205, 1970.

Behavioral Neurology

Chapter 1

SEIZURE DISORDERS

It is difficult to provide a simple, concise, and yet all-encompassing definition of epilepsy. Definitions that rely on clinical phenomena usually encompass loss of consciousness and tonic and clonic movements. Though these are components of grand mal seizures, both are absent in some forms of epilepsy. In focal motor seizures, for example, consciousness may not even be impaired. In other forms of epilepsy, such as focal sensory, petit mal, or psychomotor seizures, abnormal movement does not necessarily occur. To avoid these difficulties in defining the clinical condition, some neurologists have anchored their definition in physiology, describing seizure states as "paroxysmal depolarization shifts" or the "repetitive discharge of a hyperexcitable aggregate of neurons." Though such electrical changes accompany seizures of any kind, they are not always reflected in the electroencephalogram (EEG), and sometimes they occur in the absence of clinically apparent seizures.

The diagnosis of epilepsy is not usually difficult despite the lack of a completely satisfactory definition of the condition. After the diagnosis has been made, however, it may not always be clear how much of a patient's behavior can be attributed to epilepsy. Even with a patient who is known to have seizures and/or whose EEG suggests an epileptic tendency, there may be disagreement among competent neurologists as to the relation of abnormal behavior to a seizure state. In such cases, a therapeutic trial of anticonvulsants may appear to resolve the medical problem, but the pragmatic definition of epilepsy as "that which responds to anticonvulsants" involves post hoc reasoning which is scientifically weak.

ETIOLOGICAL CONSIDERATIONS

Idiopathic versus Symptomatic

Epilepsy traditionally has been divided into two broad etiological categories: symptomatic and idiopathic. The term symptomatic epilepsy is applied to seizure disorders with an identifiable cause, such as encephalitis, tumor, trauma, or known metabolic disease. In these conditions, seizures are considered to be a symptom of another disease. The term "idiopathic" epilepsy literally means seizure disorders that arise spontaneously and exist in the absence of other diseases of the nervous system. This term is too broadly used when applied to all convulsive disorders in which no cause has yet been identified, irrespective of the age or family history of the patient. Used indiscriminately, "idiopathic epilepsy" becomes a subterfuge when a clinician cannot make a clear-cut diagnosis. Used properly, the term probably should refer to "inherited" epilepsy, which usually begins in childhood or adolescence; here, a positive family history is most helpful in making a reliable diagnosis. In older patients with negative family histories, epilepsy "of unknown cause" should be labeled as such, and the onus for incomplete diagnosis placed on the doorstep of the clinician, not on the patient's genes.

It must be recognized that the concept of idiopathic epilepsy is artificial. The epilepsy is surely the result of a physiological dysfunction, but the biochemical or neuroanatomical locus of the abnormality is not yet known. In this sense, idiopathic epilepsy is "symptomatic," that is, it is a symptom of an unknown abnormality. A high proportion of the relatives of patients with idiopathic epilepsy have abnormal EEG's, yet most of these persons never have clinical seizures. Some patients who have idiopathic epilepsy also show other symptoms of brain dysfunction and have a history of events known to be associated with brain damage. Acquired brain damage may promote expression of the genetic trait, and to the extent that it does, the resulting seizures are "symptomatic" of brain damage. It is also true that even in symptomatic epilepsy the mechanism by which identifiable lesions cause seizures is not well understood. Not every patient with a brain tumor, for example, has seizures. In all epileptic patients, whether they have idiopathic or symptomatic epilepsy, seizures are not constant, even though the lesion may be constantly present and the EEG consistently abnormal. It seems likely, in such cases, that other factors prevent seizures from occurring all the time. The complexity of these factors is implied by the great variety of circumstances that can precipitate seizures in susceptible individuals (see Table 1-1).

Though no single factor has been identified as the primary cause of convulsive disorders, some factors are known to influence the seizure threshold (Tower, 1960). These include the availability of

Table 1-1
Factors That May Precipitate
Seizures in Susceptible Individuals

Factors
Hyperventilation
Sleep (usually within the first 30 minutes or shortly before awakening)
Sleep deprivation
Sensory stimuli
Flashing lights
Reading, Speaking, Coughing, Laughing
Touch, Pain
Sounds (music, bells, etc.)
Trauma
Hormonal changes
Menses, Puberty
ACTH, Adrenal steroids
Fever
Emotional stress
Drugs
Phenothiazines, Analeptics
Tricyclic mood elevators
Antihistamines, Alcohol withdrawal
Anticonvulsant overdose

prime energy substrates such as glucose and oxygen, the ability of the brain to utilize them, the metabolism of amino acids and acetylcholine, the activity of the sodium pump, and the distribution of cations within the nerve and at the cell membrane.

The patient's age at the onset of seizures gives an important clue to etiology. Seizures beginning before the age of six months usually reflect birth injury, congenital defect of the nervous system, metabolic errors, or infectious disease. Seizures beginning between the ages of two and twenty are usually "genetic" in etiology (i.e., idiopathic). When seizures have their initial onset after the age of thirty-five years, vascular disease, or tumor, is likely. Seizures seldom begin between the ages of twenty and thirty-five. When they do, trauma, drug abuse (particularly alcohol), and infection are common causes. Idiopathic epilepsy does not usually begin between these ages, but it may. Sometimes patients forget about convulsive episodes that occurred ten to twenty years earlier. Whenever possible, the history should be confirmed by interviews with the patient's parents or other individuals familiar with his early years. Despite this reservation, it is a good rule to assume that any seizures beginning after the age of twenty probably result from some identifiable, possibly progressive, condition, which should be diligently investigated.

GENETICS

It has been a long-standing clinical observation that epilepsy is more common among close relatives of epileptics than in the general population, in which the incidence is probably close to 1 percent. More recently, it has become quite clear that the genetic element in epilepsy is not a simple one, since the incidence of the disease in first-degree relatives of epileptics is much lower than would be expected in an autosomal dominant disorder (50%) and the incidence in siblings of epileptics is lower than would be predicted for an autosomal recessive condition (25%). Nonetheless, a dominant mode of inheritance for epilepsy with incomplete penetrance was postulated in an early paper by Lennox et al. (1940)

on the basis of the electroencephalographic traits of the relatives of epileptics. In a series of papers on centrencephalic (petit mal) epilepsy, Metrakos and Metrakos (1961) reported that the prevalence of convulsions among the near relatives of patients with petit mal epilepsy was high: 13 percent of parents were affected, and 13 percent of siblings. In more distant relatives, the prevalence was lower. This finding indicates that there is a strong hereditary tendency in centrencephalic epilepsy, but it does not reveal the actual mode of inheritance. Further data from the same study on electroencephalographic traits have conclusively demonstrated a dominant pattern of inheritance. Between the ages of 4½ and 16½, approximately 45 percent of the siblings of epileptics demonstrated the typical 3 cycles per second (cps) spike-and-wave abnormality. After 16½ years, there was a sharp decline in this abnormality; and before the age of 2½ years, only 6 percent had it. Of 40 siblings of epileptics between the ages of 4½ and 7½, exactly 20 or 50 percent, had the spike-and-wave abnormality (Metrakos and Metrakos, 1961). This is what would be predicted if the electroencephalographic abnormality were transmitted as an autosomal dominant trait. Thus, the 3-cps, spike-and-wave abnormality is the expression of an autosomal dominant gene with a very low penetrance rate at birth, which rises to nearly complete penetrance for ages 4½ to 7½ and declines to almost zero after the age of forty. The study by Metrakos and Metrakos also revealed that the electroencephalographic abnormality was not always associated with convulsions; only about 25 percent of those with the electroencephalographic abnormality actually had clinical seizures.

Acquired brain damage may be another factor that determines which individual with the genetic trait actually becomes epileptic. Reviewing prenatal and perinatal hospital records of epileptic children, Lilienfeld and Pasamanick (1954) found an increased incidence of complications of pregnancy, birth, and neonatal development compared with nonepileptic siblings. On the basis of this evidence, they suggested that brain damage often caused epilepsy even in children with a hereditary epileptic tendency.

Bray and Weiser (1964) studied focal and temporal lobe epilepsy associated with focal, temporal, or central electroencephalographic discharges. They found the same hereditary pattern that Metrakos and Metrakos had demonstrated in petit mal epilepsy. Diffuse electroencephalographic abnormalities, such as bilaterally synchronous spikes or combinations of spikes and slow wave discharges, were found in almost half the close relatives of the index cases. Both groups found that the closer the relative, the higher the prevalence of seizures and abnormal EEG's. Bray and Weiser's index cases were homologous for type and location of the electroencephalographic abnormality but not for seizure type. Like Metrakos and Metrakos, Bray and Weiser demonstrated a dominant genetic trait that is age related, with a low penetrance in early childhood that rises to approximately 50 percent in middle childhood and then declines in adult life. On the basis of these studies, it seems likely that idiopathic epilepsy is transmitted by an autosomal dominant gene in which the penetrance varies with the age of the individual and the expressivity is determined in part by the presence of brain damage.

Mothers of epileptics are more frequently epileptic than fathers of epileptics (Annegers et al., 1976). This probably does not reflect the influence of some sex-linked genetic trait but rather may stem from the adverse effect of epilepsy and anticonvulsant medications on the male libido and sexual performance. A similar situation exists among the parents of schizophrenics (see p. 123).

Twin studies have buttressed the view of the dominant inheritance of idiopathic epilepsy. Lennox (1951) found the concordance rate for seizures in the monozygotic twins of epileptics to be 85 percent as compared with 27 percent in dizygotic twins, whereas Inouye (1960) found the rates to be 54 percent and 7 percent, respectively. Inouye also found a concordance rate for electroencephalographic abnormalities of 77 percent in the monozygotic twins and 22 percent in the dizygotic twins. Similar results were reported by Marshall et al. (1962).

No study has shown a concordance rate for seizures or electroencephalographic abnormalities in monozygotic twins greater than 85 percent. The question of why the theoretically expected rate of

100 percent for monozygotic twins has not been reached is of great interest. Though the age of the nonindex twins at the time of the study and the completeness of the criteria used to determine monozygocity may influence the concordance rate, the presence of acquired brain damage in one twin is the factor most likely to cause nonconcordance in some monozygotic pairs. The presence of brain damage in one monozygotic twin might lower his seizure threshold enough to allow expression of the inherited epileptic gene. There is an increased incidence of neurological complications in multiple-birth children, and it is not unreasonable to expect that acquired brain damage would be expressed as epilepsy only in a damaged twin. Such an explanation would be consistent with the findings of Lilienfeld and Pasamanick (1954).

The high rate of epilepsy among blacks (Shamansky and Glaser, 1979) is almost certainly the result of social factors that influence the prevalence of acquired brain damage. Though full-term infants of both races with normal body weight do not differ with respect to brain weight, adult white males and females have significantly higher brain weight than black males and females (Ho et al., 1981). There appears to be a disproportionate number of preterm and low birth weight infants among the poor black population. Contributory factors may include poor prenatal care, smoking, drinking and drug use, malnutrition, teenage pregnancy, low income, and low educational status (Reed and Starky, 1977).

The National Health and Nutrition Examination Survey (Mahaffey et al., 1982) has shown elevated blood lead levels in 18.6 percent of poor black children six months to five years old. The elevated levels in blacks of all socioeconomic levels or places of residence represented a greater than expected racial difference that is as yet unexplained. Clinical studies have linked "subtoxic" (< 30 μg %) blood lead levels with psychological deficits and behavioral disorders in young children. Though disputed by some (Ernhart, Landa, and Schell, 1981), the positive findings of others (Needleman et al., 1979; Yule et al., 1981) are supported by a growing body of experimental and clinical studies. EEG studies in children have shown that slow wave voltage during sensory conditioning varies as a linear function of blood lead levels and that levels below the 30 μg percent range alter CNS function (Otto et al., 1981).

CLINICAL CLASSIFICATION (See Table 1-2)

Generalized tonic/clonic (grand mal) seizures are characterized by total loss of consciousness and stereotyped motor activity. Initially, there is a tonic stage during which the body stiffens and breathing stops. This is followed by a clonic phase characterized by rhythmic shaking of the extremities and trunk. This sequence may last for a minute or two and is sometimes repeated. After the convulsions stop, there is a postictal depression of consciousness including drowsiness, confusion, headache, and somnolence, which may last from a few minutes up to a day or two. About 50 percent of patients experience some sort of aura, which usually precedes the attack. An aura is an integral part of the seizure. In fact, an aura must be considered to be a seizure even when it is not followed by a grand mal attack. Usually, it is an ill-defined sensation of not feeling well; sometimes it is essentially a complex partial (psychomotor) seizure. Patients with focal lesions in the cortex are apt to have an aura that can be related to the damaged area. Usually, auras are of several seconds' duration, but generalized motor seizures may be preceded by prodromal periods of several hours' or even days' duration during which the patient does not feel well or is confused.

The tonic phase of a grand mal seizure coincides with the generalized synchronous spikes on the EEG. The clonic stage is characterized by grouped spikes separated by slow waves. During the postictal phase, low voltage slow waves are seen (Fig. 1-1). In about half the cases of grand mal seizure, the interictal waking EEG is normal. In the remainder, paroxysmal features including spikes, sharp activity, and slow wave bursts may be seen. If EEG's are recorded during sleep, abnormalities not seen in the waking EEG may be recorded, but 25 to 30 percent will still be normal. Grand mal seizures may occur in the absence of any structural de-

Table 1-2
Comparison of Traditional and International
Classifications of Epilepsy

Traditional	International
	I. Partial Seizures (seizures beginning locally)
Focal motor (incl. Jacksonian)	A. With elementary symptomatology (generally without impairment of consciousness)
Focal sensory	1. with motor symptoms
	2. with special sensory or somatosensory symptoms
	3. with autonomic symptoms
	4. compound forms
	B. With complex symptomatology (generally with some impairment of consciousness)
Temporal lobe	1. with impairment of consciousness only
Psychomotor	2. with cognitive symptomatology
Limbic	3. with affective symptomatology
	4. with psychosensory symptomatology
	5. with psychomotor symptomatology (automatisms)
	6. Compound forms
	C. Partial seizures, secondarily generalized
	II. Generalized Seizures (bilaterally symmetrical without known local onset with loss of consciousness)
Petit mal (centrencephalic)	A. Absence
Grand mal	B. Tonic/clonic
Grand mal	C. Tonic
Grand mal	D. Clonic
Minor motor	E. Bilateral epileptic myoclonus
Minor motor	F. Atonic
Minor motor	G. Akinetic
Minor motor	H. Infantile Spasms
Minor motor	I. Myoclonic
	III. Unilateral
	IV. Unclassified

fect but may also be seen in patients with generalized or focal cerebral disease.

ABSENCE (petit mal, centrencephalic) SEIZURES are characterized by "absence," a loss of awareness during which there is no motor activity other than blinking or a rolling up of the eyes. The epi-

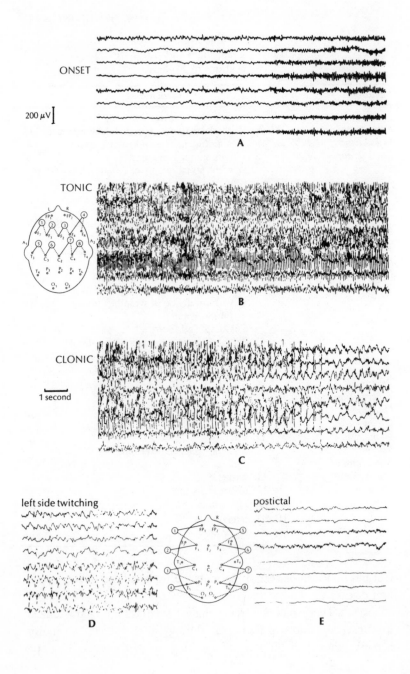

ONSET

200 μV

TONIC

CLONIC

1 second

left side twitching

postictal

A

B

C

D

E

sodes are brief, usually lasting less than 10 seconds. Patients do not fall to the ground and there is no postictal depression. These seizures occur in children and are rarely seen in anyone over fifteen years old. Of patients with this form of epilepsy, 50 to 75 percent do not have other types of seizures. The electroencephalographic pattern associated with petit mal seizures (in 90% of cases) is the 3-cps, spike-and-wave discharge (Fig. 1-2) (Loiseau et al., 1983). The EEG is seldom normal in the interictal state, and it is especially sensitive to overbreathing. The term petit mal is often mistakenly applied to other forms of seizures, particularly psychomotor seizures, though some automatisms may be present in absence attacks.

Fig. 1-1
GRAND MAL SEIZURE WITH FOCAL FEATURES;
FOCAL SEIZURE AND POSTICTAL PHASE

A.   The patient, a 36-year-old man with posttraumatic epilepsy, had a generalized seizure during the recording. Irregular sharp waves from lines 1 and 5 are seen in the first EEG page (top). This abnormal activity derives from the left frontal and temporal regions. The background rhythms elsewhere are fairly normal. Generalized spiking then develops in all regions.

B.   The second EEG page coincides with the tonic phase of the seizure. There is generalized, high-voltage spiking mixed with movement artifact from which it cannot be clearly distinguished.

C.   The third EEG page coincides with the clonic phase of the convulsion and contains grouped spikes separated by slow waves. This feature of the record is best developed in lines 1, 2, 5, and 6, all of which are recorded from the left hemisphere. Clonic movements, though generalized, were more prominent in the right arm and right leg.

D and E.   These two EEG pages are from another adult patient who had a right cerebral lesion. D was recorded during the clonic phase of a left focal seizure. Grouped spikes, separated by slow waves, can be seen in the right hemisphere. In the left hemisphere, slow waves predominate. During the postictal phase (E), there is a depression of amplitude and low-voltage slow waves in the leads from the right hemisphere, which can be compared with the somewhat irregular but more normal activity in the left hemispheric leads. During this portion of the recording, the patient had a Todd's paralysis of his left arm and left leg.

Ref Ipsi Ear

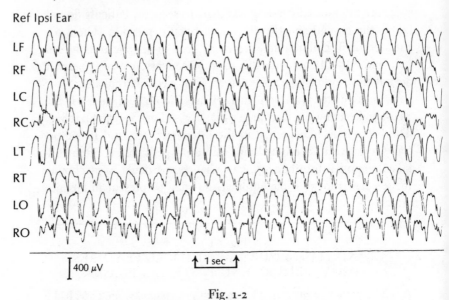

Fig. 1-2

The EEG of a seven-year-old boy with a history of typical "absence" (petit mal) attacks usually lasting 5 to 20 seconds. The record shows generalized 3-cps, spike-and-wave activity. In this illustration the spike-and-wave complexes are better developed in the left hemisphere. LF left frontal, RF right frontal, LC left central, RC right central, LT left temporal, RT right temporal, LO left occipital, RO right occipital. Each electrode is referred to the ipsilateral ear.

It has been thought that petit mal seizures result from a discharging focus in diencephalic structures. This might explain the bilaterally synchronous onset of the spike-and-wave discharge and the close timing of the mirrored waves in homologous regions of the two cerebral hemispheres in petit mal, hence the term "centrencephalic" seizures. This view was substantiated to some extent by the finding that electrical stimulation of the thalamus in cats at 3 cps produces clinical and electroencephalographic phenomena similar to those of petit mal epilepsy (Hunter and Jasper, 1949). This classic experiment led to the hypothesis that an abnormal thalamic "pacemaker" exists in patients with petit mal. Similar clinical and electroencephalographic changes, however, have been produced in cats and monkeys by symmetrically placed epileptogenic foci in the cerebral cortex. In these experiments, a primary thalamic role in the production of epileptic phenomena was ruled out (Marcus and Watson, 1968). Thus, it remains unclear whether the thalamus is the major anatomical locus of abnormality in petit mal seizures. The condition may be the result of a genetically determined, diffusely altered state of excitability of cerebral dendrites, synaptic terminals, and/or cell bodies.

PARTIAL SEIZURES (focal motor, sensory) may be motor or sensory or both. In patients over the age of ten years, they usually indicate focal disease in the side of the brain opposite the affected side of the body. Focal seizures may occur in the so-called "Jacksonian march," which starts in the distal part of one extremity and moves proximally. The seizures are not necessarily associated with unconsciousness, but generally, when they advance to both sides of the body, consciousness is lost (Fig. 1-1D, 1-1E). In the postictal phase, a phenomenon known as "Todd's paralysis" often occurs. This is a transient paralysis of the affected part of the body, which may indicate a structural abnormality of the cerebrum on the opposite side. Todd's paralysis that follows grand mal seizures may have the same focal significance. Certain metabolic disturbances may give rise to focal seizures in the absence of any structural abnormality. Among these disturbances are hypoglycemia and hypocalcemia. Children in their first decade may have focal seizures in the absence of focal brain lesions.

MINOR MOTOR SEIZURES are a category of epilepsy in which motor activity may be less dramatic and less prolonged than in other types, but the disorder of the central nervous system associated with them is not necessarily minor. Minor motor seizures may be divided into three kinds:

INFANTILE SPASMS are massive myoclonic spasms that basically consist of a sudden flexion or extension of the body and often begin with a cry. These spasms may resemble an exaggerated Moro reflex. They usually begin between three and seven months of age and are associated with an electroencephalographic pattern called

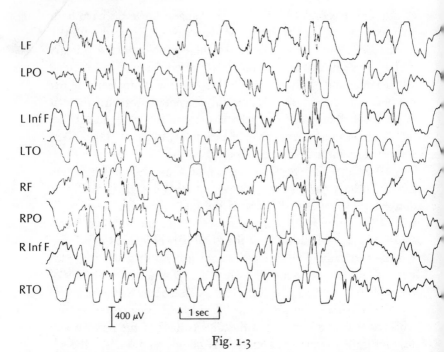

LF

LPO

L Inf F

LTO

RF

RPO

R Inf F

RTO

$\lceil$ 400 μV   ↑ 1 sec ↑

Fig. 1-3

The EEG record of an 8½-month-old girl with infantile spasms. The diagnosis of tuberous sclerosis had been entertained on the basis of the family history. The record shows large slow waves and spikes, which occur asynchronously and synchronously. Abnormal electrical activity is seen in all brain regions. LF left frontal, LPO left parietooccipital, L Inf F left inferior frontal, LTO left temporo-occipital.

hypsarhythmia. This is a maximally abnormal EEG in which diffuse slow waves and spikes occur in a multifocal asynchronous pattern in all leads (Fig. 1-3). Nine of every ten children with infantile spasms become seriously retarded.

One of the striking aspects of this form of epilepsy is that conventional anticonvulsant therapy usually has no effect. In the late 1950s, ACTH (adrenocorticotropic hormone) came into use to control infantile spasms, and there were initial reports of success. The EEG was "normalized" within days, the seizures stopped, and there was an apparent improvement in mentation. Follow-up studies indicated that, whereas ACTH often alleviates infantile spasms and "normalizes" the EEG, it has no effect on ultimate retardation in the majority of cases, though by limiting the number of postictal depressions, it does seem to brighten the patient intellectually. In isolated instances, early successful treatment has been correlated with satisfactory intellectual development, but the role of the hormone or the control of the seizures in preserving intellect in such cases is not clear.

It is now known that many conditions can cause infantile spasms. Almost all of them have in common one characteristic: they seriously disrupt nervous system function. Diseases as diverse as phenylketonuria, hypoglycemia, subdural effusions, encephalitis, and congenital malformations of the nervous system all have been known to cause infantile spasms. These seizures, therefore, should be looked upon as the response of an immature nervous system to a serious insult, and the accompanying retardation is considered to result from the same insult. Generally, infantile spasms gradually resolve or else develop into some other clinical form. As the children grow older they often appear autistic. The reason ACTH is usually effective with infantile spasms irrespective of the disease causing them is not at all clear, since in older children and adults, ACTH and adrenal steroids tend to be epileptogenic rather than the reverse (Bower and Jeavons, 1961).

In an AKINETIC SEIZURE, the child appears to fall to the floor passively and without warning; his antigravity muscles seem to have relaxed. These spells may be of very short duration, and after two or three seconds, the child may get up quickly without any postictal depression. Akinetic seizures, however, are probably not actually akinetic, but myoclonic; they often result from active flexion of the neck and hips. The fall forward in the standing or sitting position may injure the head and face (Fig. 1-4). Until such seizures can be controlled with medication, these patients must sometimes wear football helmets for protection. Akinetic spells usually first occur in children between one and seven years of age. Though these seizures may be seen in association with petit mal epilepsy

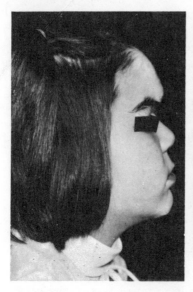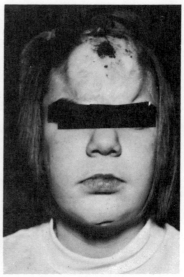

Fig. 1-4

An eight-year-old, educably retarded child with "akinetic" seizures that started at twenty months of age after an attack of encephalitis. Myoclonic flexion of her head and trunk over the years resulted in multiple facial injuries, with chin, lip, nose, and forehead scarring.

or as a manifestation of idiopathic epilepsy, most cases are associated with brain damage and have a poor prognosis for normal intellectual development. They may thus be considered a counterpart of infantile spasms in an older age group.

Akinetic seizures are often associated with an EEG pattern of spike-and-wave discharge that differs in frequency and form from the typical petit mal pattern. Hence, it is referred to as an "atypical" spike wave (Fig. 1-5).

MYOCLONIC JERKS involving smaller muscle groups than the flexors and extensors of the hips may occur alone or as a prodrome to a grand mal seizure. In either case, they may also be a part of a mild idiopathic seizure disorder and are not necessarily an ominous sign. Myoclonic jerks occasionally occur in healthy individuals as

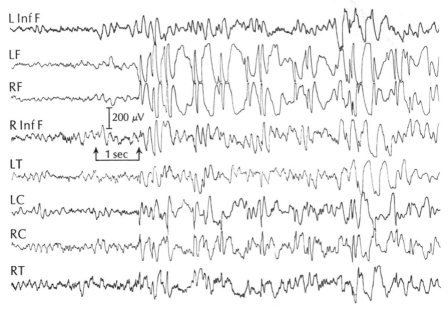

L Inf F

LF

RF

R Inf F   200 μV

LT   ↑ 1 sec ↑

LC

RC

RT

Fig. 1-5

EEG record of a mentally retarded 4½-year-old boy with grand mal
seizures, psychomotor seizures, and akinetic spells. There is a strong
family history of epilepsy. The record shows spikes, polyspikes, and
atypical spike and wave combinations mainly in the frontal region
which occur abruptly on a fairly normal background.

they are falling asleep. This sleep myoclonus is a normal phenomenon. Myoclonic jerks are not always associated with nonprogressive
disorders, however. They occur in degenerative, infectious and
progressive diseases, such as myoclonus epilepsy of Unverricht, subacute sclerosing panencephalitis (Dawson's encephalitis), storage
diseases, and certain metabolic disorders (i.e., uremia).

The terms COMPLEX PARTIAL, PSYCHOMOTOR SEIZURES, and TEM-
PORAL LOBE EPILEPSY are used synonymously. Though such identification of these seizures with the temporal lobe is an oversimplifi-
cation, like many oversimplifications, it is largely correct: discharges
that produce complex partial seizures usually but do not always

originate in deep, medially placed limbic nuclei in the temporal lobe, which consists of the amygdala, uncus, and hippocampus. They may also arise from virtually any other part of the limbic system, not all of which is located in the temporal lobe (see Ch. 2). In addition, other areas of the nervous system may be the source of these discharges; they may arise from subcortical, frontal, diencephalic, or upper brainstem regions and then spread through one or both temporal lobes. In most cases, however, electrical activity spreads to the temporal lobes so that the characteristic electroencephalographic abnormality is temporal spiking (Fig. 1-6), unilaterally or bilaterally. Nonetheless, there are no pathognomonic electroencephalographic configurations that make a diagnosis of complex partial seizures absolutely certain, and the resting EEG may be normal.

Fig. 1-6

The EEG record of a forty-six-year-old man with psychomotor seizures. There are well-localized, left anterior temporal spikes. L Ant T left anterior temporal.

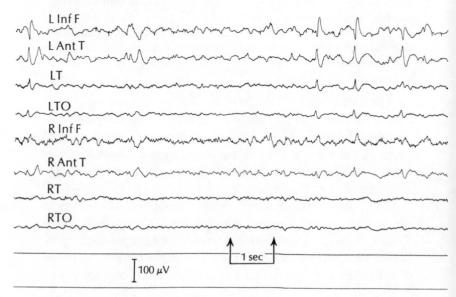

Manifestations of complex partial seizures usually fall into three categories: subjective experiences, automatisms, and postural changes. Autonomic changes also occur. The SUBJECTIVE FEELINGS (cognitive, psychosensory, affective symptoms) include forced, repetitive, and disturbing thoughts, alterations of mood, sensations of impending disaster and anxiety, as well as inappropriate familiarity or unfamiliarity (déjà vu, jamais vu). Some patients have episodes of depersonalization, dreamlike states, or sensations like those occurring in alcoholic intoxication. Metamorphopsias include visual distortions, such as macropsia and micropsia. Auditory distortions, olfactory and gustatory hallucinations, and abdominal pain are some of the more common sensory experiences. Abdominal pains associated with complex partial seizures may be so severe as to simulate an acute abdominal emergency, and in some cases, exploratory laparotomies have been performed.

The AUTOMATISMS of complex partial seizures are much more difficult to recognize as ictal events that the tonic/clonic stages of grand mal seizures. They tend to be repetitive and often are such oral activities as lip-smacking, chewing, gagging, retching, or swallowing. Some patients may perform a variety of complicated acts that seem to blend with normal behavior. Usually the behavior is inappropriate. The repetition of a phrase over and over again and the buttoning and unbuttoning of clothing are common. A few patients may assume bizarre positions resembling those of catatonic schizophrenia. These positions are held for varying periods of time. Some patients have fugue states. Fortunately, outbursts of directed, aggressive behavior are extremely rare, but when these outbursts lead to violence, they often present neurologists and psychiatrists with difficult medicolegal questions concerning the responsibility of an individual for his actions. Though the behavior of patients during complex partial seizures tends to be automatic, it may be influenced by environmental factors. Such an influence can be seen in the case of a patient who had a psychomotor seizure while he was waiting in line at the hospital pharmacy to have his anticonvulsant prescription filled. It was a hot day and he was frustrated by the long wait. During the seizure, or possibly during the postictal confusional period following it, he shoved past the people who were in front of him until he came to the pharmacist's window where he stood, mumbling incoherently, until his wife led him away. After a minute or two of confusion, his sensorium cleared.

Sometimes it is quite difficult to distinguish behavior caused by complex partial seizures from episodic aberrations caused by postictal confusion, intoxication, sociopathy, anxiety, pavor nocturnus, narcolepsy, migraine, transient global amnesia, malingering, postconcussion state, hysteria, or psychosis. In making this distinction, several questions regarding the patient's history are helpful: (1) Does the patient have a history of generalized seizures? (2) Is there a positive family history of epilepsy? (3) Is there a history of events known to be associated with seizures such as brain injury? (4) Does the patient describe subjective alterations typical of psychomotor seizures? (5) Has he been observed performing any of the characteristic automatisms? (6) Was he confused during the episode? (7) Is the patient's memory for events that occurred during the episode impaired? Though memory for the early events of the seizure may seem relatively well preserved, such memories are nearly always incomplete or incorrect. (8) Did the patient experience a postictal depression? Though such a depression is almost always present, it may be mild, and close questioning is often necessary to elicit a positive history. After the seizure, this depression may be manifest as only a brief period of fatigue, when the patient may wish to lie down, perhaps complaining of a headache or of not feeling quite normal. (9) Has he had other lapses during which he engaged in nearly identical behavior? Motor activity tends to be stereotyped in psychomotor epilepsy (Table 1-3).

In some cases of complex partial epilepsy, there may be prolonged episodes of abnormal behavior lasting for hours or days, though epilepsy is very rarely manifested solely as a prolonged behavioral disturbance. When considering episodic and especially patterned behavioral abnormalities—even when they are prolonged— the clinician should include some form of associated seizure disorder in his differential diagnosis.

Table 1-3
Features That Help To Distinguish Behavior During
Complex Partial Seizures (CPS) from Other Behaviors

Aberration	History of Generalized Seizures	Family History of Epilepsy	History of Traumatic Events Known To Induce Seizures	Subjective Experiences of CPS That Are Typical	Automatisms	Confusion	Memory Impaired for Episode	Post-Episode Fatigue	Repeated Episodes of Same Behavior	Epileptic EEG
Complex Partial Seizures	+	+	+	+	+	+	+	+	+	+
Postictal state	+	+	+	+	+	+	+	+	+	+
Intoxication			+(often)	+(often)				+	+	
Sociopathy				+(often)			+(often)		+	
Anxiety					+		+	+	+	
Pavor nocturnus					+(rare)	+		+	+	
Migraine				+(rare)		+(rare)	+			+
Transient global amnesia			+			+	+			
Malingering										
Postconcussion state						+	+	+		
Hysteria					+(often)				+	
Psychosis					+(often)				+	
Narcolepsy					+	+(rare)	+	+	+	

In addition to the above factors that may help in establishing a diagnosis of psychomotor epilepsy, the EEG and the response to anticonvulsant therapy may be useful. The EEG may help to confirm the suspicion that an active seizure state exists. It also provides information that helps determine whether a disorder is diffuse, lateralized, or focal in origin. The characteristic abnormality in psychomotor seizures is an anterior temporal spike focus. Repeating the test during sleep or using nasopharyngeal or sphenoidal leads will reveal abnormalities in some patients, but the incidence of normal records remains relatively high (see p. 26). Depending on the criteria used for the diagnosis of epilepsy, normal sleep records may be seen in roughly one-third of epileptic patients. For this reason, activating agents such as metrazole and Megimide have been used to induce electroencephalographic changes in patients suspected of being epileptic. Though this is often successful, results must be interpreted cautiously, since these drugs, even in low doses, may induce changes in some nonepileptic persons. If a normal EEG does not rule out psychomotor epilepsy, neither can the diagnosis of epilepsy be sustained merely on the basis of an abnormal record, since 10 to 15 percent of the general population have abnormal EEG's. These abnormalities, however, are usually not of a paroxysmal or an epileptiform type (see p. 25).

The use of a pharmacological response to establish a clinical diagnosis is difficult at best, and often impossible, yet a trial of anticonvulsant therapy, starting with diphenylhydantoin or carbamazepine, may sometimes provide useful diagnostic information. In such therapeutic trials, increasing doses should be given until either the seizures stop or signs of an overdose develop. The determination of the serum concentration of anticonvulsants is a useful guide to the adequacy of a therapeutic trial. Nystagmus is usually the first sign of toxicity with diphenylhydantoin, but not always. Other signs of toxicity include slurred speech, ataxia, lethargy, difficulty concentrating, and dysmnesia.

There are unfortunately no firm criteria for making a definite diagnosis of epilepsy, especially complex partial (psychomotor) epilepsy. Reports of the frequency and duration of particular manifestations of complex partial seizures are misleading and involve circular reasoning about the presence of these manifestations. For example, if an investigator regards automatisms as necessary for the diagnosis and he defines this as a meaningless movement of hand and mouth lasting a short period of time during which the patient is out of contact with the environment, his report that such brief automatisms occurred in 90 percent of cases of complex partial epilepsy should not necessarily lead us to discard this diagnosis in another case that is unaccompanied by such brief automatisms (Theodore, Porter, and Penry, 1981).

THE EEG AND THE DIAGNOSIS OF EPILEPSY

The term epileptiform has been applied to any paroxysmal discharge containing spikes or sharp waves, either localized or generalized. Such discharges are usually but not always associated with epilepsy. In a study of 6497 unselected, nonepileptic patients Zivin and Ajmone-Marsan (1968) found spikes and sharp waves in only 2.2 percent. In this group of patients with paroxysmal discharges, seizures eventually developed in 15 percent. In another study, focal spikes were found in 1.5 percent of 1000 carefully selected normal children (Petersen, Olofsson, and Sellden, 1968). In 242 children whose EEG's showed spike foci, Trojaborg (1968) found that 82 percent were epileptic, that another 13 percent without epilepsy had structural brain disease, and that only 5 percent were without any clear-cut evidence of brain disease, most of whom were diagnosed as having "behavior disorders." Clearly, epileptiform discharges are usually associated with epilepsy, but it is also possible to have an epileptiform EEG and not have epilepsy.

If an epileptiform EEG cannot fully establish the diagnosis of epilepsy, neither does the finding of a normal interictal EEG rule out the possibility of epilepsy. Ajmone-Marsan and Zivin (1970) reviewed 1824 EEG's from 308 epileptic patients who ranged in age from less than one to sixty-four years. Each patient had at least three recordings. Waking and sleep records were obtained for all, as well as responses to hyperventilation and photic stimulation. At the first examination, epileptiform activity was present in only 56 percent of patients. In subsequent recordings an additional 26 percent of patients showed such activity. Nonetheless, 18 percent of the patients had at least three consecutively negative recordings. Only 30 percent had epileptiform activity in all recordings.

The age of the patient at the time of the EEG and at the onset of seizures influenced the incidence of epileptiform tracings. When the EEG was recorded from children less than ten years old, approximately 80 percent had positive first recordings; but in subsequent decades there was a decline in the rate of positive recordings. Among those with seizures developing after the age of 30, there were several times the number of negative EEG's than repeatedly positive records. The type of epilepsy influenced the rate of positivity. Epileptiform EEG's were seen in almost 95 percent of patients with "absence" attacks. However, the authors of this important study failed to state how they established the diagnosis of epilepsy and this failure probably underlies some of their more surprising findings: that 98 percent of patients with seizures arising in the temporal lobe had an epileptiform EEG at some time and therefore that complex partial seizures correlate better with the EEG than any other clinical seizure type! This conclusion is probably unwarranted. Even though a high correlation between psychomotor-temporal lobe epilepsy and positive EEG has been duplicated many times (Currie, Heathfield, Henson et al., 1971; Glaser, 1967; Gibbs and Gibbs, 1952), this flies in the face of the common clinical experience that epileptiform EEG abnormalities in complex partial seizures are discovered in patients with complex partial seizures *less* often than in patients with most other clinical types of epilepsy. Indeed, it is known that a person can have symptomatic complex partial seizures with epileptiform activity recorded from the amygdala or hippocampus while the surface EEG is within normal limits *during the attack.* It would seem possible that in all these reports of the interictal EEG characteristics of complex partial seizures, the diagnosis of epilepsy was to some degree dependent on the EEG. In other words, the EEG was used as a diagnostic tool in establishing the diagnosis of complex partial seizures. If the EEG were not abnormal, the authors may have felt they could not sustain the diagnosis of epilepsy. The high correlation of epileptiform patterns with complex partial seizures in these reports, then, may reflect the great difficulty that clinicians face in establishing that diagnosis.

Because epileptiform features are especially critical for the diagnosis of complex partial seizures in the ordinary practice of neurology, but are difficult to uncover in patients suspected of having complex partial seizures, special recording and activating techniques have been devised. These include nasopharyngeal recordings, sphenoidal recordings, sleep deprivation, and sleep EEG's.

Unfortunately, nasopharyngeal electrodes are prone to artifacts that seriously reduce their utility. The most troublesome of these are the spikelike discharges produced by contractions of the nasopharyngeal muscles (Bickford, 1979). There is a difference of opinion concerning the usefulness of nasopharyngeal leads; some experienced electroencephalographers hold them to be useful only rarely (Louis et al., 1982). The basic question is: "How often does one see epileptiform discharges in the nasopharyngeal electrodes in a patient suspected of complex partial seizures when such discharges are completely missing from the surface recordings?" The answer to this question is not fully available for nasopharyngeal, sphenoidal, sleep deprived, sleep, or even depth recording. The usual response of encephalographers is "occasionally."

Sphenoidal leads give essentially the same information that nasopharyngeal leads are supposed to provide, but with much less of a problem caused by artifactual activity. The difficulty of positioning them in the proper location and the need for a surgical procedure to insert them has resulted in their use only in a few specialized clinics.

Sleep activation is least complicated in its interpretation when natural sleep is recorded. Many laboratories encourage a patient to drift off into sleep after obtaining an initial recording in the waking state. Most EEG activation occurs in the drowsiness or slow-wave phases during which it appears that there is a lower cerebral resistance to the synaptic spread of convulsive potentials.

Thus in slow-wave sleep, discharges that are limited during wake-fulness to deep structures such as the limbic structures now spread to cortical regions. It is not clear how often sleep recording, or sleep recording following sleep deprivation, uncovers abnormalities that are not at all present in the waking record.

Sleep deprivation per se provides an additional degree of activation compared with sleep unrelated to deprivation. Mattson et al. (1965) showed that an additional 34 percent of known epileptic patients activated significantly following sleep deprivation than with sleep alone. For this reason sleep records are usually done after a period of sleep deprivation.

The sampling problem inherent in any standard electroencephalography lasting 45 to 60 minutes is obvious. For this reason 24-hour ambulatory cassette EEG's have been introduced. This is the EEG equivalent of Halter monitoring for cardiac diseases; and it has proven to be quite useful, nearly doubling the incidence of epileptiform abnormalities as compared with standard EEG's in epileptic patients. In the initial tests of the cassette technique, the patients studied were known to have some epileptiform features by means of the much more elaborate eight-channel cable telemetry with video recording of the patient and his EEG for 24 to 72 hours (Ebersole and Leroy, 1983).

The EEG manifestations of complex partial seizures may be minimal or not pathognomonic, and even with telemetry it may be difficult to distinguish seizures from pseudoseizures. The postictal elevation of serum prolactin may represent a biochemical marker of complex partial seizures as it does for generalized tonic/clonic seizures (Prichard et al., 1983).

PSEUDOSEIZURES

The differentiation of hysterical seizures and true epilepsy is very difficult. Despite common wisdom to the effect that tongue biting, incontinence, injuries, and seizures during sleep do not occur in pseudo-grand mal seizures, there are no firm clinical criteria for the diagnosis of hysterical seizures. Self-harm may occur with hysterical attacks (Ferriss, 1972; Rossen, 1974; Standage, 1975; and Cohen and Suter, 1982) and urinary incontinence is common (Freud, 1949; Riley and Brannon, 1980).

Cohen and Suter (1982) found that of 51 patients with pseudoseizures, two reported self-injury, 13 reported urinary incontinence, 12 reported tongue lacerations and two reported spells in sleep. The diagnosis of hysterical seizures was established by initiating and terminating an attack with suggestion and saline injection during EEG monitoring without any change in the record during the attack. This activation test induced urinary incontinence twice and tongue laceration once.

The 51 patients with hysterical attacks comprised 6 percent of all patients aged 10 to 60 admitted to the hospital during the study period. Females represented 78 percent and two-thirds of the 51 were between 20 and 35 years of age. Seven were prisoners. None of the patients had more than one type of stereotyped hysterical attack. Evidence of past or present neurological disease existed in 12 patients. EEG's were normal in 32, mildly abnormal in 13, and clearly abnormal in 6. Six of the 51 patients were considered to have both hysterical and true seizures. One of these had a normal EEG but a history consistent with alcohol withdrawal seizures. Three other patients may have had childhood seizures.

A higher prevalence of coexistent organic neurological disorders (44%) and true epilepsy (37%) was reported in a group of 41 patients with "convincing evidence of psychogenic seizures" at Johns Hopkins (Krumholz and Niedermeyer, 1983). These findings are suspect because the criteria for the diagnosis of psychogenic seizures were not presented and only 13 patients had EEG's during psychogenic seizures. Sixty percent of the seizures were "major." In 34 percent, they resembled complex partial, absence, or partial attacks.

Using an EEG technique with suggestion to induce seizures, Lesser and his colleagues (1983) found that 50 of 79 patients referred to the Cleveland Clinic for differentiation between psychogenic and epileptic attacks had pseudoseizures. Five (10%) of these had both psychogenic seizures and true epilepsy. Eight patients had epileptiform records but either no psychogenic seizure was recorded or a definite decision could not be made. Amongst patients with known epilepsy, between 10 and 20 percent have experienced psychogenic seizures (Ramani et al., 1980; King et al., 1982; and Desai et al., 1979).

Underlying most of these data is the assumption that the surface EEG is the touchstone for determining the organicity of a seizure. Cohen and Suter added more stringent criteria by demanding that an attack be induced by suggestion and terminated by placebo, but even they relied heavily on the surface EEG as the ultimate criterion. It is known that spiking discharges associated with behavioral changes can be recorded from the hippocampus and amygdala while the surface recording is not epileptiform. Unknown are the answers to the questions: "How many epileptics have seizure bursts recorded in depth electrodes with clinical manifestations who show no simultaneous epileptiform surface abnormalities?" "How many of the bursts recorded in depth electrodes that are accompanied by clinical seizure activity are unassociated with epileptiform activity recorded on the surface?" If the prevalence of such combinations were high, a nonepileptiform EEG record obtained during an episode of questionable behavior would not convincingly rule out the diagnosis of epilepsy.

PRINCIPLES OF THERAPY

The major principles of therapy for epilepsy are simple. Initially, a single drug should be used at a moderate dosage. The dosage should then be increased until either the seizures are controlled or signs of toxicity appear. If it is not possible to control seizures at nontoxic doses, a second drug should be added. A word of caution is called for here. If an epileptic patient begins to manifest behavior that is deemed undesirable by either the physician or the family, there is a tendency to interpret this behavior as part of the seizure problem and to increase the anticonvulsant medication. In an attempt to bring the behavior under control, drug dosages may be increased enough to produce a toxic state that worsens the behavior and may lead to another increase in the medication, and so on. Frequently, the only intervention that need be made at this point is to reduce medication. The development and utilization of tests to determine the blood levels of the various medications, particularly phenytoin, phenobarbital, primidone, ethosuximide, and carbamazepine, has mitigated this problem. The determination of serum levels is of great help in determining whether a patient is taking his medicine as prescribed and whether more or less need be administered. Aside from the usual symptoms of toxicity with phenytoin (cerebellar symptoms, nystagmus, ataxia, sedation, euphoria) when the serum level of the drug is above 20 μg/ml, various psychiatric symptoms such as dementia, depression, and psychosis may develop. In some instances, seizures even increase in frequency. Milder behavioral symptoms that are commonly described by patients with high phenytoin blood levels include feelings of lower energy levels and initiative and decreased sociability and ability to concentrate.

Occasionally, complete seizure control is not possible without some degree of toxicity. In such cases, the functional capacity of the patient should determine what an acceptable degree of seizure control is. Among adult epileptics, grand mal seizures are generally the easiest to control, and complex partial seizures are the most difficult.

Since the introduction of phenytoin (diphenylhydantoin) in the 1930s, only a few new drugs, carbamazepine (Tegretol), valproic acid (Depakene), and clonazepam (Clonapin), have become available for the treatment of generalized motor, focal, and complex partial seizures. Carbamazepine has essentially the same spectrum of clinical usefulness as phenytoin, and it also has very similar side effects (Troupin, 1976). Dipropylacetate (valproic acid, Depakene) is most useful for generalized seizures (mainly uncomplicated tonic/clonic spells, absence and myoclonic) and has achieved a wide vogue (Delgado-Escueta et al., 1983; Wilder et al., 1983). The rare development of fatal hepatic complications resembling Reye's syndrome and pancreatitis has dampened our enthusiasm for it. Clonazepam (Clonapin), a benzodiazepine, is most helpful in myoclonic seizures. It has broader efficacy, but sedation is common at therapeutic levels and markedly limits its usefulness.

Our knowledge of and ability to use these anticonvulsant drugs has improved tremendously, and an understanding of their pharmacokinetics has been of great practical value to the practicing physician. Buchthal and others (1960) and other researchers have demonstrated that a good correlation exists between serum levels of anticonvulsants, seizure control, and the effects of overdose. The technology to determine serum levels of anticonvulsants represents, in our opinion, the most important advance in seizure therapy since the introduction of phenytoin.

When serum phenytoin and phenobarbital levels were first measured in the Epilepsy Center at Yale, it was found that in almost half the patients the levels were below the therapeutic range, though all patients were prescribed what was considered an adequate dose. Noncompliance was the main reason for this, but serial monitoring of serum levels was of great help in dealing with the problem. Over the course of two years, 48 patients followed at the Epilepsy Center experienced a steadily decreasing number of seizures when their anticonvulsant dose was adjusted to yield therapeutic levels in their serum, with the frequency of seizures per year falling from 210 to 75 (McElligott, 1974).

In some instances, individual differences in drug metabolism explain undermedication. The standard dosage of phenytoin is usually 300 mg/day, but this is often too low. In rare cases, 500 mg is too low, and in two patients whom we have seen personally, 700 mg were necessary to produce serum levels of 10 to 20 μg/ml. Recent reports by Ramsey and co-workers (1976) indicate that during pregnancy, gastrointestinal malabsorption of phenytoin may affect seizure control adversely. One woman who required 400 mg of phenytoin and 150 mg of phenobarbital to maintain her serum levels in the therapeutic range before and after pregnancy needed 1200 mg of phenytoin and 240 mg of phenobarbital during pregnancy. In addition, other drugs can affect anticonvulsant blood levels; isoniazide, chloramphenicol, dicumerol, disulfiram, or sulthiame, for example, can markedly increase diphenylhydantoin levels (Goodman and Gilman, 1975). There is some evidence, however, that anticonvulsant agents such as carbamazepine and, more recently, dipropylacetate can lower phenytoin serum levels (Mattson, 1976).

It has been the practice of most physicians to prescribe anticonvulsants in divided doses, and patients have been advised to take their medications three and even four times a day. Pharmacokinetic analysis based on blood levels indicates that this is usually an irrational way of prescribing medication in adults (though children may require it) and often works to the detriment of seizure control, since patients are more likely to forget their medication when it must be taken so frequently. In addition, midday doses can be inconvenient and embarrassing for adults at work. The half-life of an anticonvulsant is the time it takes for the serum level of an anticonvulsant to drop to half its steady-state level after it has been discontinued (see Table 1-4). Drugs with half-lives of more than 24 hours seldom need to be given more than once a day. As can be seen in Table 1-4, phenytoin, phenobarbital, and ethosuximide have half-lives of over 24 hours.

Measurements of blood levels have also provided information on how to begin therapy rationally. For some time it has been known that, when phenytoin is started orally, it takes 5 to 10 days for the blood level to rise to the therapeutic range. In the past, it had often been assumed that phenobarbital levels were achieved more quickly, but this is not the case. When a patient is given 1 to 2 mg/kg of phenobarbital orally, it takes almost three weeks to achieve steady-state levels in the therapeutic range. When double the ordinary dose is given for four days, the time required to achieve therapeutic levels is reduced to four days (Aird and Woodbury, 1974). To achieve therapeutic levels even more rapidly, 10 mg/kg of phenytoin or phenobarbital administered orally or intravenously results in levels of 15 to 30 μg/ml within a few hours. Table 1-2 summarizes some of the important features of the major anticonvulsant drugs. Though all these drugs may cause some degree of sedation at therapeutic levels, only the barbiturates and clonazepam regularly induce it.

Table 1-4
Commonly Used Anticonvulsants

Drug	Usual Daily Adult Dose (mg)	Thera-peutic Blood Level (μg/ml)	Days to Achieve Steady State (mainte-nance dose)	Adult Blood Half-Life (hours)	Major Indi-cations
Phenytoin (Diphenylhydantoin)	300–400	10–20	5–10	24–36	Generalized motor, focal motor and sensory, complex partial
Phenobarbital	90–120	15–30	14–21	96	Same
Primidone[a]	750–1000	5–15	2–4	8	Same
Phenobarbital (derived)		15–30	14–21	96	
Carbamazepine	800–1000	4–8	2–4	12	Same
Ethosuximide[b]	750–1000	40–100	5–6	60	Absence, myoclonic
Clonazepam	1–3	.03–.06	4–5	24	Myoclonic
Valproic acid	750–1000	50–90	1–3	8	Generalized motor, absence, myoclonic

Acetazolamide (Diamox) is a carbonic anhydrase inhibitor and may be effective in all seizure disorders, especially in myoclonic, atonic, akinetic seizures. High doses (30 mg/kg) are often necessary for seizure control.

Diazepam (Valium) has been effective in some minor motor seizure disorders when used orally, but it is most effective when used intravenously in the treatment of status epilepticus, where it has become the drug of choice, sometimes in combination with intravenous phenytoin.

Trimethadione (Tridione), a fairly toxic compound, is used in absence, myoclonic, atonic, and akinetic seizures, if other drugs fail.

Paraldehyde, chloral hydrate, Amytal, and the short-acting barbiturates are sedatives and are used only in status epilepticus.

Steroids and ACTH are sometimes used in infantile spasms and juvenile minor motor seizures. In other types of seizures, and at other ages, they are epileptogenic.

SURGERY IN EPILEPSY

There are very few seizure disorders that will not respond to some combination of medications, but a small number of unfortunate individuals suffer from severe seizures that cannot be controlled by medical therapy. For such cases, there are several major surgical approaches, and they all seem to be effective in certain cases. The most widely used approach involves the actual removal of epileptic brain tissue. When there is focal onset of seizures, the removal of tissue in the involved area can provide seizure control when other measures fail (Davidson and Falconer, 1975). When seizures are multifocal, this approach is unlikely to benefit patients.

Clearly, then, the discovery of a focal lesion is a critical factor in the success of surgery. Some centers that perform surgical excisions of epileptogenic foci rely on surface recording, nasopharyngeal and/or sphenoidal leads. Other centers routinely perform depth electroencephalography, despite the increase in risk and expense that this entails. Depth EEG has the potential to alter the surgical decision in half of the patients who are candidates (Spencer, 1981). In a recent report of 32 patients from a center that studies all potentially operable patients with depth recordings, 16 had unlocalized scalp EEG's. Three of these on depth recording had a consistent focal onset (Spencer et al., 1982). Of 15 with localized scalp EEG's, depth recordings revealed multiple foci in three patients and inaccurate localization of the focus on scalp recording in four more. Thus, scalp recording was inaccurate for localization in 10 of 32. When depth EEG consistently revealed a focal seizure onset and this was used to determine the site of surgical resection,

---

The Ketogenic Diet is used in difficult cases of myoclonic, atonic, akinetic seizures, though it is somewhat complicated and unpalatable. It may stop seizures in 50 percent of cases in which all drugs have failed to do so.

[a] Primidone is used primarily for control of complex partial seizures. Its major metabolite is phenobarbital.

[b] Ethosuximide is used almost exclusively in children.

good to excellent results were obtained in 12 of 13 patients. The seven patients with unlocalized seizures (less than 80% of seizures arising from one location) who underwent surgery had only fair to poor surgical results (Spencer et al., 1982).

The content of complex partial seizures has predictive value in determining the success of anterior temporal lobectomy in controlling intractable seizures. Nineteen of 20 patients whose seizures consisted of initial motionless staring, stereotyped automatisms, and reactive quasi-purposeful movements during periods of impaired consciousness stopped having attacks two to eight years after anterior temporal lobectomy. In contrast, all 11 patients who had seizures that started with complex automatisms but no initial motionless stare continued to have incapacitating seizures after surgery (Walsh and Delgado-Escueta, 1984).

Commisurotomy is another approach. Here, the corpus callosum and sometimes other tracts that connect the right and left hemispheres are severed. Reeves and Wilson (1976) have reported results with commisurotomy that seem to be typical of the hundred cases or so in which the operation has been performed since it was introduced about 10 years ago. Of their patients, three gained excellent seizure control, two improved, three remained the same or got worse, and one died shortly after the operation. As with most new surgical procedures, these operations were all performed on high risk or "last resort" cases. Consequently, little correlation with overt lesions or type of seizure has been possible. In general, the best results have been obtained in patients with infantile hemiplegia, with a shrunken, scarred hemisphere that serves no function other than to cause generalized seizures. When such patients fail to respond to anticonvulsant therapy, removal of the damaged hemisphere (hemispherectomy) can effectively control seizures, but commisurotomy is the more conservative surgical procedure because it prevents seizure activity from spreading from the damaged to the normal hemisphere.

In 1973, Cooper et al. introduced a third surgical approach to control epilepsy in a report of the effect of cerebellar stimulation via implanted electrodes upon seizures. Seven patients who had seizures despite "adequate therapy" were given such implants. Before surgery, three patients had psychomotor, three had grand mal, and one had focal seizures. After surgery, four had virtually complete control of seizures, two had markedly improved control, and one was unchanged. The stimulation was given through each of several electrodes for a 10-minute period several times a day for up to eight months. Unfortunately, the blood levels of anticonvulsants had not been estimated preoperatively for any of these patients, so the assumption of adequate medical therapy before the operation is unconfirmed.

Considerable experimental work has been done on the effect of cerebellar stimulation on seizures, but the data are conflicting and difficult to interpret (Myers et al., 1975). Suffice it to say that some investigators have shown termination of seizures in association with cerebellar stimulation, others have shown enhancement of seizures, and some have shown both. Although extremely interesting, this mode of therapy must still be regarded as of unproven value.

PERSONALITY, INTELLECTUAL DETERIORATION, AND PSYCHOSIS IN EPILEPSY

It is well known that different areas of the hippocampus, particularly Ammon's horn, are especially susceptible to reduction of energy production by such conditions as asphyxia, carbon monoxide poisoning, respiratory failure, and hypoglycemia (Green, 1964). Possibly as a consequence of this susceptibility, the hippocampus has the lowest seizure threshold of all the cortical regions. A loss of neurons in this region is commonly seen in the brains of epileptics, and it is thought that such changes result, at least in part, from the anoxia associated with seizures (Margerison and Corsellis, 1966). But these lesions in the hippocampus may also give rise to seizures, particularly psychomotor seizures, as well as to a variety of behavioral disturbances (Ounsted et al., 1966). The fact that there are lesions in these cases makes it reasonable to suppose that some form of deterioration of intellect and personality might occur in epilepsy and that such changes would be more often associated with psychomotor epilepsy than with other forms of seizure disorder.

Traditionally, many personality characteristics have been attributed to epileptics. They have been described as paranoid, preoccupied with religion, prone to aggressive outbursts, pedantic, egocentric, perseverating (sticky), and obsessive. Very few patients combine all these traits, which clearly are also present in other conditions. But a relatively consistent personality profile has been reported in patients with complex partial seizures (Bear and Fedio, 1977).

To measure intellectual deterioration in epileptics it would be necessary to control many factors, such as the age of the patient at onset of seizures, the duration of epilepsy, the clinical form of epilepsy (including the etiology and presence or absence of brain damage), the presence of other diseases, the social class and intelligence of the patient before disease onset, the drug used and its dosage and the blood level, the frequency of seizures, and, finally, the length of time between the last seizure and the examination. It hardly need be said that the perfect study has yet to be done.

On the Wechsler Adult Intelligence Scale (WAIS), most epileptic patients have scores in the normal range, but the scores do tend to cluster around the lower end of the range (Rodin, 1968). These data are consistent with the theory that deterioration may occur in epilepsy but give no information concerning the effects of repeated seizures and of different types of seizures upon the epileptic.

Obviously, longitudinal studies are preferable in ascertaining intellectual deterioration, but very few have been done. Using the Wechsler Intelligence Scale for Children (WISC), Rodin (1968) studied the intellectual development of 58 epileptic children with follow-up testing after two years. He found that seizures were indeed related to a decrease in the IQ, particularly on the performance scale. Deterioration was unrelated to the presumed etiology of seizures or to the presence of brain damage, and it occurred mostly in patients who initially had an above average IQ. Rodin concluded that patients with complete seizure control did very well compared to those with incomplete seizure control, but patients who had many seizures did not necessarily do poorly, as compared with those who had fewer seizures. Though Rodin emphasized that deterioration was not necessarily permanent, but rather reflected the state of affairs at the moment the patient was tested, his study showed quite clearly that incomplete control of seizures shows a statistically significant correlation with IQ deterioration.

Similar findings were recorded by Chaudhry and Pond (1961), who studied the role of major and minor seizures in intellectual and social deterioration of children. Twenty-eight epileptic children who showed intellectual and social deterioration by serial testing and observation were compared with an equal number of epileptics who were matched for age, sex, type of epilepsy, and brain damage but who showed no deterioration. In the first group, seizures were more frequent, the response to anticonvulsant medication was poorer, and abnormal electroencephalographic records were more common. No significant difference between the two groups was found at the ages at which brain damage had been sustained, the age of the patient at onset of epileptic attacks, the site or extent of brain damage, the amount or duration of anticonvulsant treatment, or the family history of epilepsy. Like Rodin, Chaudhry and Pond emphasized that the deterioration in social and intellectual functioning was not always permanent; they also put forward the hypothesis that some "subclinical" form of seizure might be responsible for the apparent worsening in the clinical status of the patients who deteriorated. In this way the authors tried to explain the phenomenon of deterioration in patients who had relatively infrequent clinical seizures. Though these studies are not conclusive, they do support the impression that poorly controlled seizures cause temporary and sometimes permanent intellectual deterioration.

A prospective study of the stability of IQ in 72 epileptic children tested within two weeks of the initial diagnosis and yearly for four years revealed no overall differences over time or in comparison with nonepileptic siblings. Eleven percent of the patients did experience a persistent drop in IQ of 10 points or more. In these, an early age of onset of seizures and the number of drugs to which the patient became toxic best predicted changes in IQ. This suggested that total seizure control, especially in younger children, should not be achieved at the price of repeated episodes of drug toxicity (Burgeois et al., 1983). The importance of anticonvulsant drug toxicity in the pathogenesis of behavioral disorders and poor seizure control in patients with intractable epilepsy was highlighted by a study of 69 such patients of whom more than half were benefited by withdrawal of sedative-hypnotic antiepileptic drugs with respect to symptoms of drug toxicity and seizure control (Theodore and Porter, 1983). The improvement of patients with intractable epilepsy on tests of cognitive, perceptual, motor, and memory functions has been specifically related to withdrawal of barbiturates and an overall reduction in the number of anticonvulsant drugs but not to reduction of seizure frequency (Giordoni et al., 1983).

The potential harmfulness of febrile seizures was suggested by a study of the intellectual status of 47 twins who were discordant for febrile convulsions; fourteen monozygotic pairs were included in the study (Schiottz-Christensen and Bruhn, 1973). The children's intellectual status was evaluated by interviewing their parents, sending questionnaires to their teachers, and administering Wechsler Intelligence tests of perceptual motor functions to the children. This testing was done by psychologists who did not know which twin had suffered febrile convulsions. Details of the birth histories were obtained from chart reviews.

Of greatest interest were the findings in the monozygotic twins; the psychological tests revealed a significant intellectual deficit (compared to the unaffected twin) in children who had experienced one or more febrile convulsions. Little cerebral dysfunction was found, however, and had the febrile convulsion group been evaluated by psychological tests alone, none would have been characterized as suffering from a brain lesion. The school records showed a tendency for lower scholastic achievement and more behavior problems in the febrile convulsion group. The clearest differentiation between the two groups, however, was on the Wechsler Intelligence Scale—a performance IQ difference of 7 points ($p = 0.001$).

In such a study, it is difficult to determine if brain damage is a cause or a result of a febrile seizure. But, in the whole group and in the monozygotic twins, in particular, no correlation was found between intellectual deficit and events in the history that could have been associated with brain damage. Birth weight, position, and order and assisted delivery and perinatal state did not correlate with the deficits in the seizure group. Events that can cause brain damage were encountered as often in the nonseizure twins as in the seizure twins. Since this study by Schiottz-Christensen and Bruhn was a particularly careful one, it could be concluded that febrile convulsions in themselves could cause cerebral dysfunction.

Children who suffer febrile convulsions also have been said to have an increased risk of developing temporal lobe epilepsy later (Lennox, 1953). This increased risk is attributed to damage to the mesial temporal structures by prolonged febrile convulsions. There is also some evidence that prompt treatment of prolonged febrile convulsions, followed by the prophylactic use of phenobarbital in adequate therapeutic doses, reduces the frequency of recurrent convulsions and mesial temporal sclerosis in children (Lennox-Buchtal, 1973).

The obvious conclusion to be drawn from these studies is that patients who have suffered one or two febrile seizures should be treated with phenobarbital to prevent future seizures, intellectual deterioration, and behavioral abnormalities. This conclusion has not been universally accepted. Hauser et al. (1977) followed 657 patients with fever-induced seizures for more than 8000 person-years to assess risks for subsequent afebrile seizures. When patients with profound, preexisting neurological deficits were excluded, only 3 percent of the remaining 632 patients developed recurrent afebrile seizures. The characteristics of the febrile seizures that increased the risk of subsequent afebrile seizures were those that suggest that brain damage preceded the initial febrile seizure: the presence of focal features and the prolonged duration of the seizure. Thus, this study casts doubt upon the epileptogenicity of brief, generalized febrile seizures that occur in children who are otherwise normal.

Nelson and Ellenberg (1976) reported that recurrent nonfebrile epileptic seizures had occurred by seven years of age in 2 percent of 1706 children who had experienced at least one febrile seizure. Of those whose prior neurologic or developmental status was abnormal and whose first seizure was longer than 15 minutes, multiple or focal epilepsy developed at a rate of 9.2 percent as compared with 0.5 percent in a control group without febrile seizures. Of those with a normal preseizure neurological status whose febrile seizure was noncomplex, epilepsy developed in only 1.1 percent, which is nonetheless a greater rate than that for children with no febrile seizures.

Nelson and Ellenberg (1977) have also presented data that indicate that febrile seizures have no adverse effect upon subsequent intellectual and academic performance. This prospective study included 431 sibling pairs of which one child had experienced at least one febrile seizure while the other was seizure free. Both children were tested with the Wechsler Intelligence Scale for Children and the Wide Range Achievement Test at age 7 years. No difference in the intelligence quotient or the frequency of learning disorders was found.

To those reports that question the harmful effect of febrile seizures must be added the increasing evidence that various types of behavioral disturbance and learning disorder in children may occur from the use of antiepileptic medications. It has been suggested that these disturbances may not always be reversible (Stores, 1975). Therefore, the question of whether, when, and how to treat febrile seizures remains unsettled.

Repeated stimulation may be harmful, however. A striking demonstration of change in the epileptogenicity of brain tissue as a result of electrical stimulation was reported by Goddard et al. (1969). Animals with electrodes permanently implanted in their brains were stimulated briefly each day with subconvulsant currents. During the first week of stimulation, there was no behavioral change or EEG afterdischarge, but during the second week, stimulation produced minimal focal seizures, and during the third week, bilateral seizures. These experiments suggested that a focus of abnormal electrical activity could be epileptogenic in surrounding, previously normal cell populations.

The effects of electroconvulsive therapy (ECT) on the development of epilepsy might be relevant to the issue of the epileptogenicity of epilepsy but no study has prospectively evaluated the onset of epilepsy in patients receiving ECT. Though the frequency of epilepsy after ECT (114 per 100,000) is five times greater than in an age-adjusted nonpsychiatric cohort, individual susceptibility rather than treatment features seems to be the determining factor (Devinsky and Duchowny, 1983).

Anoxia has been frequently suggested as the basic mechanism in epileptic deterioration. There is no doubt that tissue anoxia can occur in all forms of epilepsy, and it could be an important factor in deterioration. One would expect anoxia to be especially important in grand mal seizures, in which excessive muscular activity and apnea coincide with a generalized increase in neuronal firing rate, which creates a metabolic demand for oxygen that cannot be met. There is reason to believe, however, that anoxia is not the only causative factor in either chronic deterioration or postictal depression (a phenomenon that may be analogous and that is easier to study). There are as yet no firm indications of what the other factors may be—an embarrassing hiatus in medical knowledge. Todd's paralysis is, for example, a temporary paralysis that may occur after generalized seizures associated with prolonged anoxia, but it may also occur after brief focal seizures during which consciousness is preserved and respiration is normal. Impairment of recent memory following electroconvulsive therapy (ECT) in many nonepileptic patients occurs even when muscular activity during the ECT-induced seizure is abolished with succinylcholine while respiration and oxygenation are artificially maintained. After many shocks, this transient deficit may become permanent in some cases.

If anoxia and such subsequent metabolic changes as buildup of carbon dioxide and lactate and fall in pH were the only factors determining postictal depression, and if epileptic deterioration were related to these factors, patients with grand mal seizures would probably demonstrate greater intellectual deficits than those with psychomotor seizures. This has not been observed (Guerrant et al., 1962). Also, some experiments have cast serious doubt on the accuracy of the theory that anoxia and other metabolic changes consequent to it are the only important factors in postictal neural dysfunction. Even when oxygenation was maintained and large accumulations of carbon dioxide and organic acids were prevented, electrically induced seizures still produced neuronal "exhaustion" in animals and humans during the postictal phase (Posner et al., 1969).

RELATIONSHIP OF SEIZURE DISORDERS TO PSYCHOSIS

The role of seizures in the development of psychiatric disorders has been even more difficult to document than the intellectual deterioration that may result from seizures, yet much has been written about the relationship between psychomotor seizures, or temporal lobe epilepsy, and psychosis. This may be explained by the widespread clinical impression that patients with psychomotor seizures are more prone to develop psychosis than are patients with other forms of epilepsy.

In a study designed to test the hypothesis that patients with psychomotor seizures have more psychiatric disorders than have patients with grand mal epilepsy or general medical chronic illnesses, Guerrant et al. (1962) studied 32 patients with psychomotor epilepsy, 26 patients with idiopathic grand mal epilepsy, and 26 patients with a variety of chronic medical illnesses that did not involve the brain. The groups were fairly homogeneous in terms of age, sex, education, and social class, but the patients with psychomotor seizures received more anticonvulsant drugs than those with grand mal seizures, and this factor was not adequately controlled. On independent evaluation by two psychiatrists, 47 percent of the patients with psychomotor seizures were diagnosed as having an organic brain syndrome on the basis of impaired memory, attention, concentration, lability of affect, and slowed speech. Only 27 percent of those with grand mal seizures and 4 percent of those with a general medical illness were diagnosed as having organic brain syndromes. Psychosis was also much more common in the group with psychomotor seizures. It was seen in 20 percent of the patients with psychomotor seizures and in only 4 percent of those with grand mal. The incidence of psychosis in the general population is about 1 percent (Srole et al., 1962). Since the patients in Guerrant's study came from a low social class, the incidence of 20 percent for psychomotor seizures may be somewhat inaccurate for the general population, but the main point is clearly made.

Standard psychometric testing by Guerrant's group, however, failed to confirm the finding of more psychiatric disorders in patients with psychomotor seizures. This discrepancy between the clinical impression of organic mental dysfunction and psychosis, on the one hand, and conventional psychological test results, on the other, has been observed by several other investigators (Small et al., 1962; Stevens, 1966). It is possible that the standard psychological tests that were used tested aspects of cognitive and other psychological functions that were not observed in the clinical interviews.

Rodin et al. (1976) reported that more behavioral abnormalities occur in patients with temporal lobe seizures than in epileptics without temporal lobe seizures; these patients were precisely matched for age, sex, and IQ. Further analysis of the data showed that the group of temporal lobe patients who suffered from more than one seizure type was responsible for the difference between temporal lobe seizure patients and the controls. When these authors compared 56 temporal lobe patients, with more than one seizure type, against 32 controls without temporal lobe seizures, who suffered from more than one seizure type, the temporal lobe patients were found to have significantly more anxiety during mental status examination, more personality disturbance on psychological testing, more psychotic tendencies on psychological testing, and a higher elevation on the paranoia scale of the Minnesota Multiphasic Personality Inventory (MMPI) test than the controls.

Though there had been many anecdotal reports linking schizophrenia and epilepsy (and occasionally even indicating their nonassociation), it was not until publication of a large study by Slater and Beard (1963) that a clear relationship between a psychosis resembling schizophrenia and epilepsy was established. Of 69 psychotic epileptics in this study, 80 percent showed evidence of temporal lobe dysfunction on the basis of a history of psychomotor seizures or temporal lobe spiking on the EEG or both. The mean age of onset of psychosis was 30 years. The mean duration of the epilepsy before the onset of psychosis was 14 years. Seizures varied from rare to frequent. All patients, however, had incomplete seizure control at the time they became psychotic. There seemed to be no relationship between the onset of psychosis and the dosage of anticonvulsant drugs. It is highly unlikely that there could have been a chance association of epilepsy and schizophrenia in these cases. The ease with which the authors were able to collect 69 cases from the population served by their hospitals, and the low incidence of schizophrenia in the first-degree relatives of these patients strongly indicated that they were suffering from something other than classic schizophrenia. Though this group did show, at various times, all the cardinal features of schizophrenia, these psychoses deviated from norms for schizophrenia in some respects. Affective responsiveness was often preserved—to an extent unusual in schizophrenia. In the later stages of the development of psychosis, the patient's personality was sometimes left essentially undamaged, which is rarely the case in the later stages of schizophrenia.

Slater and Beard, however, felt that the psychosis could not be symptomatically differentiated from ordinary schizophrenia without reference to historical material. In fact, two-thirds of the patients who had previously come into contact with independent psychiatrists were diagnosed as schizophrenic. Slater and Beard's study strongly suggests that epileptic psychosis can exist as a clinical entity that is etiologically distinct from schizophrenia. Furthermore, the study supports the contention that patterns of abnormal activity in the temporal lobe and its limbic projections predispose an individual to a schizophrenialike psychosis. This hypothesis has been supported by other studies of psychotic epileptics (Pond, 1957; Glaser et al., 1963; Flor-Henry, 1969, 1972).

Other mental abnormalities have been reported to coexist with epilepsy, and especially with complex partial seizures. The association of seizures with depression, hysteria, and aggressiveness has been less impressively documented, however, than the schizophrenialike psychosis of epilepsy. The evidence for such an association is essentially limited to case reports. It appears, however, that the risk of suicide attempts is five times higher in epileptics than in the general population and about 10 percent of epileptic patients take antidepressant drugs (Hawton et al., 1980 and Ojemann et al., 1983).

Some authors have commented on the tendency of some patients to become psychotic when seizures are controlled and vice versa (Pond, 1957; Flor-Henry, 1969; Reynolds, 1971). The studies that have systematically directed attention to this observation are in some disagreement.

Comparing 50 temporal lobe epileptics with psychosis to 50 such epileptics without psychosis, Flor-Henry (1969) found that the number of psychomotor seizures observed was inversely related to psychosis. His psychotic patients had fewer psychomotor seizures, or none at all, yet the incidence of major convulsions and the type of medication and dosage was similar in each group. Neurological signs and abnormal EEG's (lateralized to the dominant hemisphere) were more prominent in the psychotic group, which seemed to suggest that qualitative differences between the groups were not controlled.

Standage and Fenton (1975) also compared a group of temporal lobe epileptics to a group of epileptics without temporal lobe symptoms using a detailed reliable psychiatric interview technique. They found the psychiatric symptoms in the two groups to be similar, as did Mignone (1970), but they did note a significant relationship to seizure frequency, as did Flor-Henry; that is, there was an inverse relationship between those with the most psychiatric symptoms and seizure frequency. They also noted that patients who had complex auras tended to also have more psychiatric symptoms.

In Slater and Beard's study, there was no relationship between the severity or frequency of major (grand mal) seizures and the development of psychosis in the great majority of the patients. In six cases, psychotic symptoms appeared when the seizure frequency was falling and in two, the seizures increased in frequency shortly before the psychosis appeared. This contradiction may be more apparent than real, however, since Slater and Beard did not study the frequency of psychomotor seizures in relation to psychosis and Flor-Henry studied only psychomotor seizures in this regard. More recent studies have indicated that psychosis in epileptics is associated with temporal lobe epilepsy in 6 of 10 cases and in these, the seizures antedated the psychosis. In three, the psychosis emerged as the seizures were being controlled. Two of these were receiving high doses of ethosuximide (see p. 49). In the others, no evident clues helped to explain the psychosis (Ramani and Gumnit, 1982).

The etiology of the schizophrenialike psychosis of epilepsy is obscure, but when patients with epileptic psychosis are studied, two clinical findings stand out: there is a history of (1) prolonged use of anticonvulsant medication and (2) an incompletely controlled seizure disorder, usually involving the limbic system, which precedes the psychosis.

Reynolds (1971) emphasized the possibility that anticonvulsant medication may cause epileptic psychosis. He presented evidence that anticonvulsants often lower serum, red blood cell, and spinal fluid folate levels. He feels that the mental changes encountered in epileptics may result from a similar depression of folate and vitamin B_{12} levels in brain tissue. There is, as yet, no direct evidence that brain levels of these vitamins are lower in psychotic epileptics than in nonpsychotic ones, nor is there general agreement that low folate levels in treated epileptics are related to either psychosis or seizure control (Norris and Pratt, 1971). A fairly conclusive study makes it appear highly unlikely that such a relationship exists (Cramer et al., 1976).

It is possible that chronic anticonvulsant therapy may have a toxic effect on mental functioning that is mediated by some mechanism other than interaction with folate or vitamin B_{12}. Actual drug toxicity does not seem likely to be a major factor in most cases of epileptic psychosis, since the amount of medication prescribed for patients is not related to either the incidence or severity of psychosis (though, of course, the prescribed dose is not necessarily the administered one because of the compliance problem). Also, it is well known that psychosis may also develop in untreated epileptics (Asuni and Pillutla, 1967).

Reynolds and Travers (1974) showed that patients with more behavioral symptoms than are usually observed did have higher serum phenytoin (diphenylhydantoin, DPH) and phenobarbital levels (though the drug levels were within the therapeutic range). This study should be repeated, and studies correlating different blood levels and psychiatric status in these patients are also indicated. These considerations emphasize the utility of serum drug level determinations in the management of patients.

A curious paradox exists in anticonvulsant therapy; ethosuximide, a drug used almost exclusively in children, can rapidly precipitate psychosis in adults (and rarely in children). The mechanism involved is unknown, but predisposition to psychosis does not appear to be a factor (Fischer et al., 1965).

In addition to drug effect, other hypotheses to explain the development of epileptic psychosis must be considered. If the psychosis were caused by epilepsy, that is, with schizophrenia developing as the direct result of epileptic discharge within the brain, seizure frequency could be correlated with the severity of psychosis, and anticonvulsants would be the treatment of choice for epilepsy and epileptic psychosis. But this is usually not the case.

It is also possible that epileptic psychosis is a psychological reaction to years of seizure episodes, during which clouded consciousness and periodic sensations of a disturbing nature, which often bear no relation to external reality, lead to the confusion of reality with subjective experience. Though this mechanism cannot be ruled out in some patients, other patients with epileptic psychosis do not experience seizures of this type. Also, the great majority of patients with psychomotor seizures, even those with frequent "twilight states," do not develop psychosis; if psychomotor epilepsy did produce psychosis in this way, controlling the seizures would be expected to improve the psychosis or to decrease the chances that it would develop.

On the basis of what is known about the limbic system, it is tempting to hypothesize that the schizophrenialike psychosis of epilepsy is the result of abnormal electrical activity in limbic structures over a number of years and that this activity may or may not be associated with frequent clinical seizures. Thus, one would hypothesize that psychosis would result from "subictal" or "interictal" discharging lesions in sensitive limbic areas of the brain; these discharges would present as atypical psychomotor seizures. The "interictal state" would be the abnormal behavioral or thought pattern; the "subictal discharge" would be the abnormal electrical firing, in the limbic system, that contributes to or actually produces the interictal state. The psychological correlate of the interictal state has been described as a fluctuating disorder of cerebral functioning, with "fluidity of thought processes, loss of trains of associations, word finding difficulties and faulty cognitive functioning" (Glaser et al., 1963; Glaser, 1964). The disorder does not usually respond to anticonvulsant therapy. Sometimes, but not usually, the psychotic disorder may be related to a specific psychological disturbance. The confusion and intellectual disorganization of the psychotic disorder more often develop gradually and seem unrelated to environmental stress. Such interictal disturbances are occasionally difficult to distinguish from psychomotor seizures. But they may persist for days, weeks, or months; they may not be associated with a clear-cut seizure, though at times they may lead to one. When this is the case a major (grand mal) seizure may seem to clear up the interictal state, and the patient may return to a more normal mental condition, at least temporarily. During the interictal state, the EEG may show unmodified rhythms, desynchronization, or a reinforced temporal abnormality; abnormal discharges may disappear (Glaser, 1964). Recording the EEG from the scalp can be misleading since it may not reveal epileptiform discharges, which can be detected simultaneously in the amygdaloid region with depth electrodes (Bickford, 1957).

The concept of subictal discharges could be used to explain a positive association or even a nonassociation of psychomotor seizures and psychosis, but some other factor must be invoked to explain the inverse relation Flor-Henry found between these two phenomena. One can only speculate about this, but the adaptive cerebral mechanisms that develop in response to a focal subictal discharge, and that tend to prevent it from spreading, may also cause in the region surrounding the focus changes that adversely affect mentation (see below, p. 62).

Taylor (1975) sheds some light on this in his report of a lower incidence of psychosis in patients with destructive tissue lesions compared to patients with postnatal mesial sclerosis lesions. This may indicate, at least in terms of psychosis, that it is better to have a nonfunctional temporal lobe than dysfunctional one. Interestingly, Taylor also reported a greater preponderance of dominant hemisphere lesions among the patients with psychosis. Flor-Henry (1969) made this same observation.

A careful psychological study of 27 children with either pure left (13) or pure right (14) temporal lobe epilepsy revealed no left-right differences in WISC, Halstead-Reitan, Achievement Test and Personal Inventory scores. Cognitive, personality, and school problems were encountered in 10 (five with left and five with right foci) and those showed lower neuropsychological test functioning than did the normally adjusted children (Canfield et al., 1984).

There is no clear answer to the question of whether subictal discharges can lead to severe abnormality of behavior and thought in patients who have never had a recognizable seizure, although it seems likely that this may occur in both adults (Ervin et al., 1955) and children (Green, 1961). The results of anticonvulsant therapy, however, are usually disappointing when temporal spikes are associated with behavioral abnormality in the absence of seizures.

The relationship of psychosis to epilepsy cannot be easily defined. The prolonged behavioral disturbances that respond to anticonvulsants (Friedlander and Feinstein, 1956; Goldensohn and Gold, 1960) seem to be manifestations of seizures. These include confusion, withdrawal, negativism, fogginess, and hostility.

The major tranquilizers, such as fluphenazine (an "alerting" phenothiazine), either alone or in combination with anticonvulsants, have been used successfully in patients with interictal psychosis (Detre and Feldman, 1963; Detre and Jarecki, 1971, and Ramani and Gumnit, 1982). Although high, or rapidly increasing, doses of phenothiazines precipitate seizures in some patients, low, or slowly increasing, doses often alleviate the psychosis, and they sometimes seem to lower the frequency of a patient's seizures, especially in patients whose seizure frequency is aggravated by anxiety. The treatment of psychosis is purely symptomatic and must proceed on a trial-and-error basis. There are as yet no carefully controlled studies that have established the effectiveness of ataractic drugs in the treatment of epileptic psychosis.

It may be extremely difficult in an individual case to distinguish ordinary schizophrenia from the schizophrenialike psychosis of epilepsy. In both conditions, the psychosis may begin in the second or third decade, and the course varies. Remission may occur in either, though both tend to be chronic. Personality and affect tend to be less abnormal in epileptic psychosis, but symptomatically, the two psychotic conditions may be virtually indistinguishable. The family history and a positive medical history of epilepsy, however, aids in the diagnosis. In ordinary schizophrenia there is a very high incidence of serious psychopathology in the immediate family of affected patients, with 10 to 15 percent of the first-degree relatives diagnosed as schizophrenic. By contrast, the incidence of schizophrenia in the family of patients with epileptic psychosis does not exceed that of the general population (Slater and Glithero, 1963). A history of epilepsy is, of course, the distinguishing feature, being positive in epileptic psychosis and negative in ordinary schizophrenia. The EEG may be of some help in the differential diagnosis, since electroencephalographic abnormalities, particularly those in which the anterior temporal regions are implicated, are characteristic of epileptic psychosis. There is an increase in frequency of abnormal EEG's in schizophrenics, and normal EEG's are not unusual in epileptic psychotics. Phenothiazines are beneficial, but anticonvulsant drugs are of only limited therapeutic usefulness in the two conditions.

Antidepressant drugs may lower seizure threshold (Trimble, 1978) yet some antidepressants like the tricyclic, imipramine, have anticonvulsant effects (Fromm et al., 1978). A comparison of tricyclics with tetracyclics in 186 depressed patients revealed that only 2.2 percent in the tricyclic group had seizures and 15.6 percent of those receiving the tetracyclic, maprofiline (Ludiomil), had seizures. All were generalized and none of the patients had preexistent epilepsy (Bryan et al., 1983). In 19 epileptics followed before and during treatment of depression with the tricyclic doxepin (Sinequan), improved seizure control was associated with doxepin use in 15 and there were increased seizures in two (Ojemann et al., 1983). It would thus appear that tricyclics are to be preferred for the treatment of depression in epileptics but there is some risk of increased seizure frequency if they are used.

The relationship between abnormal sexual behavior and epilepsy has often been noted but rarely studied. Gastaut and Collomb (1954) reported hyposexuality in two-thirds of 36 temporal lobe epileptics but found that it was infrequent in patients with other types of epilepsy. A striking feature of this hyposexuality is poverty of sexual drive rather than impotence. The condition seems to follow the onset of seizures. Sexual drive does not develop in psychomotor epilepsy beginning in childhood, and sexual interest diminishes after the onset of psychomotor epilepsy in adults. A study by Taylor (1969) of 100 psychomotor epileptics before and after temporal lobectomy confirmed the findings of Gastaut and Collomb. Only 14 patients had a satisfactory sexual adjustment, preoperatively. Postoperatively, the sexual adjustment in these 14 was still normal, it improved in 22 other patients, and worsened in another 14. Fifty patients maintained the same poor adjustment. Those patients who improved also experienced the greatest relief from seizures.

The relationship between epilepsy and impotence has also been studied. Hierons and Saunders (1966) reported 15 cases of impotence unrelated to diminished libido in patients with temporal lobe lesions. It is not clear whether their report reflected the selection of patients studied or accurately represented the psychosexual adjustment of all patients with temporal lobe epilepsy. It is not uncommon for sexual problems to appear in any chronically ill patient. But the experimental evidence that relates sexual function to the limbic system is a further reason to expect some sort of sexual dysfunction in psychomotor epilepsy. Destructive lesions in the amygdala have given rise to indiscriminate hypersexuality (Kluver and Bucy, 1939) and stimulation of limbic structures has given rise to erections (MacLean and Ploog, 1962). "Sexual seizures" have been noted in temporal lobe epileptics but are quite rare (Currier et al., 1971). Sexual automatisms have more recently been identified with frontal foci (Spencer et al., 1983).

Other studies have suggested a relatively high incidence of various sexual deviations among temporal lobe epileptics (Kolorsky, et al., 1967). Since the studies have been far from conclusive, this cannot be considered a clinical fact. Clearly, most sexual deviates do not have seizures. A heightening of heterosexual activity appears to be exceedingly rare after the onset of psychomotor seizures.

BEHAVIORAL SIGNIFICANCE OF ABNORMAL ELECTROENCEPHALOGRAMS IN THE ABSENCE OF SEIZURES

During the laboratory evaluation of a psychiatric patient, it is not uncommon to find an abnormal EEG when there is no evidence of overt seizures. As one might expect, the relationship between an abnormal EEG and behavior disturbance in nonepileptic patients is even more difficult to define than it is in epileptic patients, primarily because the major variables are very difficult to control.

How sure can a clinician be that a patient with a behavior disturbance and an abnormal EEG does not have a seizure disorder? The criteria for such a judgment are almost never explicitly stated. Hill (1957) has reported that a high percentage of schizophrenic patients show such paroxysmal abnormalities in their EEG's as synchronous spikes, spike-and-wave complexes (usually in the 4- to 5-cps range), and slow wave bursts. Some of these patients actually did have demonstrable seizures, and some of them therefore might have had epileptic psychosis. The criteria listed on page 22 may help differentiate behavior caused by complex partial seizures from neurotic or psychotic behavior.

Defining the limits of normality in the EEG is also a major problem. There is no doubt that spikes, spike-wave discharges, focal slowing with phase reversal, and paroxysmal activity during wakefulness are abnormal. But, there remains a question about theta rhythms intermixed with a dominant alpha pattern, prolonged slowing after hyperventilation, or even 14 and 6 positive spikes, all of which are often seen in normal adolescents. Do these have clinical significance, or are they merely maturational deviations from the norm that the individual will outgrow? These questions cannot as yet be answered. In patients who drink heavily or who have taken tranquilizers or other medication, electroencephalographic abnormalities may represent the effect of these drugs or withdrawal from them (Table 1-5). The electroencephalographic abnormalities seen in some "psychopathic" patients with a history of aggressive behavior may possibly be secondary to brain damage. Hostile behavior often elicits hostile reactions, and head injuries are quite commonly sustained during fights by patients who habitually start them. Thus, brain damage and electroencephalographic abnormalities in aggressive patients may be the result, not the cause, of the emotional disturbance. Yet, keeping this in mind, there remains considerable evidence correlating electroencephalographic abnormalities with certain psychiatric symptoms.

In a large series of unselected, nonepileptic psychiatric patients it was possible to differentiate those with abnormal EEG's from those with normal EEG's on the basis of their symptoms (Tucker et al., 1965). Symptoms that are classically associated with schizophrenia were significantly more common in the psychiatric patients with abnormal EEG's. These included impaired associations, flattened affect, religiosity, persecutory and somatic delusions, auditory hallucinations, impaired personal habits, and destructive-

Table 1-5
Effect of Commonly Used Drugs on the Electroencephalogram

Drug[a]	EEG Changes Effect on Basic Frequencies	Synchronization	New Waves	Persistence after Drug Discontinued
Phenothiazine	slowing; sometimes beta	increased	high voltage; sharp	6–10 weeks
Tricyclics	increased beta	increased	sharp	?
Barbiturates	increased beta; slowing	increased in low doses; decreased in high doses	spindles	3–6 weeks
Meprobamate	increased beta	increased	spindles	3–6 weeks
Benzodiazepines	increased beta	increased	Fast; sharp	3–6 weeks

[a] All the above drugs but the barbiturates tend to increase preexisting dysrhythmias. Withdrawal from high levels of barbiturates and meprobamate can induce increased slowing, synchronization, and paroxysmal activity and may produce seizures.

Source: Fink, 1963; Ulett et al., 1965.

assaultive behavior. The group with abnormal EEG's also exhibited symptoms classically associated with neurological diseases. These included time disorientation, perseveration, recent memory difficulty, and headaches. Neurotic and depressed patients had roughly the same incidence of abnormal EEG's as the general population (18%).

The incidence of EEG abnormality among "psychopaths" and children with serious behavior disorders is over 50 percent. In schizophrenic patients, the incidence is 24 to 40 percent (Ellingson, 1955; Hill, 1963; Williams, 1969). Nevertheless, the diagnosis of brain damage, epilepsy, or psychosis cannot be made on the basis of electroencephalographic criteria alone, and the meaning of electroencephalographic abnormalities in the absence of seizures or clinical symptoms cannot always be determined.

CURRENT STATUS OF RESEARCH ON THE ORIGIN, SPREAD, AND CESSATION OF SEIZURE ACTIVITY

The main questions about seizures that have yet to be fully answered are: What causes them to start? What causes them to spread? What causes them to stop?

There is some evidence that denervation hypersensitivity might be one mechanism by which brain damage, caused by a tumor or scar, for instance, could result in excessive activity by groups of cortical neurons (Echlin, 1959); it is well known that structures deprived of their normal innervation become supersensitive to their transmitter. The difficulties inherent in studying recurring chronic seizures in animals, however, have led to the use of acute models of epilepsy for the most part. Most of the experimental work has involved the use of agents that cause a neuronal population to become epileptogenic. After such agents as penicillin, strychnine, or cobalt have been applied, electroencephalographic spikes develop. Such EEG spikes are the hallmark of epilepsy and are episodic, of brief duration, and reversible. Once the agent has been applied, they occur in a rather random fashion without an obvious precipitating cause, but they can also be triggered by a wide variety of stimuli, such as direct electrical stimulation, flashing lights, and certain sounds.

The recording of the EEG from the brain's surface indicates that the cortical spikes represent dendritic potentials, not propagated axonal impulses (action potentials). These dendritic or postsynaptic potentials (PSP's) are much longer and much smaller than action potentials, and they do not act on an all-or-none basis. That is, the dendrites hyperpolarize or depolarize relative to the amount of transmitter present; the more transmitter, the greater the effect.

When a nerve impulse (action potential) arrives at the axon terminal, calcium as well as sodium ions enter the neuronal cell. The calcium releases packets (quanta) of neurotransmitter by means not fully understood. These quanta diffuse across the small synaptic cleft to the dendritic membrane, arriving almost simultaneously at the dendrite, changing its ionic permeability. Depending upon the kind of interaction that occurs, and whether the permeability to one or several ions increases or decreases, there may be a depolarization or hyperpolarization of the dendritic membrane. When the effect of a transmitter is to depolarize the dendrite, it is called an excitatory postsynaptic potential (EPSP). When the effect is to hyperpolarize the dendrite, it is called an inhibitory postsynaptic potential (IPSP). If the combined effect of these EPSP's and IPSP's is to depolarize the postsynaptic cell to "threshold," an action potential is propagated along its axon. Each neuron has several thousand dendrites and axonal arborizations and terminals. Most dendrites are far removed from the portion of the cell that generates an action potential and thus, under ordinary circumstances, have little effect on firing.

Recordings from single cells in an epileptogenic neuronal population that is producing cortical EEG spikes after the application of an agent like penicillin have revealed prolonged, large depolarizations called paroxysmal depolarization shifts (PDS's). The EEG spike and PDS in single cells occur almost simultaneously in a focus of epileptic activity. So intimately is the PDS associated with the EEG spike that it is considered the hallmark of an epileptic cell.

What causes the paroxysmal depolarization shift (PDS)?

Two hypotheses that are not mutually exclusive have been proposed to explain the PDS. The first contends that the PDS in a neuron results from an abnormal heightened synaptic drive (Ayala et al., 1973). In other words the PDS is, at least to some degree, a large EPSP (Prince, 1968; Johnston and Brown, 1981).

According to the second hypothesis, the pathophysiological changes underlying the PDS reflect a qualitative epileptogenic change in the individual neuron. Neurons in hippocampal slices generate PDS-like bursts normally, without the application of a convulsant agent, thus suggesting that burst firing is an intrinsic neuronal property (Schwartzkroin and Prince, 1977). This PDS burst is followed by a period of hyperpolarization. Further analysis of this bursting phenomenon has revealed that there is a delicate balance between calcium and potassium conductances. A large inward calcium current is responsible for generating the depolarizing bursting activity in hippocampal neurons. A slow, delayed outward potassium current is responsible for the subsequent hyperpolarization. This outward potassium current is activated by the calcium that enters the cell. Stimulation leads to calcium influx, which causes depolarization; calcium activates potassium efflux and this leads to hyperpolarization.

Disruption of this balance by an epileptogenic drug or by the equivalent of a heightened synaptic drive via electrical stimulation that increases calcium inward current or decreases potassium outward current would lead to more bursting activity in cells that normally "burst" and could initiate bursting in other cells (Hotson and Prince, 1980). It has also been speculated that the opposite may be true; a drug that reduces calcium conductance or augments potassium conductance would be expected to "stabilize" the neuron and prevent epileptogenic firing. There is evidence that phenytoin reduces calcium influx during stimulation and increases resting intracellular ionic calcium levels, possibly increasing potassium conductance (Pincus et al., 1980).

In what part of the nerve cell does bursting activity originate? Experiments have shown that dendrites are capable of producing calcium-mediated action potential spikes which appear in the dendrites before they appear at the soma. This sequence suggests that the drive for firing in bursting cells is generated by calcium currents in the dendrite. This view has been integrated with recent information about the effects of penicillin on IPSP activity to develop a new theory of how convulsants and certain clinical conditions produce epileptic activity.

Many convulsant agents (penicillin, bicuculine, picrotoxin) block the inhibitory effect of GABA, a transmitter that increases chloride conductance. The increase in chloride conductance usually hyperpolarizes cells and this results in an IPSP.

Any agent such as penicillin that blocks IPSP's encourages the transmission of dendritic bursting toward the soma and ultimately to the initial segment of the axon (this is the part of the axon that must be depolarized for neuronal firing to occur). Normally dendritic currents do not reach the soma because they dissipate while traveling toward the soma and are shunted away by the hyperpolarization that accompanies this increase in conductance. Penicillin prevents this shunting associated with IPSP's and allows dendrites to have a profound effect upon the soma, triggering multiple discharges at the initial segment. In effect, blocking the IPSP's causes an electrotonic shortening of the cell so that the dendrite-to-soma distance is decreased. After the application of penicillin onto cells that do not normally burst, even normal excitatory synaptic input could be the trigger for the dendrite-initiated epileptic firing of the cell. Any factor that tended to synchronize or increase the intensity of afferent input would also increase firing.

The concept that calcium-mediated spikes in dendrites underlie natural bursting phenomena may explain the special epileptogenicity of the hippocampus as compared with the neocortex. Calcium spikes and bursting cells have only been seen in hippocampal cells, never in neocortex. Possibly epileptogenicity in the neocortex is more dependent upon a synchronous orthodromic drive, while epileptogenicity in the hippocampus is more the result of an intrinsic epileptogenic propensity.

It is important to emphasize that the PDS is not an isolated event, but is often followed by hyperpolarization of the membrane. This sequence of prolonged depolarization (PDS) followed by hyperpolarization is characteristically seen in neurons in a focus during the interictal state.

It is thought that hyperpolarization in the PDS-hyperpolarization sequence is very important in maintaining the focus as a relatively localized event, and preventing spread. When intracellular recordings from cells in the region surrounding the seizure focus are made, only hyperpolarization is seen. The earliest sign of an impending generalized seizure is the progressive loss of the period of hyperpolarization that follows each PDS, and the loss of the hyperpolarization in surrounding cells. After the PDS, oscillations are superimposed upon the gradually developing tonic depolarization. These occur in increasingly longer trains, becoming more frequent and finally reaching the firing level of these postsynaptic cells; spiking occurs (many action potentials begin to fire), and the seizure begins. Then, the membrane gradually repolarizes, the firing ceases, and the seizure ends.

From this sequence of events, it appears that loss of inhibition (i.e., loss of hyperpolarization) is the primary change that determines the spread of activity from a focus. What is it that occasionally causes inhibition to fail? If we could answer this question, we might understand why generalized seizures are intermittent even when the brain damage that presumably gives rise to them is constant. Possibly, the many stimuli known to precipitate seizures in susceptible individuals act upon the inhibitory mechanisms.

Extracellular potassium concentration may also be important in determining epileptogenesis. During neuronal activity, sodium enters nerve cells and potassium leaves them. With very small extracellular space, it is possible that, during periods of intense neuronal activity, a significantly high concentration of extracellular potassium could accumulate adjacent to the neurons. Extracellular potassium accumulation has been shown to occur during stimulation in invertebrate preparations (Orkand et al., 1966) and in the mammalian cortex (Hotson et al., 1973). Such an accumulation of potassium in the extracellular space could depolarize the nerve cells to make them more excitable. In experiments in which the ventricle over the hippocampus was perfused, a relationship between an increase in extracellular potassium and epileptogenesis was indicated (Zuckermann and Glaser, 1968). Though this may be an important mechanism of epileptogenesis in the hippocampal region, experiments in which the extracellular potassium concentration in penicillin epileptogenic foci of neocortex in the cat was measured cast doubts upon the theory that the extracellular potassium level is a critical factor in the initiation or termination of neocortical ictal episodes (Futamachi et al., 1974).

Even less is known about why seizures end. In some cases, physiological changes related to oxygen lack may be important in producing "neuronal exhaustion." In other cases, a build-up of interstitial potassium to the point at which depolarization block occurs may be important, or seizures might be brought to an end by recovery of inhibition through changes in neuronal activity patterns. The latter is generally considered to be the most likely explanation, since seizure termination is usually associated with the repolarization of cells and a membrane hyperpolarization (inhibition) that lasts for many seconds. During hyperpolarization, the cells stop firing and surface brain potentials are suppressed (Ayala et al., 1970).

The widespread inhibition that follows seizures and continues during the interictal state might influence the behavioral and thought patterns of epileptics. If excessive inhibition were to have an etiological role in epileptic psychosis, for example, it might be easier to understand how control of seizures, perhaps by enhancing inhibition, could cause the psychological condition to worsen and vice versa.

REFERENCES

Aird, R. B. and D. M. Woodbury. *The Management of Epilepsy:* C C Thomas, Springfield, Ill., 1974, p. 278.

Ajmone-Marsan, C. and L. S. Zivin. Factors related to the occurrence of typical paroxysmal abnormalities in the EEG records of epileptic patients. *Epilepsia* 11:361, 1970.

Annegers, J. F., W. A. Hauser, L. R. Elveback, et al. Seizure disorders in offspring of parents with a history of seizures—A maternal-paternal difference. *Epilepsia* 17:1, 1976.

Asuni, T. and V. S. Pillutla. Schizophrenia-like psychoses in Nigerian epileptics. *Brit. J. Psychiat.* 113:1375, 1967.

Ayala, G. F., H. Matsumoto, and R. J. Gumnit. Excitability changes and inhibitory mechanisms in neocortical neurons during seizures. *J. Neurophysiol.* 33:73, 1970.

Ayala, G. F., M. Dichter, R. J. Gumnit, et al. Genesis of interictal spikes. New knowledge of interictal spikes. New knowledge of cortical feedback systems suggests a neurophysiological explanation of brief paroxysms. *Brain Res.* 52:1, 1973.

Bear, D. M. and P. Fedio. Quantitative analysis of interictal behavior in temporal lobe epilepsy. *Arch. Neurol.* 34:454, 1977.

Bickford, R. G. New dimensions in electroencephalography. *Neurology* 7: 469, 1957.

Bickford, R. G. Activation procedures and special electrodes. In: *Current*

Practice of Clinical Electroencephalography, ed. D. Kass and D. D. Daly, Raven Press, New York, p. 269, 1979.

Bourgeois, B. F. D., A. C. Prensky, H. S. Palkes, et al. Intelligence in epilepsy: A prospective study in children. *Ann. Neurol.* 14:438, 1983.

Bower, B. R. and P. M. Jeavons. The effect of corticotrophin and prednisolone on infantile spasms with mental retardation. *Arch. Dis. Child.* 36:23, 1961.

Bray, P. F. and W. C. Wiser. Evidence for a genetic etiology of temporal-central abnormalities in focal epilepsy. *New Eng. J. Med.* 271:926, 1964.

Bryan, G. E., E. E. Marsh, B. Jabbari, et al. Incidence of seizures in patients receiving tricyclic and tetracyclic antidepressants. *Ann. Neurol.* 14: 153, 1983.

Bucthal, F., O. Svensmark, and P. J. Schiller. Clinical and electroencephalographic correlations with serum levels of diphenylhydantoin. *Arch. Neurol.* 2:624, 1960.

Camfield, P. R., R. Gates, G. Ronen, et al. Comparison of cognitive ability, personality profile, and school success in epileptic children with pure right versus left temporal lobe EEG foci. *Ann. Neurol.* 15:122, 1984.

Chaudry, M. R. and D. A. Pond. Mental deterioration in epileptic children. *J. Neurol. Psychiat.* 24:213, 1961.

Cohen, R. J. and C. Suter. Hysterical seizures: Suggestion as a provocative EEG test. *Ann. Neurol.* 11:391, 1982.

Cooper, I. S., I. Amin, and S. Gilman. The effect of chronic cerebellar stimulation upon epilepsy in man. *Trans. Amer. Neurol. Assoc.* 98:192, 1973.

Cramer, J. A., R. H. Mattson, and J. Brillman. Folinic acid therapy in epilepsy. *Fed. Proc.* 35:582, 1976.

Currie, S., K. W. G. Heathfield, R. A. Henson, et al. Clinical course and prognosis of temporal lobe epilepsy: A survey of 61 patients. *Brain* 94: 173, 1971.

Currier, R. D., S. C. Little, J. F. Suess, and O. J. Andy. Sexual seizures. *Arch. Neurol.* 25:260, 1971.

Daly, D. D. Use of the EEG for diagnosis and evaluation of epileptic seizures and non-epileptic episodic disorders. In: *Current Practice of Clinical Electroencephalography.* (ed.) D. W. Klass and D. D. Daly, Raven Press, New York, 1979.

Davidson, S. and M. A. Falconer. Outcome of surgery in 40 children with temporal lobe epilepsy. *Lancet* 1:260, 1975.

Delgado-Escueta, A. V., D. M. Tremain, and G. O. Walsh. The treatable epileptics. *New Eng. J. Med.* 308:1508, 1983.

Desai, B. T., R. Porter, and J. K. Penry. The psychogenic seizure by video tape analysis: A study of 42 attacks in six patients (Abs.). *Neurology* 29:602, 1979.

Detre, T. and R. G. Feldman. Behavior disorder associated with seizure states: pharmacological and psychosocial management. In: *EEG and Behavior,* G. H. Glaser, ed., Basic Books, New York, 1963, p. 366.

———— and H. G. Jarecki. *Modern Psychiatric Treatment.* J. B. Lippincott, Philadelphia, 1971.

Devinsky, O. and M. S. Duchowny. Seizures after convulsive therapy: A retrospective case survey. *Neurology* 33:921, 1983.

Ebersole, J. S. and R. J. Leroy. An evaluation of ambulatory cassette EEG monitoring. II. Detection of interictal abnormalities. *Neurology* 33:8, 1983.

Ebersole, J. S. and R. J. Leroy. Evaluation of ambulatory cassette EEG monitoring. III. Diagnostic accuracy compared to intensive inpatient EEG monitoring. *Neurology* 33:853, 1983.

Echlin, F. A. The supersensitivity of chronically isolated cerebral cortex as a mechanism in focal epilepsy. *Electroenceph. Clin. Neurophysiol.* 11: 697, 1959.

Ellenberg, J. H. and K. B. Nelson. Febrile seizures, tested intelligence and learning disorder. *Neurology* 27:342, 1977.

Ellingson, R. J. Incidence of EEG abnormality among patients with mental disorders of apparently nonorganic origin. Critical review. *Amer. J. Psychiat.* 111:263, 1955.

Ernhart, C. B., B. Landa, N. B. Schell. Subclinical levels of lead and developmental deficit—A multivariate following reassessment. *Pediatrics* 67: 911, 1981.

Ervin, F. A., W. Epstein, and H. E. King. Behavior of epileptic and non-epileptic patients with "temporal spikes." *Arch. Neurol. Psychiat.* 74:488, 1955.

Ferriss, G. S. The recognition of non-epileptic seizures. *South Med. J.* 52: 1557, 1972.

Fink, M. Quantitative EEG in human psychopharmacology: Drug patterns. In: *EEG and Behavior*, G. H. Glaser, ed., Basic Books, New York, 1963, p. 177.

Fischer, M., G. Korskjaer, and E. Pedersen. Psychotic episodes in Zarondan treatment. Effects and side effects in 105 patients. *Epilepsia* 6:325, 1965.

Flor-Henry, P. Psychosis and temporal lobe epilepsy. *Epilepsia* 10:363, 1969.
———. Ictal and interictal psychiatric manifestations in epilepsy: Specific or non-specific? *Epilepsia* 13:773, 1972.

Freud, S. Collected papers, Vol. 2. Hogarth, London, 1949.

Friedlander, W. J. and G. H. Feinstein. Petit mal status: Epilepsia minoris continua. *Neurology* 6:357, 1956.

Fromm, G. H., H. B. Wessel, J. D. Glass, et al. Imipramine in absence and myoclonic-astatic seizures. *Neurology* 28:953, 1978.

Futamachi, K. J., R. Mutani, and D. A. Prince. Potassium activity in rat cortex. *Brain Res.* 75:5, 1974.

Gastaut, H. and H. Collomb. Etude du comportement sexuel chez les épileptiques psychomoteurs. *Ann. Medicopsychol.* 112:657, 1954.

Gibbs, F. A. and E. C. Gibbs. *Atlas of Electroencephalography*, 2nd ed., Addison-Wesley, Reading, Mass., 1952.

Giordani, B., J. C. Sackellares, S. Miller, et al. Improvement in neuropsychological performance in patients with retractory seizures. *Neurology* 33: 489, 1983.

Glaser, G. H., R. J. Newman, and R. Schafer. Interictal psychosis in psychomotor temporal lobe epilepsy: an EEG-psychological study. In: *EEG and Behavior*, G. H. Glaser, ed., Basic Books, New York, 1963, p. 345.

————. The problem of psychosis in psychomotor temporal lobe epileptics. *Epilepsia* 5:271, 1964.

Glaser, G. H. Limbic epilepsy in childhood. *J. Nerv. Ment. Dis.* 144:391, 1967.

Goddard, G. V., D. C. McIntyre, and C. K. Leech. A permanent change in brain functioning resulting from daily electrical stimulation. *Exp. Neurol.* 25:295, 1969.

Goldensohn, E. S. and A. P. Gold. Prolonged behavioral disturbances as ictal phenomena. *Neurology* 10:1, 1960.

Green, J. B. Association in behavior disorder with electroencephalographic focus in children without seizure. *Neurology* 11:337, 1961.

Green, J. D. The hippocampus. *Physiol. Rev.* 44:561, 1964.

Guerrant, J., W. W. Anderson, A. Fischer, M. R. Weinstein, R. M. Jaros, and A. Deskins. *Personality in Epilepsy.* C C Thomas, Springfield, Ill., 1962.

Gutnick, M. J. and D. A. Prince. Effects of projected cortical epileptiform discharges on neuronal activities in ventrobasal thalamus of the cat; ictal discharge. *Exp. Neurol.* 46:418, 1975.

Hauser, W. A., J. F. Annegers, and L. T. Kurland. Febrile convulsions: Prognosis for subsequent seizures. *Neurology* 27:341, 1977.

Hawton, K., J. Fogg, and P. Marsack. Association between epilepsy and attempted suicide. *J. Neurol. Neurosurg. Psychiat.* 43:168, 1980.

Hierons, R. and M. Saunders. Impotence in patients with temporal lobe lesions. *Lancet* 2:761, 1966.

Hill, D. Electroencephalogram in schizophrenia. In: D. Richter, ed., *Schizophrenia: Somatic aspects.* Pergamon Press, London, 1957, p. 33.

————. The EEG in psychiatry. In: J. D. N. Hill and G. Parr, eds. *Electroencephalography.* Macmillan, Oxford, 1963, p. 368.

Ho, K., U. Roessman, L. House, et al. Newborn weight in relation to maturity, sex and race. *Ann. Neurol.* 10:243, 1981.

Hotson, J. R., G. W. Sypert, and A. A. Ward. Extracellular potassium concentration changes during propagated seizures in neocortex. *Exp. Neurol.* 38:20, 1973.

Hotson, J. R., and D. A. Prince. Penicillin and barium-induced epileptiform bursting in hippocampal neurons: Actions on $Ca++$ and $K+$ potentials. *Ann. Neurol.* 10:11, 1980.

Hunter, J. and H. H. Jasper. Effects of thalamic stimulation in unanesthetized animals: The arrest reaction and petit mal-like seizures, activation patterns and generalized convulsions. *Electroenceph. Clin. Neurophysiol.* 1:305, 1949.

Inouye, E. Observations on forty twin index cases with chronic epilepsy and their co-twins. *J. Nerv. Ment. Dis.* 130:401, 1960.

Jasper, H. H., A. A. Wird, and A. Pope (Eds.). *Mechanisms of the Epilepsies.* Little, Brown, Boston, 1969.

Johnston, D. and D. H. Brown. Giant synaptic potential hypothesis for epileptiform activity. *Science* 210:294, 1981.

King, D. W., B. B. Gallagher, A. J. Murvin, et al. Pseudoseizures: Diagnostic evaluation. *Neurology* 32:18, 1982.

Kluver, H. and P. C. Bucy. Preliminary analysis of functions of the temporal lobes in monkeys. *Arch. Neurol. Psychiat.* 42:979, 1939.

Kolorsky, A. K. Freund, J. Machek, and O. Polak. Male sexual deviations. *Arch. Gen. Psychiat.* 17:735, 1967.

Krumholz, A. and E. Niedermeyer. Psychogenic Seizures: A clinical study with follow-up data. *Neurology* 33:498, 1983.

Lennox, W. G. The heredity of epilepsy as told by relatives and twins. *JAMA* 146:529, 1951.

————. Significance of febrile convulsions. *Pediatrics* 11:341, 1953.

————, E. L. Gibbs, and F. A. Gibbs. Inheritance of cerebral dysrhythmia and epilepsy. *Arch. Neurol. Psychiat.* 49:1155, 1940.

Lennox-Buchtal, M. Febrile convulsions: A reappraisal. *Electroenceph. Clin. Neurophysiol.* 32:Suppl:1, 1973.

Lesser, R. P., H. Leuders, and D. D. Dinner. Evidence for epilepsy is rare in patients with psychogenic seizures. *Neurology* 33:502, 1983.

Lilienfeld, A. M. and B. Pasamanick. Association of maternal and fetal factors with the development of epilepsy. *JAMA* 155:719, 1954.

Loiseau, P., M. Pestre, J. F. Dartigues, et al. Long-term prognosis in two forms of childhood epilepsy: Typical absence seizures and epilepsy with rolandic (centrotemporal) EEG foci. *Ann. Neurol.* 13:642, 1983.

Louis, A., J. C. White, and J. W. Langston. Nasopharyngeal Electrodes: Are they worth the trouble? *Ann. Neurol.* 12:95, 1982.

MacLean, P. D. and D. W. Ploog. Cerebral representation of penile erection. *J. Neurophysiol.* 25:29, 1962.

Mahaffey, K. R., Annest, J. L., Roberts, J., et al. National estimates of blood lead levels: United States 1976-1980: Association with selected demographic and socioeconomic factors. *New Eng. J. Med.* 307:573, 1982.

Marcus, E. M. and C. W. S. Watson. Symmetrical epiloptogenic foci in monkey cerebral cortex. Mechanisms of interaction and regional variations in capacity for synchronous discharges. *Arch. Neurol.* 19:99, 1968.

Margerison, J. H. and J. Corsellis. Epilepsy and the temporal lobes. *Brain* 89:499, 1966.

Marshall, A. G., E. O. Hutchinson, and J. Honisett. Heredity in common diseases: A retrospective survey of twins in a hospital population. *Brit. Med. J.* 1:1, 1962.

Mattson, R. 1977 (unpublished data).

Mattson, R. H., K. L. Pratt, and J. R. Calverley. Electroencephalograms of epileptics following sleep deprivation. *Arch. Neurol.* 13:310, 1965.

McElligott, R. F. *An analysis of the Epilepsy Center at the Veteran's Administration Hospital, West Haven, Connecticut*, Master's thesis, Yale University School of Medicine, 1974.

Metrakos, K. and J. D. Metrakos. Genetics of convulsive disorders: II

Genetic and encephalographic studies in centrencephalic epilepsy. *Neurology* 11:474, 1961.

Mignone, R. J., E. F. Donnelly, and D. Sadowsky. Psychological and neurological comparisons of psychomotor and nonpsychomotor epileptic patients. *Epilepsia* 11:345, 1970.

Myers, R. R., K. J. Burchiel, J. J. Stockard, and R. G. Bickford. Effects of acute and chronic paleocerebellar stimulation on experimental models of epilepsy in the cat; studies with enflurane, pentylenetetrazol, penicillin and chloralose. *Epilepsia* 16:257, 1975.

Needleman, H. C., C. Gunroe, A. Leviton, et al. Deficits on psychologic and classroom performance of children with elevated dentine lead levels. *New Eng. J. Med.* 300:689, 1979.

Nelson, K. B. and J. H. Ellenberg. Predictors of epilepsy in children who have experienced febrile seizures. *New Eng. J. Med.* 295:1029, 1976.

Norris, J. W. and R. F. Pratt. A controlled study of folic acid in epilepsy *Neurology* 21:659, 1971.

Ojemann, L. M., P. N. Friel, W. J. Trejo, et al. Effect of dosage on seizure frequency in depressed epileptic patients. *Neurology* 33:646, 1983.

Orkand, R. K., J. G. Nicholls, and S. W. Kuffler. Effect of nerve impulses on the membrane potential of glioma cells in the central nervous system of amphibians. *J. Neurophysiol.* 29:788, 1966.

Otto, D. A., V. A. Benignus, K. E. Muller, et al. Effects of age and body lead burden on CNS function in young children. I. Slow cortical potentials. *Electroenceph. Clin. Neurophysiol.* 52:229, 1981.

Ounsted, C., J. Lindsay, and R. Norman. Biological Factors in Temporal Lobe Epilepsy. William Heinemann Medical Books Ltd., London, 1966.

Petersen, I., O. Erg-Olofsson, and U. Selder. Paroxysmal activity in EEG of normal children. In: *Clinical Electroencephalography of Children*, eds. P. Kellaway and I. Petersen. Grune & Stratton, New York, 1968, p. 167.

Pincus, J. H., Y. Yaari, and Z. Argov. Phenytoin: Electrophysiological effect at the neuromuscular junction. *Adv. Neurol.* 27:363, 1980.

Pond, D. A. Psychiatric aspects of epilepsy. *J. Ind. Med. Prof.* 3:1441, 1957.

Posner, J. B., F. Plum, and A. Posnak. Cerebral metabolism during electrically induced seizures in man. *Arch. Neurol.* 20:388, 1969.

Prichard, P. B., III, B. B. Wannamaker, J. Sagel, et al. Endocrin function following complex partial seizures. *Ann. Neurol.* 14:27, 1983.

Ramani, V. and R. J. Gumnit. Intensive monitoring of interictal psychosis in epilepsy. *Ann. Neurol.* 11:613, 1982.

Ramani, V. and R. J. Gumnit. Management of hysterical seizures in epileptic patients. *Arch. Neurol.* 39:78, 1982.

Ramani, V., Quesney, F. F., and Olson, D., et al. Diagnosis of hysterical seizures in epileptic patients. *Am. J. Psychiat.* 137:705, 1980.

Ramsey, R. E., J. Wilder, R. Strauss, and L. J. Willmore. Status epilepticus during pregnancy: Effects of gastrointestinal malabsorption on phenytoin kinetics and seizure control. *Neurology* 26:344, 1976.

Reed, D. M. and F. J. Staley. *The Epidemiology of Prematurity.* Urban and Schwarzenberg, Baltimore, 1977.

Reeves, A. G. and D. H. Wilson. Forebrain commissurotomy for the relief of intractable seizures. *Neurology* 26:343, 1976.

Reynolds, E. H. Anticonvulsant drugs, folic acid metabolism, fit frequency and psychiatric illness. *Psychiat. Neurol. Neurochirg.* 74:167, 1971.

—— and R. D. Travers. Serum anticonvulsant concentrations in epileptic patients with mental symptoms. *Brit. J. Psychiat.* 124:440, 1974.

Riley, T. L. and W. L. Brannon. Recognition of pseudoseizures. *J. Fam. Pract.* 10:213, 1980.

Rodin, E. A. The prognosis of patients with epilepsy. C C Thomas, Springfield, Ill., 1968.

——, M. Katz, and K. Lennox. Differences between patients with temporal lobe seizures and those with other forms of epileptic attacks. *Epilepsia* 17:313, 1976.

Rossen, R. Electroencephalographic studies in idiopathic epilepsy, idiopathic syncope, and related disorders in a U.S. Naval Hospital. *Am. J. Psychiat.* 107:391, 1974.

Schiottz-Christensen, E. and P. Bruhn. Intelligence, behavior and scholastic achievement subsequent to febrile convulsions: An analysis of discordant twin pairs. *Develop. Med. Child. Neurol.* 15:565, 1973.

Schwartzkroin, P. A. and D. Prince. Penicillin in dual epileptiform activity in the hippocampal *in vitro* preparation. *Ann. Neurol.* 1:463, 1977.

Shamansky, S. L. and G. H. Glaser. Socioeconomic characteristics of childhood seizure disorders in the New Haven area: An epidemiologic study. *Epilepsia* 20:457, 1979.

Slater, E., A. W. Beard, and E. Glithero. The schizophrenia-like psychosis of epilepsy. *Brit. J. Psychiat.* 109:95, 1963.

—— and E. Glithero. The schizophrenia-like psychosis of epilepsy: Genetical aspects. *Br. J. Psychiat.* 109:103, 1963.

Small, J. G., V. Milstein, and J. R. Stevens. Are psychomotor epileptics different: *Arch. Neurol.* 7:187, 1962.

Spencer, S. S. Depth electrode encephalography in selection of refractory epileptics for surgery. *Ann. Neurol.* 9:207, 1981.

Spencer, S. S., D. D. Spencer, P. D. Williamson, and R. H. Mattson. The localizing value of depth electroencephalography in 32 refractory epileptic patients. *Ann. Neurol.,* 12:248, 1982.

——. Sexual automatisms in complex partial seizures. *Neurology* 33:527, 1983.

Srole, I., et al. *Mental Health in the Metropolis.* McGraw-Hill, New York, 1962.

Standage, K. F. The etiology of hysterical seizures. *Can. Psychiat. Assoc. J.* 20:67, 1975.

Standage, K. G. and G. W. Fenton. Psychiatric symptom profiles of patients with epilepsy. *Psychol. Med.* 5:152, 1975.

Stores, G. Behavioral effects of antiepileptic drugs. *Develop. Med. Child. Neurol.* 17:647, 1975.

Suter, C. Medical-legal aspects of EEG. Presentation course at American EEG Society, 34th Annual Meeting, Boston, 1980.

Taylor, D. C. Sexual behavior and temporal lobe epilepsy. *Arch. Neurol.* 21:510, 1969.

————. Factors influencing the occurrence of schizophrenia-like psychosis in patients with temporal lobe epilepsy. *Psychol. Med.* 5:249, 1975.

Theodore, W. H., R. J. Porter, and J. K. Penry. Complex partial seizures: A videotape analysis of 108 seizures in 25 patients. *Proc. A.N.A.* 106: 108, 1981.

Theodore, W. H .and R. J. Porter. Removal of sedative-hypnotic antiepileptic drugs from the regimen of patients with intractable epilepsy. *Ann. Neurol.* 13:320, 1983.

Tower, D. The neurochemistry of epilepsy: Seizure mechanism and their management. C C Thomas, Springfield, Ill., 1960.

Trimble, M. Non-monoamine oxidase inhibitor antidepressant and epilepsy: A review. *Epilepsia* 19:241, 1978.

Trojaberg, W. Changes in spike foci in children. In *Clinical Electroencephalography in Children*, P. Kellaway, ed. Grune and Stratton, New York, 1968.

Troupin, A. S., L. M. Ojemann, L. M. Halpern, et al. Carbamazepine (Tegretol)—A double bind comparison and phenytoin (Dilantin). *Neurology* 26:342, 1976.

Tucker, G. J., T. Detre, M. Harrow, and G. H. Glaser. Behavior and symptoms of psychiatric patients and the electroencephalogram. *Arch. Gen. Psychiat.* 12:278, 1965.

Ulett, G. A., A. F. Heusier, and T. J. Word. The effect of psychotropic drugs on the EEG of the chronic psychotic patient. In: *Applications of Electroencephalography in Psychiatry: A Symposium*, W. P. Wilson, ed. Duke University Press, Durham, 1965, p. 241.

Walsh, G. O. and A. V. Delgado-Escueta. Type II complex partial seizures: Poor results of anterior temporal lobectomy. *Neurology* 34:1, 1984.

Wilder, B. J., E. R. Ramsey, J. Murphy, et al. Comparison of valproic acid and phenytoin in newly diagnosed tonic-clonic seizures. *Neurology* 13: 1474, 1983.

Williams, D. Neural factors related to habitual aggression. *Brain* 92:502, 1969.

Yule, W., R. Lansdown, I. B. Millar, et al. The relationship between blood lead concentration, intelligence and attainment in a school population: A pilot study. *Dev. Med. Child. Neurol.* 23:567, 1981.

Zivin, L. and C. Ajmone Marsan. Incidence and prognostic significance of "epileptiform" activity in the EEG of non-epileptic subjects. *Brain* 91: 751, 1968.

Zuckermann, E. C. and G. H. Glaser. Hippocampal epileptic activity induced by localized ventricular perfusion with high potassium cerebral spinal fluid. *Exp. Neurol.* 20:87, 1968.

Chapter 2

LIMBIC SYSTEM
AND VIOLENCE

The limbic system is a meeting place for the disciplines of psychiatry and neurology. More of a philosophic concept than a discrete anatomical or physiological system, it is the ring of gray matter and tracts bordering the hemispheres in the medial portions of the brain that play a role in emotions. Phylogenetically, many of the areas designated as the limbic system are among the oldest portions of the cortex; in lower creatures these structures largely subserve smell and have traditionally been called the rhinencephalon. But, since all regions designated "limbic" are not related to olfaction, and since other brain regions in addition to the limbic system play a role in emotional functioning, the term has been criticized (Brodal, 1981). Our rationale for the continued use of the term "limbic system" rests on the corresponding results of stimulation and ablation studies demonstrating consistent interrelationships of its various components, on the importance of these components to emotional functioning, and, not least on the wide usage of the term by clinicians, physiologists, and anatomists.

It was Papez (1937) who first pointed out that the limbic system was possibly related to emotion and behavior and visceral reactivity. He regarded the hippocampus as a regulator of hypothalamic centers concerned with emotional responses. On the basis of his observations of patients with rabies (which affects the hippocampus and causes emotional and behavioral changes, such as anxiety and paroxysms of rage and terror), Papez predicted that following stimulation of the hippocampus, there could be prolonged active discharges in its own structures which resulted in very little spread to neocortical areas because of the interconnections between the limbic system components. He predicted that these "reverberating circuits" of discharge within the limbic system would produce marked alterations in the subjective emotional life of an individual. In effect, Papez proposed an anatomical and physiological substrate for the intense affective reactions and instincts that are customarily the domain of much psychiatric theory and research.

At the time Papez published his paper on the limbic system, Freudian theory was in wide vogue. The idea of a phylogenetically ancient, deep, central portion of the nervous system that influenced behavior and thought not under conscious, neocortical control was consistent with some Freudian concepts of instinctual drive. The reasoning went something like this: The sense of smell in lower animals seems to be closely associated with memory, instinct, and emotion, for it is often smell that alerts an animal to danger and provokes fear, flight, or fighting, as well as sexual arousal and mating. Smell and memory in such animals must be related functions, since it is important for lower animals to remember the associations of particular smells. The autonomic nervous system must be closely related to the rhinencephalon, since such autonomic responses as pupillary dilation, piloerection, increased heart rate, and increased blood flow to skeletal muscles occur in response to environmental circumstances in which an animal must fight or flee or prepare for mating. Though the sense of smell is no longer as important to human life, it is postulated that these rhinencephalic structures and the limbic system in man are still involved with emotions, memory, and visceral responses and that disturbances of the limbic system disrupt them.

ANATOMY

The gray matter components encompassed by the term "limbic system" include those in the anterior and medial portions of the temporal lobe and those outside the temporal lobe. Limbic components in the temporal lobe include the amygdala, hippocampus (both the gyrus hippocampus and its medial portion, the hippocampal formation, which is sometimes called Ammon's horn), and the uncus. Limbic components outside the temporal lobe include the mamillary bodies, anterior nucleus of the thalamus, gyrus cingulus, nuclei of the septum, portions of the midbrain tegmentum (interpeduncular nucleus, lateral midbrain area of Nauta, central gray and ventral tegmental nucleus of Gudden), habenula, and subcallosal and supracallosal gyri. The major tracts interconnecting these regions include the fimbria, fornix, mamillothalamic tract, anterior commissure, stria terminalis, stria medullaris, median forebrain bundle, and diagonal band of Broca (see Figs. 2-1, 2-2A, 2-2B).

In order to conceptualize this system, it may be helpful to recall that many of the medial structures of the brain have the shape of a large C, with one end in the anterior temporal lobe and the other in or near the septal region. Among the limbic components that have this form are: (1) the gyrus cingulus, (2) the fimbria-fornix-mamillary body pathway; (3) the stria terminalis, which connects the amygdala and the septal area; and (4) the supracallosal gyrus and longitudinal striae, which connect the hippocampus region with the septal region. Other tracts with a curved shape are the median forebrain bundle, which connects the septal nuclei with the midbrain tegmentum, and the stria medullaris, which connects the septal region with the habenula (Fig. 2-1). The anterior commissure is a tract that laterally connects the right and left amygdala. The diagonal band of Broca also runs laterally to connect the septum with the amygdala. The tracts that connect the gray matter of the limbic system generally contain both afferent and efferent fibers (Figs. 2-1, 2-2A, 2-2B).

The richness of interconnections among regions of the limbic system can only partly be appreciated by the account above; actually not all the interconnections are known. Each amygdaloid nucleus appears to have direct connections, most of which are reciprocal, with the other amygdaloid nucleus, olfactory bulb, septal nuclei, hypothalamus, thalamus, habenula, midbrain, and hippo-

Fig. 2-1
THE LIMBIC SYSTEM

AC–Anterior Commissure, ANthal–Anterior Nucleus of the thalamus, CG–Central Gray matter of the midbrain, DBB–Diagonal Band of Broca, G–Gudden's deep tegmental nucleus, HAB–Habenula, HYPO–hypothalamus, IPN–Interpeduncular Nucleus, LMA NAUTA–Lateral Midbrain Area of Nauta, lat olf str–lateral olfactory stria, med olf str–medial olfactory stria, MFB–Median Forebrain Bundle, MAM B–mamillary Bodies, Stria Med–stria medullaris, stria term–stria terminalis.

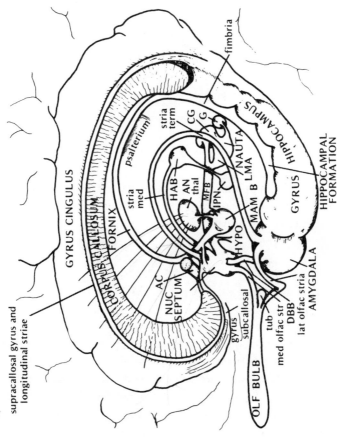

supracallosal gyrus and longitudinal striae

fimbria

GYRUS CINGULUS

Psalterium

stria term

CG

G

stria med

CORPUS CALLOSUM

FORNIX

HAB

AN thal

MFB

IPN

NAUTA

MAM B LMA

HIPPOCAMPUS

AC

HYPO

GYRUS

NUC SEPTUM

HIPPOCAMPAL FORMATION

gyrus subcallosal

tub

med olfac str

DBB

lat olfac stria

AMYGDALA

OLF BULB

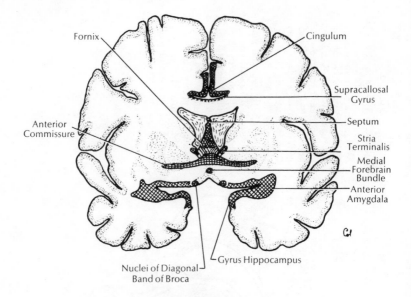

Fig. 2-2A
THE LIMBIC SYSTEM:
ANTERIOR CORONAL SECTION

campus. The hippocampus has connections with the mamillary bodies, anterior thalamic nucleus, gyrus cingulus, septum, midbrain regions, and amygdala.

PHYSIOLOGICAL PSYCHOLOGY

Efforts to determine the function of the various components of the limbic system have involved stimulation and ablation studies in animals and to some extent in man. These have yielded evidence that these components influence memory, learning, emotional states (including anxiety, rage, placidity, and alertness), visceral and endocrine responses, and behavior, particularly aggressive, oral, and sexual activity. It is not possible to define the function of each of the components of the limbic system because none of them acts as a center for a particular function. All of the limbic system is more or less associated with all of the functions enumerated above. As Papez predicted, there is a strong tendency after stimulation of limbic components for prolonged afterdischarges, which spread throughout the limbic system with comparatively little involvement of the neocortex (MacLean, 1952, 1954).

The specific aspects of behavior demonstrated by stimulation and ablation studies in the limbic system are of great theoretical interest to both psychiatrists and neurologists, since the behavioral and cognitive alterations produced by experiments in animals closely resemble human responses that are so often considered to be "functional." Stimulation of the hippocampus of cats results in apparent bewilderment and anxiety, together with intense attention to something the animal seems to sense in the environment.

Fig. 2-2B
THE LIMBIC SYSTEM:
POSTERIOR CORONAL SECTION

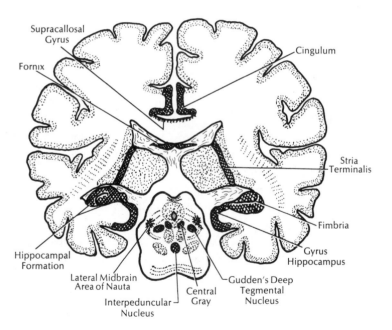

Such phenomena have been considered alerting and defensive reactions, resulting perhaps from hallucinations induced by the stimulation. Amygdalar stimulation may produce similar reactions.

Bilateral hippocampal destruction leads to recent memory loss with prevention of new learning in both animals and man. Destruction of other components of the limbic system also produces deficits in recent memory. Bilateral ablation of the anterior gyrus cingulus and bilateral division of the fornices produce similar deficits.

Stimulation of portions of the amygdala produce rage reactions in animals. Similar reactions have been seen after stimulation of the midbrain gray matter or the placement of destructive lesions in the septum. Stimulation of the amygdala in animals has provoked reactions that have been interpreted as reflecting feelings of fear. Sensations of fear have also been described in conscious human beings while this region was stimulated during surgery. Chewing, gagging, licking, retching, swallowing, bladder contractions, respiratory, pulse, and blood pressure increases, and increased secretion of ACTH have all been produced by amygdalar stimulation as well as stimulation elsewhere in the limbic system. Such phenomena are quite similar to the manifestations of psychomotor epilepsy. This clinical similarity and the characteristic anterior temporal spikes seen in the EEG of patients with psychomotor epilepsy led some clinicians to apply the term "limbic epilepsy" to such seizures (Fulton, 1953).

The bizarre behavioral alterations (e.g., docility, loss of natural fear, compulsive oral activity, and heightened indiscriminate sexual activity) noted by Kluver and Bucy (1939) after bilateral removal of the amygdaloid nuclei and overlying hippocampal cortex provided further evidence for the limbic system's role in these functions. Similar changes have been noted in man after bilateral temporal lobectomies, which, if performed somewhat caudal to the amygdala, also produce profound memory loss, particularly for recent events.

Considering the relationship between the limbic system and emotions, it might be predicted that diseases involving limbic components would cause emotional disorders. This does seem to be the case in psychomotor-temporal lobe epilepsy, as noted above. It also seems to be so in other conditions that involve limbic components.

Malamud (1967) studied 18 patients with intracranial neoplasms of the limbic system. All had originally been diagnosed as having psychiatric disorders. Ten were thought to be schizophrenics, four were depressed, one was manic, and the others appeared to be severely neurotic. Eleven of the patients had psychomotor seizures.

Subacute and chronic forms of viral encephalitis tend to affect the medial portions of the temporal lobes, which are associated with the limbic system (Glaser and Pincus, 1969; Himmelhoch et al., 1970). Such forms of viral encephalitis characteristically give rise to behavioral symptoms that are often suggestive of psychiatric disorders. Early in the course of subacute encephalitis, this may be the cause of diagnostic confusion; the disease has commonly been mistaken for schizophrenia, hysteria, or depression. The behavioral alterations seen in these patients probably are the result of both irritation and destruction of limbic components.

Gibbs (1951) found that psychiatric disorders were three times more common in patients with anterior temporal seizure foci than in those with seizure foci located elsewhere in the brain.

In patients being examined for epilepsy, electrical stimulation of the amygdala and the hippocampus after placement of chronic, implanted electrodes has produced brief alterations that mimic psychomotor seizures and persist only during the passage of current and the limited afterdischarge (Stevens et al., 1969). After such stimulation, however, mood and thought disturbances of psychotic proportions may persist for hours.

THE LIMBIC SYSTEM AND VIOLENT BEHAVIOR

Experiments on animals and a large accumulation of data on human beings have indicated that violence may be a symptom of a disturbance of brain function. Since Bard's experiments in 1928, it has been clear that brain lesions, decortication, and lesions in the region of the hypothalamus can produce marked alterations in emotional reactivity. Rage reactions in cats, which include arching of the back, piloerection, snarling, biting, and scratching, are seen when the entire cortex, basal ganglia, and most of the thalamus have been removed. The rage phenomena of decorticate cats are directed responses to a variety of environmental stimuli that do not elicit rage reactions in the normal animal. It has been assumed that the decorticate animal is not capable of subjective emotion, and accordingly, the reaction described above has been called "sham rage." But, this assumption that subjective emotion is a function of portions of the nervous system that had been removed in such animals may not be entirely justified, and it would be a mistake to make too much of the distinction between visible emotional reaction and subjective feeling on the basis of present information.

Removal of the neocortex, leaving the hippocampus, amygdala, hypothalamus, and brain stem intact, does not change the basic personality of the cat. It purrs and responds to affection. But, tail pinching or other stimuli that might elicit mild manifestations of anger in the normal cat will, in the decorticate animal, lead to a ferocious, directed attack. Destruction of the ventral medial nucleus of the hypothalamus has produced permanently ferocious animals. Stimulation of portions of the amygdala, posterior hypothalamus, or midbrain also may enhance aggressive hunting behavior in which the animal will go to great lengths to make an attack upon some object it would normally avoid or ignore, such as a larger animal or a toy. Stimulation of other components of the limbic system may stop attack behavior, and bilateral amygdalectomy makes ferocious animals permanently placid (Kluver and Bucy, 1939); yet occasionally, the reverse has been reported.

Placid, amygdalectomized animals can be made fierce by producing lesions of the ventral medial nucleus of the hypothalamus. Rats made savage by lesions in the septal region can be made tranquil by an amygdalectomy. Violent behavior in cats, monkeys, and humans may result from the electrical stimulation of several components of the limbic system. Destruction of these regions or stimulation of other limbic components can inhibit such behavior (Mark and Ervin, 1970).

The evidence from animal experiments that suggests a relationship between the neocortex, limbic system, and brainstem and violence is voluminous. Many observations and experiments have been contradictory, and one may select evidence from them to support almost any reasonable argument. It seems likely that the complex actions and subjective feelings involved in violent aggressiveness must be mediated by extensive collaboration among many parts of the brain (Brodal, 1981). It remains clear, however, that stimulation or destruction of discrete structures within the nervous system can lead to marked alterations in behavior ranging from violence to placidity. It is also clear that the amygdala, hippocampus, and other limbic structures are particularly sensitive in this regard.

VIOLENCE IN CHILDREN

Despite the accumulation of research data linking violence to brain dysfunction, not enough is known about human violence to justify dogmatic categorization. Repeated violence is committed by very few (Wolfgang, 1972) and is encountered not only in the lower classes (Elliot, 1982). If such acts were committed by those with evidence of abnormalities of cerebral functioning as reflected in the neurological examination, psychological testing, or EEG, it would shift the focus of investigations into the causes of violence from the social environment to the individual brain. Is there something neurologically different about violent individuals which might explain why they are violent?

To address this question, Lewis et al. (1977) studied a group of juvenile offenders incarcerated in a "reform" school in Connecticut. The study sample consisted of 97 boys all of whom were evaluated by a neurologist and a psychiatrist. Psychological tests and an EEG recording were performed in almost all. After all data had been collected, each child was placed in a category ranging from 1 to 4 on the basis of the total past history and records, not merely the current charge, those children rated 1 or 2 constituting the "less violent" group and those rated 3 or 4 constituting the "more violent" group. In the more violent group ($n = 78$), 31 percent had both minor and major neurologic signs. Forty-four percent had major neurological signs; 71 percent had minor neurological signs; and 81 percent had either minor or major signs. In the less violent group ($n = 19$), none had both minor and major signs. Twelve percent had major neurologic signs, 35 percent had minor neurologic signs, and 41 percent had minor or major signs. Each of these differences between the groups was statistically significant. For the purposes of this analysis major neurologic signs were considered to include a history of generalized seizures, an abnormal EEG, and an abnormal head circumference and/or Babinksi signs. Minor neurological signs included choreiform movements and the inability of the subject to skip.

Symptoms suggesting complex partial seizures were quite common amongst the 97 delinquent boys and there was a significant positive correlation between the numbers of such symptoms and the degree of violence ($p < .001$).

Two clinicians agreed that 18 of the boys (19%) had most likely suffered complex partial seizures on the basis of their having had experienced well-documented episodes, observed by others, of lapses of fully conscious contact with their environment. These episodes were followed by periods of confusion, fatigue, or sleep for which the subject's memory was impaired or absent. Fourteen of the 18 boys who were considered to have experienced complex partial seizures at some time had abnormal EEG's, and one subject with a normal EEG had a well-documented history of generalized seizures. All 18 were in the more violent group, and 8 had a history of generalized seizures.

On the basis of historical data, it seemed highly probable that five of the subjects had committed violent acts during a seizure, though in no case was EEG/video monitoring performed on the subjects. All five of the youngsters who were considered to have performed violent acts during seizures had also been violent at times when seizures were clearly not occurring.

Intelligence as measured on the WISC indicated a tendency for the less-violent children to function somewhat better intellectually but overall differences between the two groups were not striking. The two groups differed significantly in reading grade, arithmetic, and the ability to remember four numbers backward, the more violent group being at a significant disadvantage in each of these variables.

The most striking difference psychiatrically between the two groups was the finding that a significantly greater proportion of very violent children had clear histories of paranoid symptomatology. Furthermore, they were significantly more likely than their less aggressive peers to be loose, rambling, and illogical in their thought processes during interviewing. Depressive symptoms were common in both groups. There was much mental illness in the families of the more violent boys and alcoholism in the fathers, but it was difficult to compare the groups as information about fathers was often unreliable.

Virtually all the subjects came from the lowest echelons of society, and most were from broken homes with multiple social problems including criminality, alcoholism, and mental illness in parents. Most of the subjects had histories of disruptive behavior that began before puberty, often dating to the first decade. One social factor strongly distinguished the more violent from the less violent children: a history of extreme physical abuse by parents or parent substitutes.

The two samples also differed significantly in their exposure to violence in that the more violent children had witnessed extreme violence directed at others, mostly in their homes, more frequently than the less violent children. Seventy-five percent of the more violent group had been abused and 33 percent of the less violent group ($p = .003$). Seventy-nine percent of the more violent group had witnessed extreme violence as compared with 20 percent of the less violent group ($p < .001$).

These data strongly suggest that extremely violent juvenile offenders differed significantly in a number of ways from their less violent delinquent peers. They were more likely to manifest both major and minor signs of neurological impairment including complex partial seizures, to have pervasive paranoid ideation, and to have suffered abuse or witnessed extreme violence.

ABUSE AND VIOLENCE

The violence experienced at home in early childhood is probably an important etiologic factor in the development of a propensity for violence. Among 2143 families in a national survey, Murray Strauss (1981) reported a 3.4 percent annual incidence of at least a single episode of very severe violence by parents toward a child. A study by Knudsen (reported at the meeting of the International Society for Research on Aggression, August 1981, at Wheaton College, Massachusetts) of approximately 4000 undergraduate students who took an introductory psychology course at the University of Iowa revealed that 7 percent had been seriously physically abused at home. This prevalence figure was obtained from students who were virtually all-white, middle-class subjects; a third were from rural, a third from urban, and a third from suburban areas. The figure would rise to 9 percent if witnessing the abuse of a sibling were included. Knudsen defined abuse as "such severe beating that medical services were necessary." The well-known prevalence of the experience of child abuse amongst parents who are themselves child abusers also supports the hypothesis that the experience of child abuse is an important etiological factor in subsequent violent behavior, but there have been no prospective studies to date on the victims of child abuse with respect to their adult behavior. It is reasonable to hypothesize that exposure to abuse early in life sets up a "template" of behavior which is often followed in later life.

BRAIN DAMAGE AND VIOLENCE

There is evidence that "minimal brain damage," now called "attention deficit disorder" (ADD) predisposes to criminal behavior, including violence.

In one prospective study Satterfield et al. (1982) obtained serious offense records on a group of 198 adolescent boys 14 to 20 years of age, of whom 110 between 6 and 12 had been diagnosed as suffering from ADD and 88 were normal adolescents. Rates of single and multiple offenses and institutionalization for delinquency were significantly higher in the ADD subjects. About half of the ADD subjects had been arrested at least once for a serious offense after the diagnosis of ADD was made. This was defined as robbery, assault with a deadly weapon, grand theft (automobile), grand theft, and burglary. Only one ADD subject had been arrested before being given that diagnosis. Offender rates did not vary significantly as a function of socioeconomic class (Tables 2-1, 2-2, derived from Satterfield).

Table 2-1
Arrest Rate for Serious Offense

Socioeconomic Class	ADD[a] $(n = 110)$ (%)	Control $(n = 88)$ (%)	
Lower	58	11	$p < .01$
Middle	36	9	$p < .05$
Upper	52	2	$p < .001$

[a] ADD = attention deficit disorder

Table 2-2
Multiple-Arrest Rate for Serious Offense

Socioeconomic Class	ADD[a] (%)	Control (%)	
Lower	45	6	$p < .011$
Middle	25	6	$p < .001$
Upper	28	0	$p < .001$

[a] ADD = attention deficit disorder

EPILEPSY, COMPLEX PARTIAL SEIZURES, THE POSTICTAL STATE, AND VIOLENCE

Abnormalities of the EEG are quite prevalent among violent prisoners. In a study of 1250 individuals in jail for crimes of aggression, Williams (1969) found abnormal EEG's in 57 percent of the habitual aggressors and in only 12 percent of those who had committed a solitary aggressive crime, after prisoners who were mentally retarded or epileptic or had sustained serious head injury were separated from the group. Of the habitual aggressors who had electroencephalographic abnormalities, the temporal lobe was involved in over 80 percent.

In a study of more than 400 violent prisoners in a large penitentiary, it was discovered that half had symptoms suggestive of epileptic phenomena, one-third had abnormal EEG's, but fewer than 10 percent had frank temporal lobe epilepsy (Mark and Ervin, 1970). It was also apparent that these people had a characteristic social history, which included multiple physical assaults, aggressive sexual behavior including attempted rape, many traffic violations, serious automobile accidents, and "pathological intoxication."

A good deal of attention has been given to the question of whether patients with generalized and complex partial (psychomotor) seizures have a propensity toward violence before, during, after or between seizures. From the review of experimental data earlier in this chapter, one might predict that such an association exists, but it has been difficult to prove.

There are several ways in which seizures and violence could be theoretically related:

1. *An episode of directed violence could be the automatism of a complex partial seizure.*

There is considerable resistance to this concept. The directed aggression reported during epileptic attacks by St. Hilaire (1980), Ashford (1980), and Mark and Ervin (1970) have been ascribed to "fear, defensive kicking and flailing" by Delgado-Escueta and his colleagues (1981), who nonetheless reported seven patients who demonstrated aggression toward inanimate objects or another person during seizures recorded with scalp electrodes. Of these seven, "one had aggressive acts that could have resulted in serious harm to another person"; yet Delgado-Escueta and associates concluded that the commission of murder or manslaughter during psychomotor automatisms was a "near impossibility." As the study of Delgado-Escueta did not select patients from a population with known aggressive behavior, violence, and psychosis and did not study any patients who were on trial for violent crimes during epileptic attacks and did not use depth electrodes for the most part, it left open the possibility that more harmful acts of aggression could characterize the automatisms of criminals with epilepsy or violence-prone patients with psychosis and epilepsy. One report of three excessively violent male patients, one of whom had experienced grand mal seizures, utilized depth electrodes implanted in and around the amygdala with continual recordings for three to seven weeks. This study conclusively demonstrated that the episodic rage attacks of all three men were associated with spiking discharges in the amygdala and that the behavior could be reproduced by stimulation. In only one patient was there a clear indication of an ictal basis of violent behavior from the surface EEG recordings (Smith, 1980).

2. *Directed violence could be an outgrowth of the encephalopathy associated with a seizure or the postictal state.*

There have been many reports of status epilepticus presenting as prolonged confusional states (Sommerville and Bruni, 1983) and at least one report of "a man who frequently enters a confused, paranoid psychotic state immediately after a (generalized) seizure and who killed his wife while in such a state" (Gunn, 1982). This report is the more impressive because its author has often written to the effect that there is "very little evidence of violent crimes being directly related to epileptic phenomena" (Gunn, 1982).

3. *Anxiety, fear, or anger could precipitate a seizure, possibly by inducing hyperventilation.*

In this way aggressive actions could cause a seizure. The confusional state associated with such a seizure or its postictal period might allow continued aggression to occur unhindered by the inhibitions that intact cortical function might bring to bear on the situation. Even if such a seizure were brief, lasting less than half a minute (Delgado-Escueta et al., 1981), the postictal period could be much longer.

4. *Brain damage that predisposes an individual to violence might also cause seizures.*

This perspective, proposed forcefully by Stevens and Hermann (1981), regards epilepsy as an epiphenomenon in relation to violence or any other behavioral deviation but identifies limbic brain damage as a critical etiologic feature in the pathogenesis of psychopathology in epileptics. The preponderance of evidence points toward the conclusion that some patients with partial epilepsy and a focus of abnormality in the temporal lobe have a vulnerability to undergo personality change (Bear and Fedio 1977; Trimble 1983), but the role of epilepsy per se in this vulnerability is moot. Possibly epileptic discharges in sensitive regions of the brain that do not result in clinical seizures can give rise to nonictal behavioral disorders, that is, to the "interictal state."

5. *Violence and epilepsy may be only serendipitously related.*

There have been many reports of an association between complex partial seizures and violence. Falconer et al. (1958) reported that 38 percent of patients with temporal lobe epilepsy showed "pathological aggressiveness." Among 666 cases of temporal lobe epilepsy studied by Currie (1971), 7 percent were found to be "aggressive." Glaser (1967) reported "aggressive behavior" in 67 of 120 children with limbic epilepsy. Serafetinides (1965) also found "aggressiveness" to be a characteristic of temporal lobe epilepsy.

On the other hand, there have also been studies that failed to demonstrate any association between psychomotor seizures and violence. In a group of 100 children with a variety of neurological problems including seizures, Ounsted (1969) reported outbursts of rage in 36. But the patients who had only psychomotor epilepsy were "uniformly intelligent and conforming children and none of

them had rage outbursts at any time." Perhaps the most important of the studies showing no association between complex partial epilepsy and violence was that of Rodin (1973), who evaluated 57 patients with psychomotor epilepsy and photographed
them during their seizures. There were no instances of ictal or
postictal aggression. A review of 700 case histories of patients in
his epilepsy clinic revealed 34 patients who had committed aggressive acts. The presence or absence of psychomotor epilepsy in these
34 patients was not a relevant variable.

The contradictions in these results may be related to varying definitions of aggression, violence, and complex partial seizures and to
the selection of patients. In some parts of the country, for instance,
a propensity toward violence in patients may affect their referral.
Violence may be dealt with by schools or the police, with or without consultation with physicians, some of whom may not be aware
of the possibility that the suspect's behavior is influenced by seizures. Also, the referral of violent epileptics to a neurology or an
epilepsy clinic may be more or less likely depending on the local
authorities.

Some seizure units with video/EEG-monitoring equipment dis-
courage the admission of episodically violent individuals since they
are unprepared to handle violent patients and fear their equipment
may be damaged. This kind of selectivity has severely limited the
number of prolonged EEG studies of violent individuals and probably has lowered the reported prevalence of violence among epileptics so monitored (Delgado-Escueta et al., 1981).

Physicians who have cared for large numbers of seizure patients
would agree that violence and aggressive acts do occur in patients
with complex partial seizures, but they would disagree as to whether
the incidence of violence in this form of epilepsy is more or less
frequent than in the epileptic or general population.

The problem of the definition of violence and aggression is important. Fighting among children, particularly boys, is certainly
not unusual (Detre et al., 1972). But it may well be that some authors, not wishing "to give epileptics a bad name," have discounted
acts of personal violence as being within the normal range and

missed a possible association between violence and complex partial seizures. Certainly, the tremendous variation in reports of this association or its absence and the general lack of clarity in defining violence and aggression suggest that methodological problems have yet to be overcome and that the studies are not comparable.

Gunn and Bonn (1971) found no difference between epileptic and nonepileptic prisoners in terms of violent behavior. In a comparative study of epileptic prisoners and hospitalized epileptic nonprisoners, Gunn (1974) noted great similarities in organic and social factors and psychiatric symptoms; the main difference was more drinking in the group of prisoners. This again raises questions about the hypothesis that violent behavior and seizures are related.

Gunn and Fenton (1971), however, noted a relatively high incidence of epilepsy in prison populations but decided that automatic behavior during actual seizures was a rare explanation for crimes committed by epileptic patients. This study did not rule out the hypothesis that nonictal violence occurs more frequently in prisoners with complex partial seizures.

How sure can one be that a violent prisoner does not in fact have complex partial seizures? The diagnosis of such seizures is not always easy to make. Among 400 prisoners with a documented history of violent assaults against other individuals, Mark and Ervin (1970) found an obvious and known history of epilepsy in 38, an incidence more than ten times that of the general population. Even more impressive was the fact that fully 50 percent of this group of 400 had experienced phenomena resembling epileptic symptoms, including altered states of consciousness, warning stages preceding their violent act and following it, sleep or drowsiness and/or lassitude. Electroencephalographic abnormalities were seen in 50 percent of the group. How are we to decide if the incidence of complex partial seizures in this group is less than 10 percent or approximately 50 percent?

The prevalence of symptoms suggesting complex partial seizures in violent individuals was shown in a study of Lewis (1976) who evaluated the psychiatric-psychological status of 285 children referred from the juvenile court and reviewed the psychiatric, medical, and electroencephalographic records of those who manifested psychomotor seizure symptoms. Of the 285 children, 18 experienced episodes of apparent loss of fully conscious contact with reality lasting from several seconds to several hours; on occasion, these episodes were observed during psychiatric interviewing or psychological testing. Four of the children had histories of the automatisms often associated with complex partial seizures, such as lip smacking and mouth movements, and four had experienced frequent episodes of déjà vu. Of the 18 children with psychomotor symptoms, eight (44%) had been arrested for crimes of extreme personal violence including two who committed murder. Furthermore, six others who were referred for milder violations, such as truancy and property offenses, had, in fact, attacked other individuals at school or at home but were charged with lesser offenses. All told, 14 of the 18 had engaged in serious acts of violence. It should be noted that violent attacks against persons constitute 8 percent of the offenses for which children are referred to the juvenile courts and 9 percent of the juvenile offenders referred for psychiatric evaluation. The incidence of arrest for violence was significantly higher in the group with psychomotor symptoms ($x^2 = 11.4$, $p < 0.001$). In the group with psychomotor symptoms, 11 of 14 EEG's were abnormal, with three demonstrating temporal foci.

It is interesting that more than 75 percent of the prisoners studied by Mark and Ervin (1970) had histories of significant periods of unconsciousness from head injury or disease and that 15 of the 18 reported by Lewis (1976) had a similar history of events known to be associated with brain injury, such as perinatal problems including infection or prematurity, serious accidents with head trauma, or other disease. These studies strongly support the concept that violence has neurological determinants.

EFFECT OF ALCOHOL

Alcohol is one of the few drugs known to precipitate or worsen episodes of violence in individuals with a past history of violent behavior (Guze and Cartwell, 1965; Detre et al., 1972). In two of the 14 violent children reported by Lewis (1976), there was a history of alcohol use that was associated with the crimes for which they were arrested. Mark and Ervin reported a history of violent acts in the prisoners they studied; these included assaults, moving traffic violations, automobile accidents, frequent drinking, and the peculiar susceptibility to alcohol called "pathological intoxication."

The state of pathological intoxication is not synonymous with ordinary drunkenness. It is a state in which the individual engages in a violent act after drinking, an act for which he will have little or no recollection. Such behavior may sometimes be elicited by small amounts of alcohol, much less than would be required for ordinary intoxication. Blood alcohol levels below 30 mg/100 ml have been recorded in these cases. Pathological intoxication is not associated with slurred speech and incoordination and may last for only a few minutes. It occurs most often when alcohol is imbibed under circumstances "conducive" to violence, that is, at a bar or a party, and it has been difficult to reproduce this state of intoxication by administering alcohol in any quantity in a laboratory setting or by intravenous injection. Those who become pathologically intoxicated, it is said, may not be chronic alcoholics, and the condition is said not to be limited to individuals with a criminal disposition. It is relatively rare, even among brain-damaged individuals. Yet 90 percent of pathological intoxication cases are associated with brain damage, epilepsy, retardation, or psychosis (Bowman and Jellinck, 1941). Electroencephalographic changes may also be associated with episodes of pathological intoxication (Thompson, 1963). There may be an interplay among environmental and organic factors in the induction of pathological intoxication, which, were it understood, might shed light on the complex relation between brain dysfunction and violence.

Some have questioned the existence of this syndrome or refer to it simply as "intoxication." Perhaps alcohol nonspecifically "makes an organic brain syndrome worse" and then precipitates violence. At the Epilepsy Center at Yale, it has not ever been possible to induce aggressive behavior or epileptiform EEG changes by administering alcohol in a clinical setting to a patient whose history suggests pathological intoxication. Nine or more patients suspected of pathological intoxication have been studied with EEG and clinical observation during the administration of alcohol toward the levels of legal intoxication (100 g/100 ml) (personal communication R. H. Mattson).

ETIOLOGY

It is likely that the "dyscontrol syndrome" described by Mark and Ervin is the same syndrome that Detre calls "explosive personality disorder" and others "criminal sociopathic personality." The combination of a characteristic past history of violent behavior with commonly associated electroencephalographic abnormalities that often involve the temporal lobe certainly suggests that the antisocial behavior may be determined or at least influenced by neurological, if not by limbic, abnormality.

Some studies have suggested that habitual acts of antisocial behavior involving physical violence are genetically determined. While the point remains very controversial, it appears that an XYY chromosome abnormality may be associated with tall stature and aggressiveness (Hook and Kim, 1970; Jacobs et al., 1971). But, this association may be distorted. In the original studies, the relationship was observed mainly in "mental-penal" institutions, whereas more recent data seem to indicate that as much as 90 percent of the XYY population remains outside mental hospitals and prisons (Gerald, 1976).

In twin studies, the concordance rates for delinquency are higher in monozygotic than in dizygotic twins; but, such evidence for a genetic influence in episodically violent behavior is not conclusive (Slater and Cowie, 1971), and the dominant view today is that an unfavorable environment in childhood is the major determining factor in episodic violence.

There is considerable evidence that associates a disruption of family life with the development of episodic violence. Troubled family life, including brutality, alcoholism, and marital discord, is such a constant feature in the background of chronically violent persons that it is possible to predict the development of delinquent behavior on the basis of certain personality and family factors. When all of the five following factors are found in two- to three-year-old children, it seems likely that delinquency can be predicted with the same degree of accuracy (90%) as it can in five- and six-year-olds (Glueck and Glueck, 1966): (1) psychopathology of either or both parents (alcoholism, delinquency, emotional disturbance, or mental retardation); (2) indifference or hostility to the child by one or both parents; (3) extreme restlessness in the child; (4) nonsubmissiveness of the child to parental authority; (5) unusual destructiveness in the child.

On the basis of this association, it would be a mistake to attribute violence in the offspring to purely environmental factors, since brutality, alcoholism, and marital discord in parents may themselves be expressions of a genetic defect. This is supported by Heston's report (1966) that criminality and other associated sociopathic disorders were significantly more prevalent in the offspring of schizophrenics raised in foster homes than in the offspring of nonschizophrenics raised in foster homes. Another factor to be considered in the association of environmental stress and violence is the effect of a violent juvenile delinquent on his parents. The child's problem may be so severe that it disrupts the life of the whole family (Bell, 1968).

On the basis of the evidence, it is not possible to determine whether "nurture" or "nature" is more important in the development of episodic violent behavior. What does seem clear, however, is that episodic violence is not a simple functional psychological disorder. Neurological determinants are present, and the syndrome cannot be reversed by any known therapeutic means. To the extent that episodic violence is a learned behavioral pattern, it is one that is learned at a very early age (Detre et al., 1972). It appears to be at least as difficult to alter episodic violence in the adult human being as it is to alter the abnormal socialization of adult monkeys that is the result of early social deprivation (Harlow, 1971).

TREATMENT OF VIOLENCE

The treatment of episodic violence is difficult. It is possible that the episodic dyscontrol syndrome, in which attacks of explosive rage unpredictably follow minimal provocation, might be the easiest to treat, particularly if the primitive, violent behavior were out of character for the individual.

Anticonvulsant and antipsychotic drugs seldom reduce violence in nonepileptic, nonpsychotic offenders (Goldstein, 1974). This is not to say that these medications may not help individual patients (Lion, 1975; Monroe, 1975: Tupin et al., 1973). According to anecdotal statements, sedating medications such as barbiturates and minor tranquilizers usually worsen violent behavior. When violence is a concomitant of bipolar depression, lithium may be effective; it has been shown to reduce aggressive behavior in a double-blind controlled study in a penal institution (Sheard et al., 1976; Marini and Sheard, 1976, 1977).

The beta-blocker propranolol has been used to prevent recurrent rage attacks in brain-damaged individuals (Schreier, 1979; Yudofsky et al., 1981; Elliott, 1977). Elliott used a starting dose of 20 mgs. t.i.d., and this was doubled every two days, rarely to more than 480 mgs. Propranolol apparently does not work in the presence of Haldol or phenothiazines and takes approximately two weeks to control violent outbursts effectively (Elliot's remarks at meeting of International Society for Research on Aggression, August 22, 1981, Wheaton College, Massachusetts).

Despite these optimistic reports, it seems intuitively unlikely that anticonvulsant, antipsychotic, or beta-blocking medications would work in individuals whose violent behavior is semiadaptive, predatory, or motivated by loyalty to a cause even if brain damage were a factor in such individuals. We would predict greater effectiveness of pharmacotherapy in brain-damaged individuals who demonstrate episodic violence that seems remarkably atypical or alien to their baseline personality. Controlled studies have yet to be done, and they face nearly insuperable ethical problems. Such research must be conducted in prison populations to control compliance and to validate behavioral data. Incarcerated individuals commonly are not regarded as being free to give informed consent to participate and studies of incarcerated minors would be even more difficult, ethically.

Psychosurgery involving stimulation or ablation of limbic areas, as described by Mark and Ervin (1970), is ethically controversial and would appear to be of limited clinical use. Psychotherapy also seems to be of limited use. In a study of juvenile delinquents (one-third of whom were violent) at a well-organized residential center, 75 percent were found to have had two reconvictions or more after release from the center (Hartelius, 1965). Roughly the same rate of recidivism has been noted in populations of untreated violent criminals (Gibbins et al., 1959).

Violent individuals are often presented to neurologists and psychiatrists not as patients but as prisoners. Physicians are not then asked what treatment would prevent future violence but rather to what extent is the individual responsible for his past violent behavior.

VIOLENCE AND RESPONSIBILITY

Our legal system generally operates under the presumption of free will. This is basically a philosophical and religious concept, not a scientific or medical one, from which it follows that people are responsible for their actions. The law recognizes, however, that the operation of free will in certain circumstances is constrained by diseases of the brain. Accordingly, certain rules including the M'Naughten, irresistible impulse, mental incapacity, and diminished responsibility, have been developed, and the plea of innocence by reason of one of these rules has become conventional for defendants charged with serious crimes. Attorneys for defendants charged with homicide, arson, and assault commonly seek to prove that their client's responsibility for his actions was significantly diminished when the crimes were committed. To buttress this opinion, attorneys turn to psychiatrists and neurologists for medical testimony. Unfortunately, free will has no measurable parameters. One assumes that genetic endowment and life experiences form our personalities and greatly influence or fully determine our responses. Where does free will enter this equation? The mingling of legal and religious concepts with science has produced a murky swamp of belief and facts that is very difficult to negotiate. For neurologists the legal question often centers around the issue of whether violence can arise from epilepsy or brain damage and whether or not the so-called episodic dyscontrol syndrome has a physiologic basis.

Until 1970 attorneys rarely used the insanity defense, and then only in cases of homicide because, if successful, it resulted in prolonged and indefinite incarceration of the criminal in a facility for the "criminally insane." A change in the interpretation of the law, which forbade the incarceration in such facilities of individuals who have become "sane," has led to the increased popularity of the "temporary insanity" defense (or the equivalent thereof) because an individual who is adjudged not guilty by reason of insanity and who has been committed must now be released as soon as he is no longer considered mentally ill (State v. Krol, 68 NJ 236, 344A, 2d 289 [1975]).

There were 53 successful uses of the insanity defense in New York State (mostly for homicide) between 1965 and 1971 and 225 successful uses of it between 1971 and 1976. The average length of stay in mental health facilities was 369 days (Kolb et al., 1978).

Individuals convicted of first-degree murder now serve an average of nine years in prison whereas those found innocent of murder by reason of diminished mental capacity or insanity serve one to three years in an institution (Singer, 1978). Yet about 20 percent of the prisoners in New York State jails are receiving psychiatric therapy. By what logic are they in prison while others are free on the basis of mental incapacity or diminished responsibility? (Carnahan, W. Remarks at meeting at International Society for Research on Aggression, 1981).

There are many types of behavioral disorders that society is prepared to tolerate, but the line is drawn at those that may harm others. The decision whether, when, and how long to incarcerate an individual who has acted dangerously in the past is not an easy one to make. Most authorities agree that it would be necessary to detain two or three times as many patients or prisoners unnecessarily in order to ensure that those who are a danger to society do not leave a hospital or prison prematurely (*Lancet* editorial, 1982). Those who are detained in a hospital may be unjustifiably deprived of their civil rights. Several such patients in the United States have been judged unconstitutionally detained and this has led to the release of many mentally ill people against the advice of their clinicians. Follow-up of these patients has shown a much lower incidence of violence than was predicted (Steadman and Keveles, 1972; Cocozza and Steadman, 1974; Thornberry and Jacoby, 1979). Unfortunately, there is also no way of predicting when repeat offenses are likely to occur and a long period of follow-up is necessary because repetition of arson, rape, and homicide may take place many years after release (Soothill and Pope, 1973; Soothill et al., 1976).

In our opinion, the preponderance of evidence indicates that episodic violence is a behavioral syndrome that mainly affects young males and that is organically determined. Since, however, the best predictor of violent, aggressive behavior is a history of violent or aggressive behavior, and since the tendency to recidivism persists at least until the fourth decade of life (Robins, 1966), it would seem reasonable to separate such individuals from society in some manner until their thirties or until some truly effective therapeutic measure is developed.

REFERENCES

Ashford, J. W., S. C. Schulz, and F. O. Walsh. Violent automatism in a partial complex seizure. *Arch. Neurol.* 37:120-122, 1980.

Bard, P. A diencephalic mechanism for the expression of age with special reference to the sympathetic nervous system. *Amer. J. Physiol.* 84:490, 1928.

Bear, D. M. and P. Fedio. Quantitative analysis of interictal behavior in temporal lobe epilepsy. *Arch. Neurol.* 34:454, 1977.

Bell, R. O. A reinterpretation of the direction of effects in studies of socialization. *Psychol. Rev.* 75:81, 1968.

Bowman, K. M. and E. M. Jellinck. Alcoholic mental disorders. *Q. J. Stud. Alcohol.* 2:312, 1941.

Brodal, A. *Neurological Anatomy in Relation to Clinical Medicine.* 3rd ed. Oxford University Press, New York, 1981.

Cocozza, J. J. and H. J. Steadman. Some refinements in the measurement and prediction of dangerous behavior. *Amer. J. Psychiat.* 131:1012, 1974.

Currie, S. Clinical course and prognosis of temporal lobe epilepsy. *Brain* 94:173, 1971.

Delgado-Escueta, A. V. Letter. Violence and epilepsy. *New Eng. J. Med.* 306:299, 1982.

Delgado-Escueta, A. V., R. H. Mattson, L. King, et al. The nature of aggression during epileptic seizures. *New Eng. J. Med.* 305:711, 1981.

Detre, T. P. and H. G. Jarecki. Modern psychiatric treatment. J. B. Lippincott, Philadelphia, 1971.

———, Kupfer, D. J. and S. Taub. The nosology of violence: Presentation at Neurological Symposium on the Neural Basis of Violence and Aggression. Houston, Texas, March 1972.

Editorial. Dangerousness. Lancet 2:1341, 1982.

Elliott, F. A. Neurological findings in adult minimal brain dysfunction and the dyscontrol syndrome. *J. Neur. Ment. Dis.* 170:680-687, 1982.

Elliott, F. A. Propranolol for the control of belligerent behavior following acute brain damage. *Ann. Neurol.* 1:489-491, 1977.

Falconer, M. A. et al. Clinical, radiological and EEG correlations with pathological changes in temporal lobe epilepsy and their significance in surgical treatment. In: *Temporal Lobe Epilepsy.* M. Baldwin and P. Bailey, eds. C C Thomas, Springfield, Ill., 1958, p. 396.

Fulton, H. H. Discussion. *Epilepsia* 2:77, 1953.

Gerald, P. S. Current concepts in genetics: Sex chromosome disorders. *New Eng. J. Med.* 294:706, 1976.

Gibbens, T. C. N., D. A. Pond, and D. Stafford-Clark. Followup study of criminal psychopaths. *J. Ment. Sci.* 105:108, 1959.

Gibbs, F. A. Ictal and nonictal psychiatric disorders in temporal lobe epilepsy. *J. Nerv. Ment. Dis.* 113:522, 1951.

Glaser, G. H. Limbic epilepsy in childhood. *J. Nerv. Ment. Dis.* 144:391, 1967.

——— and J. H. Pincus. Limbic encephalitis. *J. Nerv. Ment. Dis.* 149:59, 1969.

Glueck, E. T. and S. Glueck. Identification of potential delinquents at 2-3 years of age. *Int. J. Soc. Psychiat.* 12:5, 1966.

Goldstein, M. Brain research and violent behavior. A summary and evaluation of the status of biomedical research on brain and aggressive violent behavior. *Arch. Neurol.* 30:1, 1974.

Guerrant, J., W. W. Anderson, A. Fischer, A. Weinstein, R. M. Jaros, and

A. Deskins.   *Personality in Epilepsy.* C C Thomas, Springfield, Ill., 1962.

Gunn, J.   Social factors and epileptics in prison. *Brit. J. Psychiat.* 124:509, 1974.

Gunn, J. C.   Epileptic homicide: A case report. *Brit. J. Psychiat.* 132:510, 1978.

Gunn, J. C.   Letter. Violence and epilepsy. *New Eng. J. Med.* 306:299, 1982.

———— and J. Bonn.   Criminality and violence in epileptic prisoners. *Brit. J. Psychiat.* 118:337, 1971.

———— and G. Fenton.   Epilepsy, automatism and crime. *Lancet* 1:1173, 1971.

Guze, S. B. and D. P. Cartwell.   Alcoholism, parole observations and criminal recidivism; study of 116 parolees. *Am. J. Psychiat.* 122:436, 1965.

Harlow, H. F., M. K. Harlow, and S. J. Suomi.   From thought to therapy: Lessons from a primate laboratory. How investigation of the learning capabilities of rhesus monkeys has led to the study of their behavioral abnormalities and rehabilitation. *Am. Scien.* 59:538, 1971.

Hartelius, H.   Study of male juvenile delinquency. *Acta. Psychiat. Scand.* 40:7, 1965.

Heston, L. L.   Psychiatric disorders in foster home reared children of schizophrenic mothers. *Brit. J. Psychiat.* 112:819, 1966.

Himmelhoch, J., J. H. Pincus, G. J. Tucker, and T. P. Detre.   Subacute encephalitis: Behavioral and neurological aspects. *Brit. J. Psychiat.* 116:531, 1970.

Hook, E. B. and D. S. Kim.   Prevalence of XYY and XXY karyotypes in 337 non-retarded young offenders. *New Eng. J. Med.* 283:410, 1970.

Hovey, J. E., M. H. NeWar, and R. Plutchik.   Characteristics of violent schizophrenic inpatients in a state hospital. Presented at ISRA meeting, August 1981, Wheaton College.

Jackobs, P. A., W. H. Prince, S. Richmond, and R. A. W. Ratecliff.   Chromosome surveys in penal institutions and approved schools. *J. Med. Genet.* 8:49, 1971.

Kluver, H. and P. C. Bucy.   Preliminary analysis of functions of the temporal lobes in monkeys. *Arch. Neurol. Psychiat.* 42:979, 1939.

Kolb, L., W. W. Carnahan, H. Steadman and J. Wright.   The insanity defense in New York. N.Y. State Dept. of Mental Hygiene, 1978.

Lewis, D. O.   Delinquency, psychomotor epileptic symtomatology and paranoid symptomatology: A triad. *Am. J. Psychiat.* 1977.

Lewis, D. O., J. H. Pincus, S. S. Shanok and G. H. Glaser.   Psychomotor epilepsy and violence in a group of incarcerated adolescent boys. *Amer. J. Psychiat.* 139:882, 1982.

Lewis, D. O., S. S. Shanok, J. H. Pincus, et al.   Violent juvenile delinquents: Psychiatric, neurological, psychological and abuse factors. *J. Amer. Acad. Child Psychiat.* 18:307, 1979.

Lewis, D. O., S. S. Shanok, and J. H. Pincus.   A comparison of the neuropsychiatric status of female and male incarcerated delinquents: Some evidences of sex and race bias. *J. Amer. Acad. Child Psychiat.* 21:190, 1982.

Lewis, D. O. and D. A. Balla. *Delinquency and Psychopathology.* Grune and Stratton, New York, 1976.

Lion, J. R. Conceptual issues in the use of drugs for the treatment of aggression in man. *J. Nerv. Ment. Dis.* 160:76, 1975.

MacLean, P. D. Some psychiatric implications of physiological studies on fronto-temporal portion of limbic system (visceral brain). *Electroenceph. Clin. Neurophysiol.* 4:407, 1952.

————. The limbic system and its hippocampal formation. Studies in animals and their possible relation to man. *J. Neurosurg.* 11:29, 1954.

Madden, D. J., J. R. Lion, and M. W. Penna. Assaults on psychiatrist by patients. *Amer. J. Psychiat.* 133:422, 1976.

Malamud, N. Psychiatric disorder with intracranial tumors of the limbic system. *Arch. Neurol.* 17:113, 1967.

Mark, V. H. and F. R. Ervin. *Violence and the Brain.* Harper & Row, New York, 1970.

Marini, J. L. and M. H. Sheard. Antiaggressive effect of lithium ion in man. *Acta Psychiat. Scand.* 55:269, 1977.

Mednick, F. A. and K. Christiansen. *Biosocial Bases of Criminal Behavior.* Chapter 1. Gardner Press, New York, 1977.

Monroe, R. R. Anticonvulsants in the treatment of aggression. *J. Nerv. Ment. Dis.* 160:119, 1975.

Ounsted, C. Aggression and epilepsy: Rage in children with temporal lobe epilepsy. *J. Psychosom. Res.* 13:237, 1969.

Papez, J. W. A proposed mechanism of emotion. *Arch. Neurol. Psychiat.* 38:725, 1937.

Robins, L. N. *Deviant Children Grown Up: Sociological and Psychiatric Study of Sociopathic Personality.* Williams & Wilkins, Baltimore, 1966.

Rodin, E. A. Psychomotor epilepsy and aggressive behavior. *Arch. Gen. Psychiat.* 28:210, 1973.

Saint-Hilaire, J. M., M. Gilbert, and G. Bouner. Aggression as an epileptic manifestation: Two cases with depth electrode study. *Epilepsia* 21:184, 1980.

Satterfield, J. H., C. M. Hope, and A. M. Schell. A prospective study of delinquency in 110 adolescent boys with attention deficit disorder and 88 normal adolescent boys. *Amer. J. Psychiat.* 139:795, 1982.

Schreier, H. A. Use of propranolol in the treatment of postencephalitis psychosis. *Amer. J. Psychiat.* 136:840, 1979.

Serafetinides, E. A. Aggressiveness in temporal lobe epileptics and its relation to cerebral dysfunction and environmental factors. *Epilepsia* 6:33, 1965.

Sheard, M. H., J. L. Marini, C. I. Bridges, et al. The effect of lithium on impulse, aggressive behavior in man. *Amer. J. Psychiat.* 133:1409, 1976.

Singer, A. C. Insanity acquittal in the 1970's: Observation on empirical analysis of one jurisdiction. *Ment. Dis. Law Rep.* 406:417, 1978.

Slater, E. and V. Cowie. *The Genetics of Mental Disorders.* Oxford University Press, London, 1971.

100   *Behavioral Neurology*

Small, J. G., V. Milstein, and J. R. Stevens. Are psychomotor epileptics different? *Arch. Neurol.* 7:187, 1962.

Smith, J. S. *Episodic Rage in Limbic Epilepsy and the Dyscontrol System.* M. Girgis and L. G. Kiloh, eds. Elsevier/North Holland, Biomedical Press, 1980, p. 255.

Somerville, E. R. and J. Bruni. Tonic status epilepticus presenting as confusional state. *Ann. Neurol.* 13:549, 1983.

Soothill, K. L. and P. J. Pope. Arson: A twenty year cohort study. *Med. Sci. Law* 13:127, 1973.

Soothill, K. L., A. Jack, and T. C. N. Gibbens. Rape: A twenty-two year cohort study. *Med. Sci. Law* 16:62, 1976.

Steadman, H. J. and G. Keveles. The community adjustment and criminal activity of the Backstrom patients 1966-1790. *Amer. J. Psychiat.* 129: 304, 1972.

Stevens, J. R. Psychiatric implications of psychomotor epilepsy. *Arch. Gen. Psychiat.* 14:461, 1966.

Stevens, J. R. and B. P. Hermann. Temporal lobe epilepsy, psychopathology and violence: The state of the evidence. *Neurology* 31:1127, 1981.

Stevens, J. R., V. H. Mark, F. Erwin, P. Pacheco, and K. Suematsu. Deep temporal stimulation in man: Long latency, long lasting psychological changes. *Arch. Neurol.* 21:157, 1969.

Straus, H. et al. *Behind Closed Doors. Violence in the American Family.* Doubleday, 1981.

Thompson, G. N. Electroencephalogram in acute pathological alcoholic intoxication. *Bull. Los Ang. Neurol. Soc.* 28:217, 1963.

Thornberry, T. P. and J. E. Jacoby. *The Criminally Insane in a Community Followup of Mentally Ill Offenders.* Chicago University Press, 1979.

Trimble, M. R. Personality disturbances in epilepsy. *Neurology* 33:1332, 1983.

Tupin, J. P., D. B. Smith, T. L. Clanon, et al. The long term use of lithium in aggressive prisoners. *Comp. Psychiat.* 14:311, 1973.

Williams, D. T., R. Mehl, S. Yudofsky, et al. The effect of propranolol on uncontrolled rage outbursts in children and adolescents with organic brain dysfunction. *J. Amer. Acad. Child Psychiat.* 1984 (in press).

Williams, D. T. Neural factors related to habitual aggression. *Brain* 92:503, 1969.

Wolfgang, M. Delinquency and violence from the viewpoint of criminality. In: *Neural Bases of Violence and Aggression.* W. S. Fields and W. H. Sweet, eds. Warren Green, St. Louis, 1975, pp. 456-493.

Yudofsky, S., D. Williams, and J. Gorman. Propranolol in the treatment of rage and violent behavior in patients with chronic brain syndrome. *Amer. J. Psychiat.* 138:218, 1981.

Zitrin, A., A. S. Nardesky, E. I. Burdock, et al. *Amer. J. Psychiat.* 133:142-149, 1976.

Chapter 3

SCHIZOPHRENIA

Schizophrenia, manifested most notably by bizarre or delusional thoughts, is often easier to diagnose than to define. Nonetheless, on the basis of a distinctive and consistent constellation of symptoms and elements in the family history, it must be considered a dysfunction of the brain. The consistency of the symptoms supports the disease concept of schizophrenia, since the clinical picture has changed little in time and varies only slightly from culture to culture (Sanua, 1969). The means of establishing the diagnosis of schizophrenia are limited exclusively to history and observation, particularly the age of onset, the clinical course, the characteristically abnormal family history, and the phenomenology of the symptoms as well as the response to treatment. There are no laboratory tests to establish the diagnosis. Largely for this reason, schizophrenia has been regarded by many clinicians as a functional disorder, the product of environmental stress. In this chapter we will present the criteria that are most helpful in establishing the diagnosis of schizophrenia and differentiating it from other conditions, and we will summarize the evidence that it is an organic dysfunction of the brain.

CLINICAL FEATURES

Age at Onset

Schizophrenia is primarily a disease of young people. Kraeplin noted that most patients were under the age of thirty-five at the time of diagnosis, a finding that has been confirmed in many studies. The first clear-cut symptoms appear before the age of twenty-five in 50 percent of the cases; onset after the age of forty is unusual (Kraeplin, 1925). Symptoms rarely begin in the first decade, but when they do, they virtually always occur in the latter half, never before the age of five. Childhood schizophrenia has often been confused with infantile autism, a condition that usually begins in the first year of life and that always appears before age five (see p. 189).

Symptoms

Though the criteria put forward by different authors for establishing the diagnosis of schizophrenia vary somewhat, Beck et al. (1962) and Hordern et al. (1968) have found over 80 percent agreement in those cases for which experienced clinicians state that they are certain of the diagnosis. One reason for the differences in the diagnostic criteria has been the attempt to identify a basic symptom or characteristic in schizophrenia to which all other symptoms are secondary, and thus to validate a specific etiologic theory of schizophrenia. Recently, there has been a marked turn to descriptive phenomenology and away from attempts to provide etiologic diagnostic classifications. Actually there is much consistency among different authors in enumerating the symptoms of schizophrenia. What differences there are relate mainly to the emphasis placed upon individual symptoms (see Table 3-1). Take, for example, the emphasis placed on delusions and hallucinations. Kurt Schneider claimed that if an individual were experiencing any hallucinations or delusions in the absence of disturbances of memory or orientation, or similar symptoms usually associated with delirium or toxic conditions, one could make a decisive clinical diagnosis of schizophrenia (Schneider, 1959) (Table 3-1). He considered such experiences to be unique to schizophrenia. Despite the importance Schneider attached to delusions and hallucinations, Bleuler regarded them as secondary and instead emphasized loose associations (Bleuler, 1950).

In the past several years this consistency among diagnostic cri-

Table 3-1
Summary of Diagnostic and Phenomenological Symptoms and Signs of Schizophrenia

First Rank Symptoms
(Schneider) (only one necessary for diagnosis)

1. *Auditory Hallucinations*
   a. Audible thoughts (voices speaking patient's thoughts aloud)
   b. Voices arguing (two or more voices arguing usually about patient—refer to patient in third person)
   c. Voices commenting on patient's actions
2. *Delusional Experiences*
   a. Bodily sensations imposed on patient by some external source
   b. Thoughts being taken from his mind
   c. Thoughts ascribed to others
   d. Diffusion of thoughts (patient's thoughts experienced as all around him)
   e. Feelings, impulses, volitional acts imposed on him or under control of external sources
3. *Delusional Perception* (private meaning of a consensually validated perception)

Diagnostic and Statistical Manual of Mental Disorders (DSM-II)
(APA, 2nd ed.) (unclear how many necessary for diagnosis)

1. *Distribution in Thinking*—alterations of concept formulation leading to misinterpretation of reality and sometimes delusions and hallucinations
2. *Mood Changes*—ambivalent, constricted, and inappropriate emotional responsiveness and loss of empathy
3. *Behavior*—withdrawn, regressive, and bizarre

Bleuler's Criteria
(Only fundamental necessary)

1. *Fundamental Symptoms*
   a. Loose associations
   b. Impaired affect
   c. Ambivalence
   d. Autism
2. *Intact Functions*
   a. Sensation and perception
   b. Orientation
   c. Memory
   d. Consciousness
   e. Motility
3. *Accessory or Secondary Symptoms*
   a. Hallucinations and delusions
   b. Catatonia
   c. Depressive symptoms

Diagnostic Criteria for Psychiatric Research
(Feighner et al.) (All necessary for diagnosis)

1. Chronic illness of at least 6 months' duration
2. Absence of depressive or manic symptoms
3. Delusions or hallucinations
4. Verbal productions that make communication difficult because logical or understandable organization lacked
5. At least three of the following:
   a. single
   b. poor premorbid social or work adjustment
   c. family history of schizophrenia
   d. no alcoholism or drug abuse
   e. onset of illness under age forty

A 12-Point Diagnostic System
(Carpenter, 1976)

1. Restricted affect
2. Poor insight
3. Thoughts aloud
4. Waking early (−)*
5. Poor rapport
6. Depressed facies (−)*
7. Elation (−)*
8. Widespread delusions
9. Incoherent speech
10. Unreliable information
11. Bizarre delusions
12. Nihilistic delusions
   *(−) indicates that absence of the criterion favors a diagnosis of schizophrenia.

Diagnostic and Statistical Manual of Mental Disorders (DSM-III)
(APA, 3rd ed.) (criteria necessary as specified for diagnosis)

A. At lease one of the following during a phase of the illness:
   1. bizarre delusions (content is patently absurd and has no possible basis in fact), such as delusions of being controlled, thought broadcasting thought insertion, or thought withdrawal
   2. somatic, grandiose, religious, nihilistic, or other delusions without persecutory or jealous content
   3. delusions with persecutory or jealous content if accompanied by hallucinations of any type
   4. auditory hallucinations in which either a voice keeps up a running commentary on the individual's behavior or thoughts, or two or more voices converse with each other
   5. auditory hallucinations on several occasions with content of more than one or two words, having no apparent relation to depression or elation
   6. Incoherence, marked loosening of associations, markedly illogical think-

ing, or marked poverty of content of speech if associated with at least one of the following:

a. blunted, flat, or inappropriate affect

b. delusions or hallucinations

c. catatonic or other grossly disorganized behavior

B. Deterioration from a previous level of functioning in such areas as work, social relations, and self-care.

C. Duration: Continuous signs of the illness for at least six months at some time during the person's life, with some signs of the illness at present. The six-month period must include an active phase during which there were symptoms from A, with or without a prodromal or residual phase, as defined below.

Prodromal phase: A clear deterioration in functioning before the active phase of the illness not due to a disturbance in mood or to a Substance Use Disorder and involving at least *two* of the symptoms noted below.

Residual phase: Persistence, following the active phase of the illness, of at least *two* of the symptoms noted below, not due to a disturbance in mood or to a Substance Use Disorder.

Prodromal or Residual Symptoms

1. social isolation or withdrawal
2. marked impairment in role functioning as wage-earner, student, or homemaker
3. markedly peculiar behavior (e.g., collecting garbage, talking to self in public, or hoarding food)
4. marked impairment in personal hygiene and grooming
5. blunted, flat, or inappropriate affect
6. digressive, vague, overelaborate, circumstantial, or metaphorical speech
7. odd or bizarre ideation, or magical thinking, e.g., superstitiousness, clairvoyance, telepathy, "sixth sense," "others can feel my feelings," overvalued ideas, ideas of reference
8. unusual perceptual experiences, e.g., recurrent illusions, sensing the presence of a force or person not actually present

Examples: Six months of prodromal symptoms with one week of symptoms from A; no prodromal symptoms with six months of symptoms from A; no prodromal symptoms with two weeks of symptoms from A and six months of residual symptoms; six months of symptoms from A, apparently followed by several years of complete remission, with one week of symptoms in A in current episode.

D. The full depressive or manic syndrome (criteria A and B of major depressive or manic episode), if present, developed after any psychotic symptoms, or was brief in duration relative to the duration of the psychotic symptoms in A.

E. Onset of prodromal or active phase of the illness before age 45.

F. Not due to any Organic Mental Disorder or Mental Retardation.

teria has increased. We have added to Table 3-1 the American Psychiatric Association's DSM-III criteria and the diagnostic criteria derived from the International Pilot Study of Schizophrenia sponsored by the World Health Association. Both these diagnostic schemata are moving closer to Feighner's previously listed diagnostic schema (Feighner et al., 1972) and away from the vagaries of DSM-II and Bleuler's criteria. The DSM-III criteria are longitudinal, rather than cross-sectional like DSM-II, requiring data from the patient's history in addition to present symptoms. Also, the diagnosis of schizophrenia can only be made in the absence of major affective symptomatology. Basically, the DSM-III criteria delineate a more chronic population of schizophrenics; they are less inclusive than the old criteria.

The greater emphasis on, and precision in, diagnosis has affected clinical psychiatry in several ways. Psychiatrists have become increasingly aware of "schizophreniform" illnesses associated with such conditions as epilepsy and normal pressure hydrocephalus, and they are questioning many of the entities that have been traditionally grouped under the broad rubric of schizophrenia. As large groups of patients with prominent catatonic symptoms are carefully examined, for example, it has become clear that there are strong family histories of affective illness and that very few of the patients meet the rigid diagnostic criteria for schizophrenia; a high proportion, however, meet the criteria for affective disorder (Morrison, 1974; Abrams and Taylor, 1974, 1976; Pope, 1979).

In addition to shifts in emphasis, there are more substantial differences among the diagnostic schemes listed in Table 3-1. Depression is considered a secondary symptom by Bleuler, yet it rules out the diagnosis according to Feighner et al. and DSM-3, and is not mentioned by Schneider. Feighner's criteria are detailed and clearly useful for research but perhaps too restricted for clinical purposes (Feighner et al., 1972; Taylor and Abrams, 1975). Schneider's criteria for diagnosis, which are used widely in England, have the advantage of not needing gradation; they are either fulfilled or not fulfilled. But the symptoms on which the diagnosis rests are neither unique nor, in our opinion, universally found in schizophrenia (Carpenter and Strauss, 1974; Taylor and Abrams, 1975). Bleuler's major criteria cannot be easily quantitated. It is not clear how many of the fundamental criteria are necessary for diagnosis or how serious a symptom must be to indicate the presence of schizophrenia; hence, the relative importance of the symptoms for diagnosis cannot be precisely assessed. As the newer American and international diagnostic criteria are more widely used, it will be interesting to see if the disparity noted in the past between the diagnosis of schizophrenia in this country and in Europe narrows (Hordern et al., 1968; Cooper, 1972).

Although most of these diagnostic schemes have high degrees of reliability in use, they are basically empirical and thus somewhat arbitrary (Endicott, 1982; Kendall, 1979). Until a more etiologically based diagnostic system is available, we believe that the most important criteria for establishing the diagnosis of schizophrenia are:

1. A thought disorder characterized by: (1) hallucinations or delusions in the absence of such known causes of these symptoms as encephalitis, hallucinogenic drugs, or epilepsy; and/or (2) some other form of conceptual disorganization.
2. An early onset of symptoms, usually in young adult life.
3. Absence of major affective symptoms.
4. Absence of major neurological deficits.
5. A progressively deteriorating course of illness or an intermittent course with remissions.
6. A history of schizophrenia in close relatives contributes but is not necessary for the diagnosis.

In most classificatory schemes of schizophrenia, thought disturbance is considered a basic symptom of schizophrenia. Though all patients may not manifest a specific type of thought disorder at all times, some defect in cognition must be present during the course of the illness. It is not difficult to recognize delusions and hallucinations, but conceptual disorganization is a less precise, more inclusive term. Many types of schizophrenic conceptual disorganization have been described (Andreasen 1979; Taylor and Abrams 1984).

LOOSE ASSOCIATIONS are, in Bleuer's view, the basis for establishing a diagnosis of schizophrenia. Loosening of associations means an absence of normal connections between expressed thoughts. An overt example of this was given by Bleuer. "My last teacher in that subject was Professor A. He was a man with black eyes. I also like black eyes. There are also blue and gray eyes and other sorts too. I have heard it said that snakes have green eyes. All people have eyes" (Bleuer, 1950, p. 17). In a milder form, the patient's thought pattern may not immediately appear to be abnormal, but after ten or fifteen minutes' conversation, one may not be quite sure what he is talking about or how he arrived at a particular point. If the examiner then pays attention to the associative pattern, he will find that the patient is constantly switching from one topic to another, often introducing new ideas that are unrelated to what has gone before.

Another abnormal pattern of thought characterized as "basic" to schizophrenia is OVERINCLUSION. This refers to the patient's apparent failure to exclude from his consciousness competing, contradictory, or merely irrelevant thoughts so that his thinking is encumbered with ideas that are insufficiently connected to his main train of thought (Cameron, 1963). Overinclusion, in our view, can be placed under the rubric of loose association.

Another defect in the thought patterns of schizophrenics has been described in what can be called the ABSTRACT-CONCRETE DIMENSION. The Russian psychologist Vygotsky felt that schizophrenic thought disorder essentially represented a loss of the ability to think abstractly and a tendency to concreteness (Vygotsky, 1962). Concreteness has been defined as an attitude that is determined by and cannot proceed beyond some immediate experience, object, or stimulus (Mayer-Gross et al., 1969). From his work on patients with organic brain injuries, Kurt Goldstein developed a similar concept of the "concrete attitude," which he applied to the problem of schizophrenic thinking. Goldstein believed that many of the peculiarities in the behavior of schizophrenics became understandable when they were considered as an expression of abnormal concreteness (Goldstein, 1944). He was quick to point out, however, that the level and type of concreteness is not identical with that seen in neurological cases, primarily because of the intrusion of idiosyncratic and personalized ideas in schizophrenic thinking (Goldstein, 1958). (See below.) Not all schizophrenics seem to be concrete or literal, and some patients, especially those with markedly paranoid features, have even been described as overly abstract.

A defect that many psychoanalysts consider basic to schizophrenia is found in the SYMBOLIC-LOGICAL DIMENSION. Schizophrenics are seen as "paralogical"; they equate the identities of subjects on the basis of identical predicates, i.e., "I am a woman, the Virgin Mary was a woman, therefore I am Mary" (Von Domarus, 1944). This position is held by such other prominent clinicians as Arieti (1955). Many of the psychoanalytic interpretations of schizophrenic language emphasize its symbolic, dreamlike nature (Sullivan, 1953).

Among the most striking of the abnormalities of thought and speech in schizophrenics is the idiosyncratic, personalized, and often bizarre character of their verbal expressions (Harrow et al., I, 1972; Tucker and Rosenberg, 1975). When it is bizarre, this quality is easily noticed, but it may be subtle and become apparent only during a formal mental status examination. The part of the examination that is especially useful for this purpose is proverb interpretation and discernment of similarities and differences. For example, when asked the meaning of "People in glass houses should not throw stones," one of our patients replied, "Because people would see me in my house and throw stones at me." Another, when asked the similarity between an apple and an orange, said, "An apple is round and symbolizes perfection but none of us can be perfect." In these responses one can see aspects of many of the disturbances of thinking mentioned above. With the mental status examination, one can determine not only personalized, bizarre, and idiosyncratic concept formation in schizophrenics but also abnormal concreteness, loose associations, and overinclusive thought. Obviously, there is much overlap in these descriptions of schizophrenic thought patterns. When examining for schizophrenia it is important to use several proverbs and similarities, since abnormal responses may occur only after several adequate answers. Disjointedness, idiosyncrasy, and bizarreness seem to be more characteristic of schizophrenia than of any other psychiatric or neurological condition. If this type of thinking is present, one must suspect schizophrenia.

In addition to the many formal verbal disturbances associated with schizophrenia, there is a clinical impression of paraphasia or word-finding difficulty that is suggestive of aphasia. Farber et al. (1983) explored this by comparing the verbal behavior of schizophrenics with that of aphasics. While observers were able to distinguish the two groups, threre was some overlap. Paraphasic-type errors were equally present in both groups, but the schizophrenics showed more illogicality, loose associations, complex word usage, and adequate auditory function.

The other "fundamental" symptoms in Bleuler's classification—disturbances of affect and ambivalence and autism—can be helpful but are not essential in diagnosing schizophrenia. AFFECT in schizophrenics is classically described as "flattened": emotional expression is absent or its range is limited. This is found to be true more frequently in chronic patients; in acute schizophrenic breaks, it is uncommon. The affect may also be "inappropriate" in that a patient can tell a happy story and appear sad or vice versa.

AMBIVALENCE is the capacity of schizophrenic patients to feel intense contradictory emotions at the same time, for instance, to express both hate and love for a person in almost the same breath: "I hate that Dr. X and want to strangle him, that wonderful man who saved my life." Neither ambivalence nor flattened affect is consistently present in schizophrenia; therefore we do not feel that either is necessary for diagnosis.

Bleuler defined AUTISM as a break with external reality, in which the patient becomes preoccupied with his inner life; this results in an incapacity to develop meaningful human relationships. External events may become so blended with subjective feelings or fantasy that the patient sees them as relating specifically to him; at this point such symptoms could be called delusional or hallucinatory. Autism in schizophrenics appears to be a behavioral result of thought disorder.

SUBTYPES OF SCHIZOPHRENIA AND PROGNOSIS

The classical diagnosis subtypes of schizophrenia (hebephrenic, catatonic, undifferentiated, etc.) as delineated in the earlier diagnostic and statistical nomenclature of the American Psychiatric Association are of little value in ascertaining prognosis or choosing therapy. Phenomenologically, they merely mean that one or the other of Bleuler's secondary symptoms is prominent. These classical subtypes thus are of little more than historical interest. A more useful distinction between "process" and "reactive" schizophrenia has had wide acceptance among psychiatrists. (Phillips, 1953; Kantor and Herron, 1966). This concept has been restated in part as a distinction between "negative" and "positive" symptoms. Patients with negative symptoms are characterized by an absence of affect and few verbal productions; they might have been referred to as "process" schizophrenics in the past. Patients with positive symptoms have hallucinations, delusions, and the more vivid florid symptoms that one associates with "reactive" schizophrenia (Andreasen, 1982A, 1982B). The distinction between "process" and "reactive" still has prognostic value.

PROCESS SCHIZOPHRENIA, which calls to mind the classical description of Langfeldt and Kraepelin, has the following characteristics: (1) Preexisting *schizoid personality*. A schizoid person is shy, oversensitive, seclusive, and avoids close competitive relations. He may always have been described as eccentric and daydream a good deal and be unable to express emotions. His social and sexual adjustment is poor. (2) *Insidious onset* that is difficult to date exactly. (3) *No clear precipitating factor* that seems serious enough to have produced psychosis.

In REACTIVE SCHIZOPHRENIA there is: (1) A relatively *acute onset* that is easily dated. The initial symptoms are separated from their time of maximal development by six months or less. (2) *Precipitat-*

ing factors that are obviously emotionally charged, such as divorce or leaving home. (3) *No preexisting schizoid personality traits* and, therefore, a better premorbid social and sexual adjustment than in process schizophrenia. Often there are prominent affective, mainly depressive, symptoms and confusion during the acute episode (Vaillant, 1964; Stephens and Astrup, 1963).

This process-reactive distinction has been validated in many studies (Philips, 1953; Kantor and Herron, 1966) and is clearly related to prognosis. Reactive schizophrenics have a good short-term and long-term prognosis; process schizophrenics have a very poor prognosis (Garmezy and Rodnick, 1959; Higgins, 1969; Harrow et al., 1969). It is of interest that the distinguishing criteria are prognostic indicators *only* in schizophrenia, not in depression or other nonschizophrenic disorders (Bromet et al., 1971; Rosen et al., 1969).

There is some question about whether the reactive form should be considered schizophrenia. Many of the characteristic features of reactive schizophrenia may be encountered in other conditions that mimic schizophrenia.

A young psychotic with prominent affective symptoms, for example, may be suffering from a primary depression, not schizophrenia (see below). Some of the florid symptoms in such a patient may be related to such secondary factors as sleep deprivation. Features typical of reactive schizophrenia, such as the acute onset of confusion and psychosis in a patient with a normal premorbid emotional adjustment, have been cited as helpful in ruling out schizophrenia in favor of some other disease process, such as subacute encephalitis (Himmelhoch et al., 1970). For these reasons, it is conceivable that process schizophrenia may be the real disease and reactive schizophrenia may be something else, perhaps a psychological reaction to stress, an adolescent adjustment process, an affective disorder, or an acute encephalopathy. This formulation is supported by Kety's finding (1976) of little schizophrenic illness among the biological relatives of patients diagnosed as having an "acute schizophrenic reaction" but much schizophrenic illness among the biological relatives of patients diagnosed as having "chronic schizophrenia." In the absence of a demonstrable biological basis for the diagnosis of schizophrenia, the relation of reactive to process schizophrenia cannot be fully defined; but, the diagnosis of schizophrenia must always be considered tenuous if there has been only a single acute psychotic break. If the disorder becomes chronic, the diagnosis of schizophrenia is more certain.

The relation of reactive schizophrenia to hysterical psychosis or what the Europeans call psychogenic psychosis is difficult in terms of differential diagnosis. Patients with hysterical personalities seem to have a high incidence of what has been called hysterical psychosis. Hirsch and Hollender (1969) describe hysterical psychosis as a "state marked by a sudden and dramatic onset, temporarily related to a profoundly upsetting event." Patients may have hallucinations and delusions, and they may engage in unusual behavior; thought disorder is transient and circumscribed, and affect is volatile rather than flat. The acute episode typically lasts one to three weeks and leaves no residual symptoms. Most clinicians have seen dramatic cases of this type, which are more common in some subcultures than in others, but the question arises as to the relation of these episodes to the psychotic disorders they resemble, especially schizophrenia. European psychiatrists make a clear distinction between schizophrenia and "psychogenic psychosis," which we call hysterical psychosis. Stromgren (1974) describes hysterical psychosis as follows: (1) the psychosis would not have arisen without some distince mental trauma, which often makes it easy to understand the etiology. (2) There tends to be a psychological predisposition, of a neurotic or psychopathic nature, to the reactions that represent hysterical psychosis, but no genetic relationship with schizophrenia exists. (3) There must be a close temporal relation between the onset of trauma and of psychosis, and the psychosis often ends shortly after the trauma does. There are no residual symptoms. Hysterical psychosis takes three common forms: (1) emotional reactions that are usually depressive, (2) alterations of consciousness or clouded states (see Ch. 6, p. 309), and (3) paranoid states and delusions. These conditions can be distinguished from schizophrenia by applying the diagnostic criteria for schizophrenia (p. 103).

The problem of establishing the relative frequency of occurrence, the etiology, and the prognosis of process and reactive schizo-phrenia has been greatly complicated by variations in the popula-tions studied. In a chronic, state-hospital population, there will be a high proportion of "process" schizophrenics. Among schizo-phrenics admitted for the first time to an acute service in either a community mental health center or a general hospital, there will be relatively few "process" schizophrenics and more "reactives." Apparently, in most of the population studies, only chronic (pro-cess) schizophrenia has been considered in the determination of prevalence rates for the disease; this accounts for the consistency of prevalence rates throughout the world, despite the fact that diag-nostic criteria are less rigorous in some countries than in others. But, the "nature versus nurture" argument regarding the etiology of schizophrenia arises partly from the confusion of an acute "re-active" psychosis with chronic schizophrenia. And for this same reason, studies of the course of schizophrenia are not necessarily comparable.

Many changes in long-term patients that have been attributed to schizophrenia may actually be caused by aspects of life in a large, poorly staffed, state hospital; these include sensory and emotional deprivation and poor nutrition. Thus, the distinction, between pro-cess and reactive schizophrenia should, if possible, be made at the onset of illness rather than after a patient has been hospitalized for many years.

Schizoaffective Disorder

The term "schizoaffective" is used to indicate the presence of both schizophrenic and affective symptoms. Much confusion surrounds this category; operational criteria for the diagnosis are given in the Research Diagnostic Criteria (Spitzer, 1978) but not in DSM-III. There are indications that it is primarily an affective disorder (Pope, 1980). From a study of 39 schizoaffective patients, their family histories, and first-degree relatives, Clayton et al. (1968) concluded that schizoaffective disorder is a genetic variant of affec-tive illness. This was supported by data from a review of 420 twin pairs selected from military veterans in which one twin, or both twins, was psychotic (Cohen et al., 1972). The concordance rate for schizoaffective disorder in this group was the same as that for manic-depressive illness (50%) and more than twice as high as that for schizophrenia.

Clayton (1982) has provided data which may demonstrate that everyone is partially correct. In a small sample of schizoaffective patients, she noted that the "manic" cases seemed closer to bipolar disorder (perhaps a more severe form) and that the "depressed" cases were a more heterogeneous group of depressed schizophrenics and patients with affective disorders primarily. Perhaps as biologic measures become available, these distinctions will become less arbitrary, but at present the category does represent a clash between clinical experience and nosological neatness.

COURSE AND NATURAL HISTORY

Kraepelin's original clinical delineation of schizophrenia as a disease entity was made primarily on the basis of its poor prognosis; he postulated that schizophrenic patients manifested a consistently progressive course over time without full recovery. Psychotic patients who recovered were not schizophrenic by definition. In recent years, this has been questioned. Manfred Bleuler, for instance, described several patterns of evolution of the disease. One pattern, which varies in severity, is characterized by gradual deterioration over time, and another pattern is episodic. In the episodic course, complete or partial remissions are punctuated by acute exacerbations (Bleuler, 1968).

Bleuler believes that the milder chronic conditions have increased in frequency and that the severe chronic conditions have diminished. This trend has been observed by others (Grinker, 1972; Remar and Hagopian, 1972), who also noted shorter psychotic episodes and less bizarre, generally more moderate symptoms. Whereas some believe this may be related to the increased use of psychopharmacological agents, others feel that it represents less repression and greater tolerance of deviance in our contemporary society and take this as evidence that schizophrenia is a culturally determined disorder.

In a study of the charts of schizophrenic patients hospitalized in 1850 and 1950, only minor differences were noted in the symptoms and course (Klaf and Hamilton, 1961). The most marked differences between the two groups were in the kind of delusions the patients had. Patients in 1850 tended to be preoccupied with religion, whereas patients in 1950 were more preoccupied with sex. The average age, the proportion of married to single patients, and the incidence of mental illness in the patients' families were the same. Though hospital stays were twice as long in the nineteenth as in the twentieth century, the percentages of cure in both centuries were the same. The remarkable similarity of the symptoms, family history, age of patients, and clinical course lends credence to the disease concept of schizophrenia rather than to a primarily environmental etiology and casts suspicions on the clinical impression that schizophrenia is becoming milder.

Though Kraepelin's view that schizophrenia has a uniformly poor outcome is distasteful to those with some therapeutic optimism, the definitive study to prove him wrong has yet to be done. Two follow-up studies of 37 years (Ciompi, 1980) and 22.4 years (Huber, 1975, 1980) have been widely cited as showing that schizophrenia may have a more favorable long-term outcome than most believe. But both of these studies have problems. Huber included many cases that would be considered schizophreniform or reactive in type. Ciompi included former hospital patients who were less than 65 years old at their first hospitalization at one Swiss hospital. This yielded a group of 1642 cases of schizophrenia, but only 389 patients (18%) survived to provide data for the follow-up examination. This clouds somewhat the "more favorable" outcome of the survivors. Ciompi noted that the average mortality in his study group of schizophrenics was almost twice as high as would be expected from a normal population of the same age. This high rate of death in schizophrenics has been noted by others (Niswander, 1963; Tsuang, 1979).

It is notable that Kraepelin studied his patients over a long period of time. Though many of these patients made short-term recoveries, they all ultimately deteriorated. Current data suggest that his prognostic view was unnecessarily gloomy for the short-term but that it may well be valid for the long-term course. The studies that have examined this point and are in disagreement with Kraepelin suffer from either of two major difficulties: many of the more recent and well-controlled studies are relatively short term, and the older studies are retrospective and accurate diagnostic data are frequently not available.

One of the main obstacles to long-term prospective studies in this country is the strong tradition of divorcing hospital treatment from outpatient treatment. The hospital psychiatrist seldom follows his patient through into outpatient treatment. This is not due to lack of interest; it is a logistical problem resulting from the fact that most schizophrenic patients are placed in large state mental hospitals, which are far from metropolitan centers. After discharge, they return to their homes in the metropolitan areas where outpatient treatment is arranged. This not only complicates patient care but makes good follow-up studies much more difficult.

Table 3-2 is a summary of some of the follow-up studies done over the years. Though one would like to think that the introduction of psychopharmacological agents has greatly affected outcome, and it is clear that improvements have certainly occurred, no "miracles" are as yet evident: In 1963, Peterson studied 177 patients treated with phenothiazines from 1956 to 1958 and showed that over the following five years one-half of the patients were not readmitted, and, for those admitted again, another half were not readmitted, and so on for each subsequent admission. Of all the patients studied, 24 per cent remained hospitalized at the end of five years (Peterson et al., 1964). Several recent studies have reconfirmed that nonpsychotherapeutic regimens (psychopharmacological agents, ECT, etc.) are the most effective form of treatment (Hogerty et al., 1974; May, 1976; Davis, 1976). But the major criteria are either rehospitalization rate or total number of days spent in the hospital. Very little has been done to evaluate the quality of

Table 3-2
Follow-up Studies of Schizophrenic Patients

Author	Dates of Study	Number of Subjects	Results	Duration of Follow-up
Bleuler 1950	1898– 1905	515	after 1st episode 60% able to support selves (mild deterioration) 22% deteriorate (severe) 18% medium deterioration (medium)	
Freyham 1955	1920– 1955	100	54% (sudden onset) out of hospital 24% (gradual onset) out of hospital	35 years
	1940– 1955	100	71% (sudden onset) out of hospital 49% (gradual onset) out of hospital	15 years
Israel 1956	1913– 1952	4,254	64.1% discharged 24% permanent hospitalization 60% of all discharged never readmitted	40 years
Mandel-brote 1970	1963– 1963[a]	63	46% discharged in 12 months 64% 1st admissions out for 2 years 26% 1st admissions out and discharged but readmitted	3 years
Roder 1970	1951– 1955	310	28% of admissions under 5 months' stay	3 years
	1956– 1960		58% of admissions under 5 months' stay	
	1951– 1952		20.8% not readmitted	
	1959– 1960		44.4% not readmitted	
Huber 1980	1945– 1973	502	22% complete remission 43% residual but no psychosis	22.4 years
Ciompi 1980	1963	289	27% recovery 20% mild	37 years

[a] Phenothiazines introduced in 1954

life of patients who are not hospitalized or of hospitalized patients during the periods they are out of the hospital. The lives of many of these patients outside the hospital probably remains dependent and sheltered (Engelhardt and Rosen, 1976). This is particularly true of those patients who meet more rigid diagnostic criteria. Winokur and Tsuang (1975) noted that meeting rigid diagnostic criteria for schizophrenia leads to a poor prognosis.

DIFFERENTIAL DIAGNOSIS

Any disease of the central nervous system or any disruption of its function (e.g., drugs, sleep deprivation) may have behavioral manifestations. The differential diagnosis rests heavily on the type of symptoms present, the mode of onset, the family history of mental illness, the medical history, and the clinical course.

Neurological Diseases

Schizophrenia is not the only condition that can cause disturbances of thinking, though it is by far the most common single cause of such symptoms in young adults. The incidence of schizophrenia in the general population is taken to be approximately 1 percent (Srole et al., 1962). Because of this high incidence there is a strong temptation to make the diagnosis of schizophrenia whenever a thought disorder is present. Schizophrenialike episodes, however, have been described in association with cerebral trauma, tumor, encephalitis, presenile degeneration and other degenerative diseases of the gray and white matter, narcolepsy, vascular disorders, and a host of metabolic or toxic disorders, such as endocrinopathies, cerebral anoxia, and hypercapnia (Davison and Bagley, 1969). Though psychoses are commonly seen in these conditions, they rarely mimic the symptoms of schizophrenia exactly; the disorientation, memory deficit, confusion, and fluctuating states of consciousness that are characteristic of some neurological diseases are seldom encountered in schizophrenia. The difficulty in differentiating schizophrenia from neurological conditions mainly arises in the initial onset of neurological disease. Most neurological diseases will either progress to overt neurological symptoms or else clear completely. So our comments deal mostly with diagnostic problems of acute onset. The mistake often made by inexperienced clinicians is to label as schizophrenic any bizarre, delusional, or mute behavior that cannot be easily explained and is not one of the traditional symptoms associated with a particular medical condition; they often overlook such signs as disorientation, dysmnesia, and such other signs of neurological disorder as tremor, myoclonic jerks, and asterixis.

In addition to disorientation and dysmnesia, there are a few simple guidelines for the differentiation of acute neurological disease from classical schizophrenia. In ACUTE NEUROLOGICAL DISORDERS there is usually: (1) A good premorbid social history. The patient does not have problems at work and his family is generally warm and supportive rather than disturbed, as is so often the case in schizophrenia (Lidz, 1968; Wynne, 1968). Sociability is characteristically preserved in most neurological disorders until a very late stage of deterioration, long after disorientation and dysmnesia have appeared. In schizophrenia, early loss of sociabiliy is common. (2) An abrupt change in personality, mood, and ability to function at work and at home of less than six months' duration. (3) Rapid fluctuations in mental status. The patient has a clouded sensorium and is disoriented one day, then completely oriented the next. Though fluctuations can also be seen in some schizophrenics, they are generally not so rapid. Even when the schizophrenic's mental status seems to clear suddenly, he will still show some signs of bizarre behavior or delusional thinking. Marked fluctuations in mental status are, in general, more characteristic of acute neurological disease than schizophrenia, but this is not necessarily true of chronic neurological disease. The fluctuations in mental status of neurological patients may also be accompanied by fluctuating motor behavior. The patient may display aggressive impulses and engage in assaultive behavior at one moment but at the next apologize profusely and try to befriend the people he has just abused. The mode of behavior during this period frequently has a "driven quality" to it, as has been described in brain-injured patients by Goldstein and Scheerer (1941) and Kahn (1934). (4) A patient with an acute neurological problem is usually unresponsive to psychiatric intervention, whether psychotherapeutic or pharmacological. Rather than controlling behavior, psychopharmacological agents may, paradoxically, precipitate a stuporous or comatose state depending on the underlying condition.

Many patients who present with bizarre behavior and mute states are shunted immediately to the psychiatrist. Even major neurological signs can be overlooked or interpreted as part of the patient's "functional" disturbance. It goes without saying that marked behavioral aberrations should not blind clinicians to neurological symptoms.

Drug Reactions

Symptoms suggesting schizophrenia are commonly seen in patients who have taken amphetamines, cocaine, LSD, mescaline, ketamine, and belladonna alkaloids. Hallucinations and psychosis may also accompany alcohol and barbiturate withdrawal. These states of intoxication and withdrawal may cause a psychosis without major disorientation (though this is rare) as well as any of the physical changes seen in the neurologically impaired. The presence of visual hallucinations, however, should always suggest the possibility of a drug reaction or a toxic or metabolic encephalopathy. Formed visual hallucinations are unusual in schizophrenia and in diseases that affect the structure of the brain (e.g., brain tumors). Auditory hallucinations, however, are common in schizophrenia and unusual in drug reactions.

Sleep Disorders

Prolonged inability to sleep may produce disorganized thought patterns and even such major distortions of reality as illusions, delusions, and hallucinations. It is possible that this happens only in individuals with a schizophrenic predisposition. Resumption of a normal sleep pattern in such individuals will resolve their symptoms quickly. Residual thought disorder persists in most schizophrenics even after normal sleep has been restored (Berger and Oswald, 1962; Detre and Jarecki, 1971).

THE GENETIC ASPECTS OF SCHIZOPHRENIA

As noted, the incidence of schizophrenia in the general population is about 1 percent. The data obtained in epidemiological surveys of schizophrenia in different countries and cultures are in agreement, and all investigators agree that the incidence is increased in families of schizophrenics and is highest in their first-degree relatives. The rate is roughly 10 to 15 percent in the parents, siblings, and children of schizophrenics. This consistency is remarkable considering the differences and imprecision of the various diagnostic criteria applied (Table 3-1).

The interpretation of these facts differs, of course. Those who believe that schizophrenia is primarily a functional disorder, and who favor an environmental explanation of its development, claim that the higher incidence in relatives is due to the exposure of children to the abnormal environment created by sick adults. Those who favor a genetic hypothesis believe that these figures reflect a genetic predisposition. Most psychiatrists in this country take the middle view that schizophrenia is a functional illness influenced by genetic factors.

Many studies of families of schizophrenics have been made. In virtually all of them, approximately half of the parents of schizophrenics displayed serious personality disorders. Lidz (1968) found that 60 percent of the patients' parents displayed "psychotic traits." Alanen (1968) reported that 63 percent of the mothers of schizophrenics were "more seriously ill than psychoneurotic." These authors favor an environmental hypothesis of the etiology of schizophrenia, but their data could equally serve to support a genetic hypothesis.

A major criticism of the view that schizophrenia is a functional disorder is that many schizophrenics do not come from an abnormal environment. In our opinion, an even stronger objection to the view that psychogenic stress or life experience can cause schizophrenia is that no one has ever identified *specific* environmental circumstances to which an increased morbidity risk of schizophrenia can be attributed. Many psychogenic theories have been proposed over the last 50 years, but no predictions of psychogenic risk factors have ever been verified. Most studies that purport to show the effect of environment on the development of schizophrenia do not include adequate control groups and do not distinguish between the effect of a schizophrenic child has on his parents' mental state and the effect the parents have on the child.

Some few jots of evidence can be interpreted as suggesting that the psychological environment plays an important role in the development of schizophrenia. Hollingshead and Redlich (1954) have shown that prevalence rates for schizophrenia are eight times higher in the lower classes (Class V) than in the highest class (I). This, it has been said, implies that the lower-class environment contains unfavorable factors that are etiologically important. It has not been possible to substantiate this interpretation of the data of Hollingshead and Redlich. A study of a national (British) sample of schizophrenics (Goldberg and Morrison, 1963), which confirmed the higher prevalence of the disease in the lower classes, found that the patients' fathers had an occupational distribution corresponding to the general population. In other words, the low social class of the patients is likely to be the result of a downward drift occurring during the premorbid phase or the insidious early stages of illness. There is abundant evidence that such a prepsychotic drift occurs (Slater and Cowie, 1971; Pollack et al., 1966; Bower et al., 1960; Prout and White, 1956).

Another finding interpreted as supporting the environmental hypothesis is that schizophrenia is more common among the mothers of schizophrenic offspring than among their fathers. This, along with descriptive studies by Alanen (1958) and others that indicate a high rate of nonschizophrenic psychiatric disturbance in the mothers of schizophrenics, has been a main pillar of support for the "schizophrenogenic mother" variant of the environmental hypothesis. According to this theory, the patient's mother causes schizophrenia by the harmful way she relates to her child. But, there are alternative explanations for the data on which this theory is based. The higher incidence of schizophrenia in mothers of schizophrenics may reflect the fact that reproductive capacity is adversely affected by schizophrenia, but women marry at an earlier age than men and tend to become schizophrenic at a later age than men. Thus, the interval between the age of marriage and onset of psychosis is greater for women than for men. Since the requirement for an active role in reproduction is greater for men than for women, schizophrenic women would be more likely to produce children than schizophrenic men, even after psychosis has developed. Very much against the "schizophrenic mother hypothesis" is evidence that the children of schizophrenic fathers run the same risk of developing the disease as the children of schizophrenic mothers (Slater and Cowie, 1971).

Twin studies have added to the evidence against the environmental hypothesis, and support the genetic. There have been eleven major twin studies of schizophrenia. These studies were done in the United States, the United Kingdom, Japan, Germany, and Scandinavia. In all but one (Tienari, 1963), the incidence of schizophrenia is much higher in monozygote than dizygotic twins of schizophrenics (Gottesman and Shields, 1966). The overall incidence of schizophrenia in the monozygotic twins of schizophrenics is 61 percent. This represents 240 concordant twins out of 409 twin pairs. In the dizygotic twins studied, there was a 12 percent concordance rate (70 out of 571 pairs). In other words, the incidence of schizophrenia in dizygotic twins is the same as in non-twin siblings of schizophrenics. The unique prospective study of Gottesman and Shields, a particularly careful one, was based on consecutive admission to outpatient and short-stay inpatient facilities over a 16-year period and thus included mild and severe cases. By adhering to strict criteria of monozygoticity and spelling out in detail the criteria on which they based their assessment of the severity of the disease, these authors overcame the major criticisms of earlier twin research in schizophrenia in their study. They found a 42 percent incidence in the monozygotic twins of schizophrenics and a 9 percent incidence in dizygotic twins. But, monozygotic concordance for severe schizophrenia was 77 percent compared to 27 percent for mild schizophrenia. The corresponding figures for the dizygotic probands were 15 and 10 percent. A recent updating of the National Council Twin Registry showed a concordance rate for schizophrenia of 30.9 percent for monozygotic twins and 6.5 percent for dizygotic twins (Kendler and Robinette, 1983).

The obvious interpretation of these facts is that schizophrenia is a genetic illness, but objections to this interpretation have been raised to this effect: since parents tend to treat monozygotic twins in an identical manner and to treat dizygotic twins differently, the harmful influence (unspecified) that derives from the psychic environment is likely to affect monozygotes in the same way but will be unequally felt by dizygotes. This hypothesis can be tested by studies of monozygotic twins (one of whom has become schizophrenic) separated in the first year of life and raised apart. Slater and Cowie (1971) reviewed all reports of such cases and found that of twelve monozygotic pairs, nine were concordant. Though these numbers are small, the high concordance rate argues strongly against a significant environmental influence in schizophrenia.

Another approach to testing the environmental hypothesis was taken in a study of the psychosocial adjustment of 47 adults born to schizophrenic mothers and permanently separated from their mothers in the first few days of life (Heston, 1966). They were compared to 50 control adults with nonschizophrenic mothers who had also been permanently separated from their natural mothers in the first few days of life. The comparison was based on a review of school, police, army, and hospital records, plus a personal interview and personality testing (MMPI). IQ testing and social-class determination were also done, and three psychiatrists independently rated the subjects. In this study, schizophrenia was significantly more prevalent in the individuals born to schizophrenic mothers. Of 47 persons with schizophrenic mothers, five were schizophrenic. No cases of schizophrenia were found in the 50 control subjects. The age-corrected rate for schizophrenia in the experimental group was 16.6 percent, a finding consistent with that of all the family studies that had been done on children raised by schizophrenic biological parents. In addition, serious psychosocial disability, that is, psychiatric diagnosis other than schizophrenia, was found in approximately half the persons born to schizophrenic mothers. An increased incidence of schizophrenia-"related" personality disorders has also been noted in the families of schizophrenic patients (Kendler, 1984). Many had been discharged from the armed forces for behavioral reasons; others had police records or a history of alcoholism. The diagnosis of sociopathic personality was more than four times as common in the experimental group, in which five times as many persons spent more than one year in a penal or psychiatric institution.

These findings have been substantiated by an independent study (Kety, 1976). In this study, 364 first-degree relatives of 33 schizophrenic adoptees and controls (nonschizophrenic adoptees) were interviewed by a man who did not know the relationship of the person he was interviewing to the adoptee. In almost all cases, the relative being interviewed did not know of the relationship or the adoptee's diagnosis. From summaries of these interviews, three independent raters made a psychiatric diagnosis. After a consensus was reached among these three psychiatrists, the subjects were divided into four groups: biological or adoptive relatives of schizophrenic index adoptees (two groups) and biological or adoptive relatives of control adoptees (two groups). The prevalence of schizophrenic illness (chronic schizophrenia, latent schizophrenia, and uncertain schizophrenia) in subjects genetically related to the schizophrenic index cases was 13.9 percent. The prevalence of schizophrenic illness among the adoptive relatives of schizophrenics was 2.7 percent, and it was 3.8 percent in all subjects not genetically related to a schizophrenic index case. The difference between the group genetically related to the schizophrenic index cases and the group not so related is highly significant. These relatives did not differ from the rest, however, with regard to mental illness other than schizophrenia.

This evidence strongly supports the genetic hypothesis of schizophrenia, but some might argue that environmental factors, such as very early mothering experiences, might still play a role in the development of schizophrenia. In Kety's study, however, there were 63 biological paternal half-siblings of the schizophrenic index cases and 64 biological paternal half-siblings of the controls. Obviously, biological paternal half-siblings do not have the same mother, neonatal mothering experience, or postnatal environment as their half-siblings with a different mother. They only had the father and his gene pool in common. Of the biological paternal half-siblings of the schizophrenic patients, 20 percent carried a diagnosis of schizophrenia as compared with 3.1 percent of the controls, a highly significant difference.

There has been doubt as to whether adoptive parents might somehow provide a "schizophrenigenic environment" for their adopted children, thus allowing the expression of a genetic tendency. There is considerable evidence to indicate that they do not. In Kety's study (1976), the incidence of schizophrenia among the adoptive parents of schizophrenics was the same as in the control population. A study comparing psychopathology in adoptive parents of schizophrenics, biological parents of schizophrenics, and controls clearly demonstrated an increase in the incidence and severity of psychopathology among biological as opposed to adoptive parents of schizophrenics (Rosenthal et al., 1968; Wender, 1968). The importance of these studies by Kety, Rosenthal and Wender, and the uniqueness of the data is attested to by the fact that others have reanalyzed the data using DSM-III criteria and, in general, have confirmed the strong genetic components cited above (Kety, 1983). There is no evidence that children born to nonschizophrenics and adopted by schizophrenics or the half-siblings of schizophrenics have an increased risk of schizophrenia. In fact, there is evidence that this does not occur (Kallman, 1946). The irrelevance of the psychosocial family environment is shown by the finding of the same high prevalence of schizophrenia in the children of monozygotic twins discordant for schizophrenia (Fischer, 1971).

These studies do more than merely support a theory about the genetics of schizophrenia. They indicate that it is a genetic disease. They offer no support for the view that the psychosocial environment plays any role in determining the risk of developing schizophrenia in individuals who are, genetically, at high risk. A *child of a schizophrenic has the same increased chance of developing the*

disease whether he is raised by his schizophrenic parent or by a
nonschizophrenic foster parent in a normal environment.

Supporters of the environmental hypothesis for the development of schizophrenia have claimed that the failure of concordance rates for monozygotic twins to reach 100 percent is evidence in favor of their position. That this is not warranted can be seen by comparing schizophrenia with epilepsy. The tendency of petit mal and other forms of epilepsy, as demonstrated by EEG studies, is genetically transmitted as an autosomal domniant trait. Yet concordance rates for clinical epilepsy in monozygotic pairs do not reach 100 percent. No one can claim that emotional factors explain this discrepancy in concordance rates for epilepsy, but acquired brain damage in one sibling often seems to be responsible. Using this analogy, and the well-established fact that multiple pregnancies result in a higher incidence of neurological complications, one can hypothesize that acquired brain damage in an individual with a genetic tendency for schizophrenia might allow full expression of the gene in that individual. If this were so, the incidence of low birth weight and factors known to be associated with brain damage would presumably be higher in the schizophrenic twin of a discordant monozygotic pair (Campion and Tucker, 1973).

This expectation has been realized in a study of fifteen such pairs by Pollin and Stabenau (1968). Of the fifteen schizophrenics, eleven had lower birth weights than their monozygotic twin, as well as disordered early feeding and sleep patterns. Two of the remaining four suffered severe early childhood illnesses (prolonged cyanosis caused by an exposure to gas in one and Rocky Mountain spotted fever in the other). There were many minor neurological abnormalities in the schizophrenic twins.

Thus, there would certainly appear to be an environmental influence in schizophrenia, if by "environmental" one means acquired brain damage and not such psychosocial factors as emotional deprivation.

The idea that brain damage might allow the full expression of a gene for schizophrenia can be invoked to explain the high incidence of neurological and electroencephalographic abnormalities seen in schizophrenic patients. Available data suggest that there might be an autosomal dominant gene for schizophrenia, as there is for petit mal epilepsy, with a penetrance that varies with the age of the individual and an expressivity that is, in large part, determined by the presence of acquired brain damage and by other genes that influence personality, adaptability, and other functions. The difference between this view and the "polygenic" theory of the inheritance of schizophrenia is slight. According to the polygenic theory, a number of genes and acquired traits determine an individual's liability to the disease. If an individual inherits many "bad" genes, he is likely to have severe schizophrenia. A milder schizophrenic condition would result if fewer bad genes were present and, in the mildest cases resulting from an even smaller number, a variety of nonschizophrenic alterations in behavior or personality could develop. The relative merits of the polygenic and single gene hypotheses have been discussed extensively by Slater and Cowie (1971), Gottesman and Shield (1972), and Reich et al. (1975).

NEUROLOGICAL ABNORMALITIES IN SCHIZOPHRENIC PATIENTS

Minor neurological abnormalities and physical anomalies are commonly found in schizophrenia (Guy et al., 1983). This is not what one would expect in a "functional" disease, and for this reason, such signs are often overlooked or considered epiphenomena. One only has to walk through the chronic wards of a large state hospital to be impressed that many of the patients suffer neurological dysfunction in terms of impaired equilibrium, gait, coordination, and even gross mental retardation. The effects of medication, malnutrition, and multiple electrical shock treatment may have something to do with these abnormalities. Certainly, many of the studies of neurological change in state hospital populations, in which both the cause for admission and original symptoms often have been long forgotten, are suspect when a high incidence of neurological findings in schizophrenics is cited. The few such studies done on acute patients, however, have also documented a significant degree of neurological dysfunction. Abnormalities include minor motor and sensory ("soft") neurological signs on physical examination, electroencephalographic abnormalities, and "organic" patterns on psychological tests. Heightened "arousal responses" have also been considered by many investigators to represent a primary neurological abnormality.

MINOR NONLOCALIZING NEUROLOGICAL ABNORMALITIES "soft signs") have been noted in many studies of acute schizophrenic adult patients (Pollin and Stabenau, 1968; Kennard, 1960; Larsen, 1964; Rochford et al., 1970) and adolescent schizophrenics (Hertzig and Birch, 1966, 1968).

Rochford examined 65 hospitalized untreated psychiatric patients for the presence of the following minor signs: (1) motor impersistence; (2) stereognosis; (3) graphesthesia; (4) extinction during bilateral simultaneous stimulation; (5) bilateral marked hyperreflexia; (6) coordination defects; (7) disturbance of balance and gait; (8) cortical sensory abnormalities; (9) mild movement disorders; (10) speech defects; (11) abnormal motor activity; (12) defective auditory-visual integration; (13) choreiform movements and adventitious motor overflow (tremor); (14) cranial nerve abnormalities, such as slight anisocoria, esotropia, auditory deficit, and visual field and retinal defects; and (15) unequivocally abnormal EEG's. He found neurological abnormalities in 36.8 percent of the psychiatric patients (all diagnostic groups). This was signicantly different from an age-matched normal control population (5%). Neurological "soft" signs were found in 65.5 percent of the schizophrenic patients. By way of comparison, there were no "soft" signs in patients with primary affective disorders. In 72.5 percent of the schizophrenics he and his colleagues studied, Pollin found at least one neurological sign (Pollin and Stabenau, 1968). The most common neurological abnormalities in Pollin's schizophrenic patients were defects in stereognosis; graphesthesia; difficulty in coordination, balance, and gait; and tremor. There was also some difficulty in the integration of auditory-visual stimuli.

In several recent studies, not only has an increased incidence of soft signs in schizophrenic patients been observed, but also a high correlation between these signs and "thought disorder," especially overinclusive thinking. The relation of neurological impairment to thought disorder is stronger than its relations to diagnostic category (Tucker et al., 1974, 1975). The main tests for these neurological impairments were specific sensorimotor portions of the Halstead-Reitan battery (e.g., finger agnosia, fingertip writing, tactile form recognition, and the tactile performance test). Davies et al. (1975) found a high correlation of neurological soft signs and behavioral symptoms in schizophrenics, especially those with paroxysmally abnormal EEG's. Quitkin et al. (1976) found more neurological soft signs in schizophrenics with premorbid asocial behavior as well as in individuals with emotionally unstable character disorders, two conditions that are generally chronic. Fish (1975) has described "neurointegrative" defects in infancy that she considers signs of "dysregulation" of maturation in neurological systems that represent a biological continuum with schizophrenic disorders in later life. The prospective study of persons at high risk for schizophrenia, particularly the offspring of schizophrenic parents, is an important area of research, not only for the evaluation of the role of the central nervous system but also for an understanding of the spectrum concept of schizophrenia (Campion and Tucker, 1973). An excellent study by Rieder (1975) is a start in this direction. Rieder compared the offspring of schizophrenics with a matched control group to find a surprising increase in the incidence of fetal and neonatal deaths among the children of schizophrenics.

Rosenbaum (1971) noted defects in schizophrenic patients with regard to weight discrimination and proprioception. He postulated that these defects are related to "insufficiently articulated proprioceptive signals . . . in schizophrenic persons." The abnormalities he found can be considered soft signs, similar to those observed in the studies cited above.

Aberrant vestibular function has been widely noted in schizophrenic patients. The vestibular system integrates sensation with motor functions and behavior. Studies made by eleven different groups over the past 50 years have all shown reduced nystagmus in schizophrenic patients in response to caloric and rotational stimulation of the vestibular system (Ornitz, 1970; Myers et al., 1973; Jones, 1983). Whereas the reduced nystagmus response is directly related to duration of illness in many studies, the relation of vestibular alterations to schizophrenia remains unclear. In some studies (Tice, 1968), auditory and visual hallucinations have followed pharmacological suppression of vestibular sensibility, but the possibility of direct toxic effects of the drugs occurring elsewhere in the brain was not ruled out. Prolonged use of psychotropic drugs may induce vestibular changes in chronic patients, which may obscure the association between vestibular defects and schizophrenia in recent studies. In the older studies, however, these psychotropic drugs were not used, since they were not yet available.

In a consideration of these vestibular dysfunctions, the report by Holzman et al. (1973) that smooth pursuit eye movements during pendulum tracking characterize schizophrenic patients and their families and thus may prove to be a genetic marker may be useful. Shagass et al. (1974) observed the same characteristic eye movements but found that they related more to psychosis in general than to schizophrenia specifically.

The theory that the behavior of schizophrenics reflects a disturbance of the sensory integrative functions of the brain gained support from a series of studies by Silverman (1968) and Buchsbaum and Silverman (1968). These studies show that schizophrenics may actually process incoming stimuli abnormally by attenuation or reduction. It is known that schizophrenics have a tendency to underestimate tactile, auditory, and visual stimuli. Though the traditional psychological interpretation of these reduction phenomena has been that they represent a defensive reaction to the schizophrenic's sense of being bombarded by stimuli, the tendency to reduce incoming stimuli may conceivably be a primary defect that produces many of the subjective phenomena common to schizophrenia and sensory deprivation (Vosburg et al., 1959). Silverman postulates that three conditions are associated with and precede such subjective phenomena: (1) sensory overload or sensory underload, (2) attentiveness to a too broad or a too narrow range of stimuli (hypo- or hyperattentiveness), and (3) a change in the neurophysiological sensory response systems. Supporting this theory is the clinical observation that accutely schizophrenic patients tend to be in a state of hyperattentiveness to stimuli (McGhie and Chapman, 1961; Chapman, 1966; Tucker et al., 1969; Harrow et al., 1972), as do individuals under the influence of LSD 25. According to Silverman's theory, the cause of schizophrenia is an inability to screen out varied internal and external stimuli. Schizophrenics seem to have a defective sensory filtering mechanism that does not allow them to focus attention on relevant stimuli (Payne, 1960; Callaway, 1970). An inability to focus attention is also one of the features of the altered state of cognitive functioning that occurs during sensory deprivation.

The gross disruptions of perceptual and sensory integrative functions produced by drugs and sensory deprivation regularly lead to psychoticlike states that are, at times, indistinguishable from schizophrenia. It has long been known that people in such isolated situations as Arctic camps and solitary prison confinement, patients in iron lungs, and survivors at sea experience a variety of disturbing subjective alterations. In fact, any environment that is unvarying and that offers only a limited range of sensory stimuli can give rise to (1) difficulty in focusing and organizing thoughts, (2) illusions and delusions, (3) a sharp sense of the need for variation in extrinsic stimuli, (4) a distortion of the sense of time passing, and (5) the hallucinatory experiences that occur during prolonged deprivation. These alterations are not limited to the period of deprivation but persist briefly after it has ended. Objects continue to appear to swirl, and shapes and lines seem distorted (Solomon et al., 1957). These perceptual experiences associated with sensory deprivation are similar to those described by schizophrenics and by patients with parietal lobe dysfunction.

There is a certain paradox inherent in this theory of the pathogenesis of schizophrenia. The inability to screen out external stimuli is presented as a primary deficit, on the one hand, and yet, on the other hand, it is suggested that alterations in cortical sensory processing produce psychosis by creating a state of sensory deprivation.

ELECTROENCEPHALOGRAPHIC DATA

Most of the available data relating electroencephalographic abnormalities to abnormal mental states were discussed in chapter 1. In regard to schizophrenia, EEG changes do not have a specific diagnostic or therapeutic significance. A "choppy" EEG (low voltage, 26- to 51-cps record) in schizophrenic patients has been reported by Davis and Davis (1939), Gibbs et al. (1938), and Hill (1957). Reports of electroencephalographic abnormality in schizophrenic patients referred at random range from 5 to 80 percent, with an average of about 25 percent (Abenson, 1970); but the vagaries of EEG interpretation and the variability in diagnosing schizophrenia obscure the meaning of these data. Patients diagnosed as catatonic schizophrenics seem to show consistently higher rates of electroencephalographic abnormality, usually manifested as nonspecific slowing. Since catatonic states are often acute and have a relatively good prognosis, one wonders if all cases so labeled are really catatonic schizophrenia. We have seen patients with seizures, toxic-metabolic encephalopathy, encephalitis, occult hydrocephalus, and left middle cerebral artery occlusion presenting with speechlessness, waxy flexibility, and other "psychotic" behavioral abnormalities; as a result, they were thought to have catatonic schizophrenia. The higher rate of electroencephalographic abnormality in catatonic schizophrenics raises some question about the diagnosis (Liberson et al., 1958; Tucker et al., 1965). There have also been reports of focal temporal lobe electroencephalographic abnormalities in schizophrenic patients, and the increased prevalence of electroencephalographic abnormalities among schizophrenics in general seems well documented (Hill, 1957; Small et al., 1964; Treffert, 1964; Tucker et al., 1965).

Frequency analyses of the EEG in schizophrenia have shown decreased variability and high mean energy content (Goldstein et al., 1963). In several studies, this stability or hyperregulation in the EEG's of schizophrenics correlated with a poor prognosis, whereas dysrhythmic records correlated with a better prognosis (Igert and

Lairy, 1962; Yamada, 1960). Many of the EEG studies of schizophrenics were complicated by the treatment given the patients. Fukuda and Matsuda (1969) found high voltage slow wave changes after five electroconvulsant treatments (ECT's) in 40 to 70 percent of patients, and in 80 to 87 percent after ten ECT's. Though they reported that almost all EEG's returned to normal in 3 days, Muscovitch and Katzelenbogen (1948) claimed that such abnormalities lasted at least 10 months. Phenothiazines and other psychotropic drugs complicate EEG studies even more; they typically cause slowing of alpha rhythms and an increase in amplitude, with superimposed sharp fast activity (Steiner and Pollack, 1965). These changes may persist from 10 weeks to 3 months after medications are stopped (Fink and Kahn, 1956; Swain and Litteral, 1960). To make interpretation more difficult, predrug EEG's have not usually been recorded. In a study of schizophrenic patients on phenothiazines, Steiner found patterns characteristic of sleep activity in 65 percent and significant amounts of diffuse delta and theta activity in 43 percent.

In summary, electroencephalographic abnormalities are seen in schizophrenics, especially catatonic schizophrenics, more often than in the general population. This statement seems valid even when allowances are made for an occasional misdiagnosis and the effect of drugs and shock therapy. It is not known whether the schizophrenic process or an underlying biochemical defect causes these electroencephalographic abnormalities. One possibility is that brain damage, which may be reflceted in the EEG, could facilitate the development of schizophrenia in individuals with a genetic tendency toward the disease.

COMPUTERIZED TOMOGRAPHY IN SCHIZOPHRENIA

Computerized tomography and more recently positron tomography have opened exciting possibilities for studying the structure and function of the central nervous system in schizophrenics. Since 1976 there have been persistent reports of ventricular enlargement, hemispheric asymmetry, and cerebellar atrophy in schizophrenic patients. Johnstone (1976), Weinberger (1979, 1980), and Golden (1980) have all shown ventricular changes in schizophrenics. They have also shown that these ventricular changes correlate with other findings such as increased neuropsychological impairment, poor response to treatment, and poor premorbid adjustment. The ventricular enlargements that these authors have demonstrated would not be called abnormal by radiologists but rather are subtle variations within the normal range. The authors also clearly stated that these changes were not present in all the schizophrenics they studied. More recent investigations have not confirmed their findings of ventricular enlargement (Jernigar, 1982; Andreasen, 1982; Woods and Wolf, 1983). Almost all the studies in this area, whatever their results, suffer from serious methodologic problems, such as: (1) The study populations have been disparate, ranging from old to young, chronic to acute, rigidly diagnosed to less rigidly diagnosed. (2) The techniques of measuring ventricular size in each study were not standardized and vary from actual manual measurements to computerized measurements; consequently, there is great variation from study to study in the incidence of abnormal findings, as well as their comparability. (3) The control populations have varied from none to reported norms in the literature, to normal populations, to neurologic patients who are referred for evaluation for headaches, and so on. Very few of these studies have compared other chronic psychiatric patients to the schizophrenic patients, and none have utilized a "blind" technique for reading CAT scans. When this comparison has been made, "significant" differences often disappear in the schizophrenic group (Weinberger et al., 1983).

Investigations of cerebral blood flow in psychiatric and neurologic disease were initiated by Kety (1948) over 35 years ago. Positron emission tomography (PET) is now being used to study schizophrenia, and this new technique is so sophisticated that we may be able to observe dynamic changes of cerebral function in schizophrenic patients during different psychopathologic states and to follow these changes through the course of illness. The PET studies seem to show that there is some decrease of blood flow in the frontal lobes of schizophrenics. Minor asymmetrical hemispheric differences were noted as well (Buchsbaum, 1982; Farkas, 1980; Bunney et al., 1983; Ariel, 1983; Mathew, 1982; Morihisa, 1983, Morstyn, 1983). All of these studies, however, have involved so few patients with such varying diagnoses and drug regimens that we must await larger studies and more standardization of the research methods.

PSYCHOLOGICAL TESTING FOR SCHIZOPHRENIA

The three types of psychological tests used most frequently in studies of schizophrenia are projective tests (e.g., Rorschach), personality inventories (e.g., MMPI), and performance tests for organicity (e.g., Halstead Organic Test Battery).

PROJECTIVE TESTS present many problems. In the first place they are usually of questionable reliability and validity. Though standardized scoring techniques have been developed, the information gained differs little from what can be learned in an interview and is, in fact, no more objective than the clinical impression in determining the presence of a thought disorder (Zubin et al., 1965). Also, it is almost impossible to distinguish neurological from psychiatric disorders with projective tests. In particular, they fail to reliably separate schizophrenics from neurological patients (Fisher et al., 1955; Dorken and Kral, 1952). Since they depend primarily on the verbal responses of patients to vague stimuli, they share the same difficulty in discrimination that the clinical interview does with regard to diagnosis.

PERSONALITY INVENTORIES usually deal with long-standing personality traits. Though helpful in raising a suspicion of chronic schizophrenia or schizoid personality, they fail to discriminate acute schizophrenia from acute neurological syndromes.

PERFORMANCE TESTS for "organicity" do not distinguish the chronic schizophrenic from the brain-damaged patient. This has been demonstrated quite clearly in two detailed studies in which the Halstead Organic Test Battery was used (Watson et al., 1968); in these studies, the "organics" could not be distinguished from the chronic schizophrenics (Lacks et al., 1970); Vega and Parsons (1967) repeated these findings.

The limited value of psychological tests in differentiating neurological causes of thought disorder from schizophrenia perhaps reflects the "organicity" of the latter disorder.

Arousal

Many studies have identified the schizophrenic as "hyperaroused," a term that refers to an abnormally heightened state of neurophysiological activity. Some feel that this state may actually cause thought disorders. The term "arousal" is not clearly defined, but, in general, it refers to a state of alertness with increased physiological measurements of the kind often associated with high levels of anxiety. These include increased galvanic skin resistance, increased muscle tension as measured by electromyography, desynchronization of the EEG with alpha suppression, and increased pulse rate. This evidence of "hyperarousal" has been speculatively linked with statements by acute schizophrenics indicating that they are "flooded" with stimuli, that is, "When I try to read something, each bit I read starts me thinking in ten different directions at once." It has been suggested that the hyperarousal leads to a "low threshold for disorganization under increasing stress" (Epstein and Coleman, 1970). The psychophysiological disorganization caused by stimulus overload is hypothesized as the primary causal factor in the thought disturbance typical of schizophrenic patients. When the physiological parameters of "arousal" are studied in samples of schizophrenic and nonschizophrenic patients, however, they correlate more closely with anxiety than with schizophrenia (Tucker et al., 1969). Consequently, hyperarousal, though frequently present in schizophrenics, is likely to be secondary to anxiety rather than a primary manifestation or cause of schizophrenic thinking.

RELATION OF NEUROLOGICAL ABNORMALITIES TO SCHIZOPHRENIA

It is unlikely that the prevalence of minor neurological abnormalities in schizophrenic patients is a fortuitous association, since most of the surveys showing a 60 to 70 percent incidence have been done on large groups of psychiatric patients with different diagnoses; also, such minor neurological findings have been *infrequently* noted in nonschizophrenic patients. The fact that the abnormalities are minor rather than major may explain why they were not reported in the early literature. In our view, these signs are minor only in their motor or sensory manifestations; we think that they reflect widespread dysfunction throughout the nervous system and often given rise to serious behavioral and intellectual abnormalities (see p. 192). Not until recent years has it become respectable to consider schizophrenia an organic disease of the brain, one that might be associated with neurological abnormalities. If this association is not fortuitous, there are of course two possibilities: that "minor" brain dysfunction could give rise to schizophrenia or that the schizophrenic process or its treatment could cause the neurological signs.

The first possibility seems plausible, since some neurological conditions produce symptoms that are characteristic of schizophrenia; the subacute encephalitides and temporal lobe epilepsy, for example, can cause a schizophrenialike psychosis. It could be that such conditions act as precipitating factors in individuals having a specific diathesis for becoming schizophrenic. But this hypothesis is not supported by family studies in cases of the schizophrenia-like psychosis of epilepsy or amphetamine psychosis. If an individual had inherited a schizophrenic tendency, however, he might well be more likely to develop the symptoms of psychosis if he had also sustained brain damage (see p. 128).

Though it is possible that the neurological abnormalities in schizophrenics may occasionally represent an organic manifestation of the schizophrenic process or its treatment, in 25 to 30 percent of schizophrenic patients, medicated and unmedicated, there are no neurological findings. To resolve the question of the meaning of neurological abnormalities in schizophrenia it would be necessary to know: (1) whether the neurological findings are present throughout the life of the patient or become evident at certain developmental stages; (2) whether these neurological findings persist during remissions of schizophrenic illness; and (3) whether the prognosis for schizophrenic patients with neurological abnormalities is poorer.

EFFECT OF EMOTIONAL FACTORS UPON SCHIZOPHRENIA

Unfavorable psychosocial factors can affect schizophrenics, as they may affect diabetics or epileptics, by augmenting illness, coloring the content of the symptoms, and increasing the frequency and severity of the symptoms. Favorable psychosocial factors can undoubtedly help schizophrenics in terms of treatment or supportive environment.

As Cannon (1915) pointed out long ago, emotional factors may cause physiological changes. Acute stress reactions may be associated with hormonal changes and increases in blood pressure, pulse rate, and respiratory rate. The clinical impression that anxiety may precipitate seizures in epileptics seems well substantiated, though the mechanisms by which anxiety affects the frequency and severity of seizures are only partly understood. There may be a "limbic reflex" in which excitatory impulses alter the resting potentials of neurons in critical regions—lowering thresholds and producing uncontrolled discharge. It is known, however, that anxiety-induced hyperventilation can precipitate seizures by causing either respiratory alkalosis or cerebral anoxia secondary to a decrease in cerebral blood flow.

The clinical impression of psychiatrists that life stresses are associated with decompensation in patients with a preexisting schizophrenic diathesis also seems fairly well substantiated, though it must be remembered that all such clinical impressions are scientifically suspect and involve post hoc reasoning. Though the basis for this remains obscure, it may involve a possible alteration of biogenic amines in critical areas of the hypothalamus and the reticular activating and limbic system. Many examples could be given of schizophrenia and indeed of other psychoses in which environmental stresses may have determined the timing, severity, and type of the signs and symptoms. It is quite another thing, however, to go on to claim, as many do, that emotional stress causes the psychotic condition.

TREATMENT

Aside from the environmental and psychotherapeutic aspects (Tucker et al., 1984) of maangement, it is unquestionable that the use of the major antipsychotic drugs (phenothiazines, thioxanthene, butyrophenones, and reserpine) is essential to the treatment of acute schizophrenics (Donaldson et al., 1983). Not only are these drugs more effective than placebos for schizophrenics (Klein and Davis, 1969), but they are also more effective than any type of psychotherapy alone (May, 1968; Grinspoon et al., 1968; May, 1976; Hogarty, 1974; May, 1981; Siris and Rifkin, 1983). In acute schizophrenia, or chronic schizophrenia with an acute exacerbation, the response to the phenothiazines is so prompt and consistent that the diagnosis is likely to be incorrect if there is not a favorable response to treatment. But in process schizophrenia—chronic and undifferentiated, simple and hebephrenic schizophrenias—there is usually no significant response to treatment.

Though there are many major tranquilizers, controlled studies show little difference in their effectiveness. The clinician should probably acquaint himself with one or two of these drugs (preferably one of the phenothiazines that is marketed in pill, elixir, and injectable form) so as to become familiar with the effects, onset of action, and side effects. Perhaps the most common error in the use of phenothiazines is not using a large enough dose (Davis, 1976; Davis et al., 1983).

Whereas the exact site of action of the major tranquilizers is unclear, their behavioral effects are slowly being defined. In a large study sponsored by the National Institute of Mental Health, these drugs were effective in controlling such associated deficits as overinclusive thinking and poor abstracting ability, withdrawal, autism, hallucinations, hostility, and uncooperativeness. The drugs were not as effective for such symptoms as blunted affect, paranoid ideas, or grandiosity, which nevertheless can sometimes be moderated with phenothiazines (Chapman and Knowles, 1964; Goldberg et al., 1965; Saretsky, 1966; Shimkunas et al., 1966).

REFERENCES

Abenson, M. H. EEG's in chronic schizophrenia. *Brit. J. Psychiat.* 116:421, 1970.

Abrams, R. and M. Taylor. Catatonia. *Arch. Gen. Psychiat.* 33:571, 1976.

────── and ──────. Manic depressive illness and paranoid schizophrenia. *Arch. Gen. Psychiat.* 31:640, 1974.

Alanen, Y. O. The mothers of schizophrenic patients. *Acta Psychiat. Scand.* Suppl. 124, 1958.

──────. From the mothers of schizophrenic patients to interactional family dynamics. In: *The Transmission of Schizophrenia*. Pergamon Press, David Rosenthal and Seymour Kety, eds. London, 1968.

American Psychiatric Association. *Diagnostic and Statistical Manual of Mental Disorders.* 2nd ed. American Psychiatric Association, Washington, D.C., 1968.

Andreasen, N. C. Thought, language and communication disorders. *Arch. Gen. Psychiat.* 36:1315, 1979.

──────. Negative symptoms in schizophrenia. *Arch. Gen. Psychiat.* 39:784, 1982.

────── and S. Olsen. Negative versus positive schizophrenia. *Arch. Gen. Psychiat.* 39:789, 1982.

──────, M. R. Smith, C. Jacoby, J. Dennert, and S. Olsen. Ventricular enlargement in schizophrenia. *Amer. J. Psychiat.* 139:292, 1982.

Arieti, S. *Interpretation of Schizophrenia.* Brunner, New York, 1955.

Beck, A. T., C. H. Ward, M. Mandelson, J. E. Mock, and J. K. Erbaugh. Reliability of psychiatric diagnosis: 2. A study of consistency of clinical judgments and ratings. *Amer. J. Psychiat.* 119:351, 1962.

Berger, R. J. and I. Oswald. Effects of sleep deprivation, subsequent sleep and dreaming. *Brit. J. Psychiat.* 108:457, 1962.

Bleuler, E. *Dementia Praecox or the Group of Schizophrenias.* Zinkin (trans.). International Universities Press, New York, 1950.

Bleuler, M. A 23 Year Longitudinal Study of 208 Schizophrenics. In: *Transmission of Schizophrenia*, D. Rosenthal and S. Kety, eds. Pergamon, London, 1968, p. 3.

Bower, E. M., T. A. Shellhamer, and J. M. Daily. School characteristics of male adolescents who later become schizophrenics. *Amer. J. Orthopsychiat.* 30:712, 1960.

Bromet, E., M. Harrow, and G. J. Tucker. Factors related to short-term prognosis in schizophrenia and depression. *Arch. Gen. Psychiat.* 25:148, 1971.

Buchsbaum, M. and J. Silverman. Stimulus intensity control and cortical evoked response. *Psychosom. Med.* 30:12, 1968.

———, D. Ingvar, R. Kessler, et al. Cerebral glucography with positron tomography. *Arch. Gen. Psychiat.* 39:251, 1982.

Callaway, E. Schizophrenia and interference. *Arch. Gen. Psychiat.* 22:193, 1970.

Cameron, N. *Personality Development and Psychopathology.* Houghton Mifflin, Boston, 1963.

Campion, E. W. and G. J. Tucker. A note on twin studies, schizophrenia and neurological impairment. *Arch. Gen. Psychiat.* 35:60, 1973.

Cannon, W. B. *Bodily Changes in Pain, Hunger, Fear and Rage.* D. Appleton, New York, 1915.

Carpenter, W. Current diagnostic concepts in schizophrenia. *Amer. J. Psychiat.* 133:172, 1976.

Chapman, L. J. and R. R. Knowles. The effects of phenothiazine on disordered thought in schizophrenia. *J. Consult. Psychol.* 28(2):165, 1964.

Chapman, J. The early symptoms of schizophrenia. *Brit. J. Psychiat.* 112:225, 1966.

Ciompi, L. Catamnestic long-term study on the course of life and aging. of schizophrenics. *Schizophrenia Bull.* 6:606, 1980.

Clayton, P. J., L. Rodin, and G. Winokur. Family history studies III: Schizoaffective disorder. *Comp. Psychiat.* 9:31, 1968.

Cohen, S. M., M. G. Allen, W. Pollin, and Z. Hrubec. Relationship of schizoaffective psychosis to manic depressive psychosis and schizophrenia. *Arch. Gen. Psychiat.* 26:539, 1972.

Davies, R., J. Neil, and J. Himmelhoch. Cerebral dysrhythmias in schizophrenics receiving phenothiazines. *Clin. Electroencephalography* 6:103, 1975.

Davis, J. Recent developments in the drug treatment of schizophrenia. *Amer. J. Psychiat.* 133:208, 1976.

———, P. Janicak, R. Snider, et al. Neuroleptics and psychotic disorders. In: *Neuroleptics,* J. T. Coyle and S. J. Enna, eds. Raven Press, New York, 1983.

Davis, P. A. and H. Davis. Electroencephalograms of psychotic patients. *Amer. J. Psychiat.* 95:1007, 1939.

Davison, K. and C. R. Bagley. Schizophrenia-like psychoses associated with organic disorders of the central nervous system: A review of the literature. In: *Current Problems in Neuropsychiatry,* R. N. Herrington, ed. Ashford, Kent, Headley Bros., 1969.

Detre, T. and H. Jarecki. *Modern Psychiatric Treatment.* J. B. Lippincott, New York, 1971.

Dorken, H. and V. A. Kral.   The psychological differentiation of organic brain lesions and their localization by means of the Rorschach Test. *Amer. J. Psychiat.* 108:764, 1952.

Endicott, J., J. Nee, J. Fleiss, J. Cohen, J. Williams, and R. Simon.   Diagnostic criteria for schizophrenia. *Arch. Gen. Psychiat.* 39:884, 1982.

Engelhardt, P. and B. Rosen.   Implications of drug treatment for the social rehabilitation of schizophrenic patients. *Schizophrenia Bull.* 2:454, 1976.

Epstein, S. and M. Coleman.   Drive theories of schizophrenia. *Psychosom. Med.* 32:113, 1970.

Farkas, T., M. Reivich, A. Alani, et al.   The application of [18F]-deoxy-2-fluro-glucose and positron emission tomography in the study of psychiatric conditions. In: *Cerebral Metabolism and Neural Functions*, J. V. Passonneau, R. A. Hawkins, W. D. Lust, et al., eds. Williams & Wilkins, Baltimore, 1980, p. 403.

Feighner, J. P., E. Robins, S. B. Guze, R. A. Woodruff, G. Winokur, and R. Munoz. Diagnostic criteria for use in psychiatric research. *Arch. Gen. Psychiat.* 26:57, 1972.

Fink, M. and R. C. Kahn.   Relation of EEG delta activity to behavioral response in electroshock. *Arch. Neurol. Psychiat.* 78:516, 1956.

Fischer, M.   Psychosis in the offspring of schizophrenic monozygotic twins and their normal cotwins. *Brit. J. Psychiat.* 118:43, 1971.

Fish, B.   Biologic antecedents of psychosis in children. In: *Biology of Major Psychosis*, D. X. Freedman, ed. Raven Press, New York, 1975.

Fisher, J., T. A. Gonda, and K. Little.   The Rorschach and central nervous system pathology. *Amer. J. Psychiat.* 111:487, 1955.

Freyhan, F. A.   Course and outcome of schizophrenia. *Amer. J. Psychiat.* 111:161, 1955.

Fukuda, T. and Y. Matsuda.   Comparative characteristics of slow wave EEG, autonomic function and clinical picture in typical and atypical schizophrenia during and following electroconvulsive treatment. *Int. Pharmacopsychiat.* 3:13, 1969.

Garmezy, N. and E. H. Rodnick.   Premorbid adjustment and performance in schizophrenia: Implications for interpreting heterogeneity in schizophrenia. *J. Nerv. Ment. Dis.* 129:450, 1959.

Gibbs, F. A., E. L. Gibbs, and W. G. Lennox.   Likeness of cortical-dysrhythmias of schizophrenia and psychomotor epilepsy. *Amer. J. Psychiat.* 95:255, 1938.

Goldberg, E. M. and S. L. Morrison.   Schizophrenia and social class. *Brit. J. Psychiat.* 109:785, 1963.

Goldberg, S. C., G. Klerman, and J. Cole.   Changes in schizophrenia psychopathology and ward behavior as a function of phenothiazine treatment. *Brit. J. Psychiat.* 111:120, 1965.

Golden, C. J., J. A. Moses, R. Zelogowski, et al.   Cerebral ventricular size and neuropsychological impairment in young chronic schizophrenics. *Arch. Gen. Psychiat.* 37:619, 1980.

Goldstein, K.   Methodological approach to the study of schizophrenia thought disorder. In: *Language and Thoughts in Schizophrenia*, J. S. Kasanin, ed. W. W. Norton, New York, 1944.

———. Concerning the concreteness in schizophrenia. *J. Abnorm. Soc. Psychol.* 57:146, 1958.

——— and M. Scheerer. Abstract and concrete behavior, an experimental study with special tests. *Psychol. Monogr.*, 53(2), Whole No. 239, 1941.

Goldstein, L., H. B. Murphree, A. A. Sugarman, C. C. Pfeiffer, and E. H. Jenney. Quantitative electroencephalographic analysis of naturally occurring (schizophrenic) and drug-induced psychotic states in human males. *Clin. Pharmacol. Ther.* 4(1):10, 1963.

Gottesman, I. I. and J. Shields. Schizophrenia in twins: 16 years consecutive admissions to a psychiatric clinic. *Brit. J. Psychiat.* 112:809, 1966.

——— and ———. A polygenic theory of schizophrenia. *Int. J. Ment. Health* 1:107, 1972.

Grinker, R. R. Changing Styles in Psychiatric Syndromes: Psychoses and Borderline States. Presented at 125th Annual Meeting, American Psychiatric Association, Dallas, Texas, May 1972.

Grinspoon, L., J. R. Ewalt, and R. Shader. Psychotherapy and pharmacotherapy in chronic schizophrenia. *Amer. J. Psychiat.* 124:1645, 1968.

Harrow, M., G. J. Tucker, and E. Bromet. Short-term prognosis of schizophrenic patients. *Arch. Gen. Psychiat.* 21:195, 1969.

———, ———, and D. Adler. I. Concrete and idiosyncratic thinking in acute schizophrenic patients. *Arch. Gen. Psychiat.* 26:433, 1972.

———, ———, and P. Shield. II. Stimulus overinclusion in schizophrenic disorders. *Arch. Gen. Psychiat.* 27:40, 1972.

Hertzig, M. A. and H. G. Birch. Neurologic organization in psychiatrically disturbed adolescent girls. *Arch. Gen. Psychiat.* 15:590, 1966.

——— and ———. Neurologic organization in psychiatrically disturbed adolescents. *Arch. Gen. Psychiat.* 19:528, 1968.

Heston, L. L. Psychiatric disorders in foster home reared children of schizophrenic mothers. *Brit. J. Psychiat.* 112:819, 1966.

Higgins, J. Process-reactive schizophrenia recent developments. *J. Nerv. Ment. Dis.* 149:450, 1969.

Hill, D. Electroencephalogram in schizophrenia: In: *Schizophrenia: Somatic Aspects*, D. Richter, ed. Pergamon, London, 1957.

Himmelhock, J., J. H. Pincus, G. J. Tucker and T. Detre. Behavioral features of subacute encephalitis. *Brit. J. Psychiat.* 116:531, 1970.

Hirsch, S. and M. Hollender. Hysterical psychosis. *Amer. J. Psychiat.* 125:909, 1969.

Hogarty, G., S. C. Goldberg, N. R. Schooler, and R. F. Ulrich. Drug and sociotherapy in the aftercare of schizophrenic patients. *Arch. Gen. Psychiat.* 31:603, 1974.

Hollingshead, A. B. and F. C. Redlich. Social stratification and schizophrenia. *Amer. Sociol. Rev.* 19:302, 1954.

Holzman, P., L. R. Proctor, and D. W. Hughes. Eye-tracking patterns in schizophrenia. *Science* 181:179, 1973.

146   *Behavioral Neurology*

Horden, A., M. G. Sandifer, L. M. Green, and G. C. Tinbury. Psychiatric diagnosis: British and North American concordance on stereotypes of mental illness. *Brit. J. Psychiat.* 114:935, 1968.
Huber, G., G. Gross, and R. Schuttler. A long term follow-up study of schizophrenia. *Acta Psychiat. Scand.* 52:49, 1975.
Igert, C. and G. C. Lairy. Intêret prognostique de l'EEG au cours de l'évolutions des schizophrènes. *Electroencephalog. Clin. Neurophysiol.* 14:183, 1962.
Israel, R. H. and N. A. Johnson. Discharge and readmission rates in 4,254 consecutive first admissions of schizophrenia. *Amer. J. Psychiat.* 112:903, 1956.
Jerinigan, T. L., L. M. Katz, J. A. Moses, and P. A. Berger. Computed tomography in schizophrenics and normal volunteers. *Arch. Gen. Psychiat.* 39:765, 1982.
Johnstone, E. C., T. J. Crow, C. D. Frith, et al. Cerebral ventricular size and cognitive impairment in chronic schizophrenia. *Lancet* 2:924, 1976.
Kahn, E. Organic driveness: A brainstem syndrome and an experience with case reports. *New Eng. J. Med.* 210:748, 1934.
Kallman, F. J. The genetic theory of schizophrenia. *Amer. J. Psychiat.* 103:309, 1946.
Kantor, R. E. and W. G. Herron. *Reactive and Process Schizophrenia.* Science and Behavior Books, Palo Alto, California, 1966.
Kendall, R. E., I. F. Brockington, and J. Seff. Prognostic implications of six alternative definitions of schizophrenia. *Arch. Gen. Psychiat.* 36:25, 1979.
Kennard, M. Value of equivocal signs in neurological diagnosis. *Neurology* 10:753, 1960.
Kety, S. Genetic aspects of schizophrenia. *Psychiat. Ann.* 6:11, 1976.
Klaf, F. S. and J. G. Hamilton. Schizophrenia—a hundred years ago and today. *J. Ment. Science* 107:819, 1961.
Klein, D. F. and J. M. Davis. *Diagnosis and Drug Treatment of Psychiatric Disorders.* Williams & Wilkins, Baltimore, 1969.
Kraepelin, E. *Dementia Praecox and Paraphrenia.* 8th Ger. ed. Livingstone, Edinburgh, 1925.
Lacks, P. B., J. Colbert, M. Harrow, and J. Levine. Further evidence concerning the diagnostic accuracy of the Halstead Organic Test Battery. *J. Clin. Psychol.* 26:480, 1970.
Larsen, V. Physical characteristics of disturbed adolescents. *Arch. Gen. Psychiat.* 10:55, 1964.
Liberson, W. T., I. W. Scherer, and C. J. Klett. Further observations on EEG effects of chlorpromazine. *Electroenceph. Clin. Neurophysiol.* 10:192, 1958.
Lidz, T. The family, language, and the transmission of schizophrenia. In: *Transmission of Schizophrenia,* D. Rosenthal and S. Ketty, eds. Pergamon, London, 1968.
Mandelbrote, B. M. and K. L. K. Trick. Social and clinical factors in the outcome of schizophrenia. *Acta Psychiat. Scand.* 46:24, 1970.

May, P. R. A. *Treatment of Schizophrenia.* Science House, New York, 1968.

May, P. Rational treatment for an irrational disorder. *Amer. J. Psychiat.* 133:1008, 1976.

May, P. R. A., H. Tuma, W. Dixon, et al. Schizophrenia: A follow-up study of the results of five forms of treatment. *Arch. Gen. Psychiat.* 38:776, 1981.

Mayer-Gross, W., E. Slater, and M. Roth. *Clinical Psychiatry.* 3rd ed. Williams & Wilkins, Baltimore, 1969.

McGhie, A. and J. Chapman. Disorders of attention and perception in early schizophrenia. *Brit. Med. Psychol.* 34:103, 1961.

Morrison, J. Catatonia. *Comp. Psychiat.* 15:317, 1974.

Muscovitch, A. and T. Katzelenbogen. Electroshock therapy, clinical and EEG studies. *J. Nerv. Ment. Dis.* 107:517, 1948.

Myers, S., D. Caldwell, and G. Purcell. Vestibular dysfunction in schizophrenia. *Biol. Psychiat.* 3:255, 1973.

Niswander, G. D., G. M. Haslerud, and G. D. Mitchell. Changes in cause of death of schizophrenic patients. *Arch. Gen. Psychiat.* 9:229, 1963.

Ornitz, E. Vestibular dysfunction in schizophrenia and childhood autism, *Compr. Psychiat.* 11:159, 1970.

Payne, R. W. Cognitive Abnormalities. In: *Handbook of Abnormal Psychology*, H. J. Eysenck, ed. Pitman, London, 1960.

Peterson, D. B., M. O. Fulton, and G. W. Olson. First admitted schizophrenics in drug era. *Arch. Gen. Psychiat.* 11:137, 1964.

Phillips, L. Case history data and prognosis in schizophrenia. *J. Nerv. Ment. Dis.* 117:515, 1953.

Pollack, M., M. G. Woerner, W. Goodman, and I. M. Greenberg. Childhood development patterns of hospitalized adult schizophrenic and nonschizophrenic patients and their siblings. *Amer. J. Orthopsychiat.* 36:510, 1966.

Pollin, W. and J. Stabenau. Biological, psychological, and historical differences in a series of monozygotic twins discordant for schizophrenia. In: *Transmission of Schizophrenia*, D. Rosenthal and S. Kety, eds. Pergamon, London, 1968.

Pope, H. G., J. F. Lipinski, B. Cohen, and D. Axelrod. Schizoaffective disorder. *Amer. J. Psychiat.* 137:921, 1980.

———. Diagnosis in schizophrenia and manic depressive illness. *Arch. Gen. Psychiat.* 35:811, 1978.

Prout, C. T. and M. A. White. The schizophrenic's sibling. *J. Nerv. Ment. Dis.* 123:162, 1956.

Quitkin, F., A. Rifkin, and D. Klein. Neurologic soft signs in schizophrenia and character disorders. *Arch. Gen. Psychiat.* 33:845, 1976.

Reich, T., R. Cloninger, and S. Guze. The multifactorial model of disease transmission. *Brit. J. Psychiat.* 127:1, 1975.

Remar, E. M. and P. B. Hagopian. Changing Clinical Syndromes: Forty-Year Perspective. Presented at 125th Annual Meeting of American Psychiatric Association, Dallas, Texas, May 1972.

Rieder, R., D. Rosenthal, P. Wender, and H. Blumenthal.   The offspring of schizophrenics. *Arch. Gen. Psychiat.* 32:200, 1975.

Rochford, J. M., T. Detre, G. J. Tucker, and M. Harrow.   Neuropsychological impairments in functional psychiatric diseases. *Arch. Gen. Psychiat.* 22:114, 1970.

Roder, E.   A prognostic investigation of female schizophrenic patients discharged from Sct. Hans Hospital, Dept. D, during the decade 1951–1960. *Acta Psychiat. Scand.* 46:50, 1970.

Rosen, B., D. F. Klein, S. Levenstein, and S. P. Shahinian.   Social competence and posthospital outcome among schizophrenic and non-schizophrenic psychiatric patients. *J. Abnorm. Psychol.* 74:401, 1969.

Rosenbaum, G.   Feedback mechanisms in schizophrenia. In: *Lafayette Clinic Studies on Schizophrenia.* Wayne State University Press, Detroit, 1971, p. 163.

Rosenthal, D., P. H. Wender, S. Kety, F. Shulsinger, J. Weiner, and L. Ostergaard.   Schizophrenics' offspring reared in adoptive homes: In: *Transmission of Schizophrenia,* D. Rosenthal and S. Kety, eds. Pergamon, London, 1968.

Sanua, V. D.   Sociocultural aspects. In: *The Schizophrenic Syndrome,* L. Bellak and L. Loeb, eds. Grune and Stratton, New York, 1969, p. 256.

Saretsky, T.   Effects of chlorpromazine on primary-process thought manifestations. *J. Abnorm. Psychol.* 71:247, 1966.

Schneider, K.   *Clinical Psychopathology.* M. W. Hamilton, trans. Grune and Stratton, New York, 1959.

Shagass, C., M. Amadea, and P. Duerton.   Eye-tracking performance in psychiatric patients. *Biol. Psychiat.* 9:245, 1974.

Shimkunas, A. M., M. D. Gyntherm, and K. Smith.   Abstracting ability of schizophrenics before and during phenothiazine therapy. *Arch. Gen. Psychiat.* 14:79, 1966.

Silverman, J.   A paradigm for the study of altered states of consciousness. *Brit. J. Psychiat.* 114:1201, 1968.

Slater, E. and V. Cowie.   *The Genetics of Mental Disorders.* Oxford University Press, London, 1971.

Small, J. G., I. F. Small, and W. R. P. Surphils.   Temporal EEG abnormalities in acute schizopherenia. *Amer. J. Psychiat.* 121:262, 1964.

Solomon, P., P. H. Leiderman, J. Mendelson, and D. Wexler.   Sensory deprivation: A review. *Amer. J. Psychiat.* 114:357, 1957.

Srole, L., et al.   *Mental Health in the Metropolis.* McGraw-Hill, New York, 1962.

Steiner, W. G. and S. L. Pollack.   Limited usefulness of EEG as a diagnostic aid in psychiatric cases receiving tranquilizing drug therapy. *Prog. Brain Res.* 16:97, 1965.

Stephens, J. H. and C. Astrup.   Prognosis in "process" and "non-process" schizophrenia. *Amer. J. Psychiat.* 119:945, 1963.

Strauss, J., W. Carpenter, and J. Bartko.   The diagnosis and understanding of schizophrenia. *Schizophrenia Bull.* 11:61, 1974.

Stromgren, E. Psychogenic Psychosis. In: *Themes and Variations in European Psychiatry*, S. Hirsch and M. Shepard, eds. University Press of Virginia, Charlottesville, 1974, p. 97.

Sullivan, H. S. Conceptions of Modern Psychiatry. W. W. Norton, New York, 1953.

Swain, J. M. and E. B. Litteral. Prolonged effect of chlorpromazine: EEG findings in a senile group. *J. Nerv. Ment. Dis.* 131:550, 1960.

Taylor, M. and R. Abrams. A critique of the St. Louis Psychiatric Research Criteria for Schizophrenia. *Amer. J. Psychiat.* 132:1276, 1975.

Tice, L. F. New drugs of 1967. *Amer. J. Pharm.* 140:4, 1968.

Tienari, P. Psychiatric illness in identical twins. *Acta Psychiat. Scand.* Suppl. 171, 1963.

Treffert, D. A. Psychiatric patient and EEG temporal lobe focus. *Amer. J. Psychiat.* 120:765, 1964.

Tsuang, M. T., R. Woolson, and J. Fleming. Long term outcome of major psychosis. *Arch. Gen. Psychiat.* 39:1295, 1979.

Tucker, G. J. and S. Rosenberg. Computer content analysis of schizophrenic speech. *Amer. J. Psychiat.* 132:611, 1975.

———, T. Detre, M. Harrow, and G. H. Glaser. Behavior and symptoms of psychiatric patients and the electroencephalogram. *Arch. Gen. Psychiat.* 12:278, 1965.

———, M. Harrow, T. Detre, and B. Hoffman. Perceptual experiences in schizophrenic and nonschizophrenic patients. *Arch. Gen. Psychiat.* 20:159, 1969.

———, R. B. Ferrell, and T. R. P. Price. The hospital treatment of schizophrenia. In: *Treatment and Care of Schizophrenia*, A. S. Bellack, ed. Grune and Stratton, Orlando, 1984.

———, E. W. Campion, P. A. Kelleher, and P. M. Silberfarb. The relationship of subtle neurological impairments to disturbances of thinking. *Psychother. Psychosom.* 24:165, 1974.

———, ———, and P. M. Silberfarb. Sensorimotor functions and cognitive disturbance in psychiatric patients. *Amer. J. Psychiat.* 132:17, 1975.

Vaillant, G. E. Prospective prediction of schizophrenic remission. *Arch. Gen. Psychiat.* 11:509, 1964.

Vega, A. and O. A. Parsons. Cross-validation of the Halstead-Reitan tests for brain damage. *J. Consult. Psychol.* 31:619, 1967.

Von Domarus, E. The specific laws of logic in schizophrenia. In: *Language and Thought in Schizophrenia: Collected Papers*, J. S. Kasamin, ed. University of California Press, Berkeley, 1944.

Vosburg, R., N. Fraser, and J. Guehl. Sensory deprivation and image formation. *Psychiat. Commun.* 4:157, 1959.

Vygotsky, L. S. *Thought and Language*. E. Hanfman and G. Vakar, eds. and trans. John Wiley, New York, 1962.

Watson, C. G., R. W. Thomas, D. Andersen, and J. Felling. Differentiation of organics from schizophrenics at two chronicity levels by use of the Reitan-Halstead Organic Test Battery. *J. Consult. Clin. Psychol.* 32:679, 1968.

Weinberger, D. R., L. B. Bigelow, J. E. Kleinman, et al. Cerebral ventricular enlargement in chronic schizophrenia. *Arch. Gen. Psychiat.* 37:11, 1980.

———, E. F. Torrey, A. N. Neophytides, et al. Lateral ventricular enlargement in chronic schizophrenia. *Arch. Gen. Psychiat.* 36:735, 1979.

Wender, P. H., D. Rosenthal, and S. Kety. A psychiatric assessment of the adoptive parents of schizophrenics. In: *Transmission of Schizophrenia*, D. Rosenthal and S. Kety, eds. Pergamon, London, 1968.

Winokur, G. and M. T. Tsuang. A clinical and family history comparison of good outcome and poor outcome schizophrenics. *Neuropsychobiology* 1:59, 1975.

Wynne, L. C. Methodologic and conceptual issues in the study of schizophrenics and their families. In: *Transmission of Schizophrenia*, D. Rosenthal and S. Kety, eds. Pergamon, London, 1968.

Yamada, T. Heterogeneity of schizophrenia as demonstrable in EEG. *Bull. Osaka Med. Sch.* 6:107, 1960.

Zubin, J., L. D. Eron, and F. Schumer. *An Experimental Approach to Projective Techniques.* John Wiley, New York, 1965.

Chapter 4

DISORDERS OF
INTELLECTUAL FUNCTIONING

The terms organic brain syndrome and dementia are applied to those acquired disorders of thinking and other cognitive functions that are believed to arise from altered structure or function of the brain and thus stand opposed to the "functional" disorders. The inadequacy of this distinction is immediately apparent: all functional disorders must be the result of disordered brain activity. In conventional use, organic brain syndrome and dementia refer to disorders of mentation caused by diseases traditionally considered to lie within the province of neurologists, and it is in this sense that we will use these terms in this chapter. The symptoms of dementia can be similar to those of amentia or congenital mental retardation, but the first term implies the loss of previously acquired mental abilities and, hence, has different diagnostic and therapeutic implications.

Neurological diseases that may cause dementia characteristically impair orientation, memory, and arithmetic ability when dysfunction is extensive, but when it is less serious, more subtle changes of personality and intellectual functioning may precede disorientation, dyscalculia, and dysmnesia. Whereas disturbances of orientation to time, place, person, numerical ability, and of memory are perhaps the hallmarks of organic brain syndromes, it is important to note that other types of dysfunction are also characteristic. Impairment of verbal and spatial abilities may become manifest in disturbances of language function, and of the ability to orient oneself or objects in space. Impairment may also be evident in personality changes and in the level of consciousness, or "vigilance," at which a patient seems to be functioning. Thus, the diagnosis of an organic brain syndrome involves an evaluation of: (1) orientation; (2) memory; (3) verbal, spatial, and numerical ability; (4) level of consciousness; (5) perception; and (6) change in personality. It is important to note that disturbances of these functions may involve only one or all areas, and when more than one area is involved, the degree of dysfunction in each may vary. The mental functions by which we characterize an organic brain syndrome are basically those we can measure. They are all part of the mental status examination (Taylor, 1981; Kaufman, 1979; Anthony, 1982; and Strub and Black, 1977).

FACTORS IN CONTENT

Three major factors determine the manifestations of an organic brain syndrome: (1) the amount of tissue destroyed; (2) the location of the lesion in the brain; and (3) the nature of the disease process. There has been a classic argument in neurology as to whether location or amount of damage is the more important factor. On one side are those who equate structure with function and attempt to identify "centers" or anatomical loci of particular functions in the brain. On the other side stand those who agree with Lashley (1929) that all cortical regions of the brain are equipotential for intelligence and that the mass of brain tissue destroyed is therefore much more important than the location of the lesion. On the basis of evidence, presented below, it is clear that anatomical specialization does exist in the human brain to some degree, but it is not sufficient to provide functional divisions for many intellectual abilities.

Amount of Destruction

Chapman and Wolff (1959) made the most extensive, systematic test of Lashley's hypothesis in human beings. Their classic study correlated the amount of brain tissue removed during the surgical removal of a tumor with the postoperative intellectual deficiency. When brain damage was not extensive (involving less than 120 gm of cortical tissue), adaptive capacities were found to be impaired even though orientation and memory remained intact. Chapman and Wolff divided the symptoms of such "minimal" brain damage into four categories. (1) Expression of needs, appetites, and drives. There is less seeking of challenges and adventure, less imagination, less desire for human association and sexual activity, along with a passive acceptance of circumstances and a lack of aspiration in brain-damaged patients. When mild, such symptoms mimic depression, and indeed, patients with slight brain damage often are depressed; the depression may be a reaction to or a manifestation of their deficit. When brain damage is severe, inability to express needs may even extend to such basics as food, shelter, and warmth. (2) Capacity to adapt for the achievement of goals. Brain-damaged individuals have a decreased ability to anticipate either dangerous or propitious circumstances, to plan, arrange, invent, postpone, modulate, or discriminate in achieving goals. Business failure or unwise sexual liaisons, for example, may occur in the course of advancing disease and may cause great distress to the patient's family, especially when he seems normal in other ways. (3) Integration of socially appropriate reactions of defense under stress and (4) capacity to recover promptly from the effects of stress. Deficits in the third and fourth categories can lead to the catastrophic reaction first noted in war veterans who had apparently recovered from brain injuries. When confronted with an arithmetic problem they once could have solved easily, patients became "dazed, agitated, anxious, started to fumble; a moment before amiable, they became sullen, evasive, and exhibited temper" (Goldstein, 1948). The "therapeutic" effect of frontal lobotomy, however, could be regarded as a manifestation of a deficit in reaction to stress. In such lobotomized patients, many of whom were incapacitated by anxiety, responsiveness to disturbing thoughts was altered by the operation. The thoughts themselves did not change—delusions and hallucinations continued—but the anxiety and the protective reactions they had formerly evoked were markedly dampened.

Region of Destruction—Frontal Lobes

Though symptoms of brain dysfunction, such as those described above, have been seen in patients with brain injury regardless of the site of the lesion, they are often associated with frontal lobe damage. This has led to the formulation of a "frontal lobe syndrome." The frontal lobes are the largest neocortical region, and much of their tissue, particularly tissue anterior to the motor region, can be removed with little or no disturbance of motor and sensory function. Bilateral frontal lobe damage can cause subtle alterations in the highest integrative functions without causing disorientation or dysmnesia. Lesions of similar extent elsewhere in the neocortex may produce the same symptom complex but, in addition, are necessarily accompanied by disorders of motility, sensory function, speech, and visual motor function; and the subtle manifestations of disordered thought, which stand alone in frontal lobe lesions, may be overshadowed by the presence of the other, more dramatic symptoms.

Though the intellectual changes that are part of the "frontal lobe syndrome" are not specific, it may be worth while to list here those additional changes that characteristically occur when the frontal lobes are damaged. There may be a prominent tendency toward inappropriate jocularity (*Witzelsucht*) as well as inappropriate ill humor. Emotional "incontinence" occurs, i.e., crying and laughing, which often alternate rapidly. Such crying and laughing, are both provoked by minimal stimuli and often are not related to feelings of sadness or mirth. Indeed, a dulling of subjective emotionality is also characteristic. Dulled responsiveness may lead to poor self-control, and an inability to understand the consequences of actions and to orient actions to the social and ethical standards of the community. When lesions are extensive, dulling may give way to torpor and apathy and sometimes to a state of "akinetic mutism," in which the patient will not respond to spoken commands or even to painful stimuli but will lie still, speechless, with open eyes. The patient looks awake and, therefore, is not considered to be in coma yet has little more cognitive function than a coma-tose person.

Some adverse reactions to neuroleptic medication may be con-fused with akinetic mutism. These include catatonic and akinetic reactions (Gelenberg, 1977; Van Putten, 1978) and a syndrome ominously called the neuroleptic malignant syndrome (Caroff, 1980). These drug reactions are characterized by a mixture of cata-tonic symptoms (waxy flexibility, reduced responsiveness, slow responses, incontinence of urine) and Parkinsonian symptoms (stiffness, bradykinesia, rigidity, and tremor). The onset is usually gradual and the symptoms do not respond to anti-Parkinson agents. The neuroleptic malignant syndrome (NMS) is manifested by lead-pipe rigidity; "plastic" akinesia; hyperthermia; altered con-sciousness (mutism, stupor, coma); and autonomic dysfunction (sialorrhea, increased heart rate, incontinence). Although only about 60 cases have been reported to date, the incidence of this condition is estimated to be 0.5 to 1 percent of those taking neuro-leptic medication. Recovery is usually complete within 5 to 10 days after withdrawal of neuroleptics, but there is a 20 percent mortality in this condition. Its occurrence has been reported with all neuro-leptics and seems to be more frequent in males, especially those over 40 years, and in patients with organic brain syndromes. There is often moderate leukocytosis and elevated creatine phosphokinase (CPK). The EEG may be indicative of a metabolic encephalopa-thy. Some patients may appear to be suffering from encephalitis, but the cerebrospinal fluid is normal. The etiology is believed to be similar to that of the hyperthermia noted after the administration of some anesthetics. Other than withdrawal of the medication and supportive therapy, there is at present no specific treatment, al-though Dantrolene and Bromocriptine are reportedly helpful (Zu-benko, 1983).

Motor signs are somewhat more specific for frontal lobe disease. When the motor portions of the frontal lobe are involved, partic-ularly areas 4 and 6 or their many subcortical connections, motor paralysis may develop. In addition, a form of increased muscle tone (*gegenhalten*) may develop. This is also called "counterpull" and is manifested by the semivoluntary resistance the patient increasingly offers to passive movement of his limbs. When the examiner attempts to extend the patient's elbow, for example, the patient will resist, and his resistance will increase as the elbow is extended farther. Forced grasping may be seen in response to tactile stimulation of the patient's palm by the examiner's fingers. When the examiner attempts to extend the patient's fingers while disengaging his own from the patient's grip, he may encounter counterpull.

Various forms of gait disorder may result from frontal lobe damage. One type that is quite similar to cerebellar ataxia may be seen in frontal lobe lesions and presumably reflects the many connections of the frontal lobe with the pons and cerebellum. Apraxia of gait may lead to loss of the ability to stand and walk, or even to sit steadily, despite a well-coordinated movement of the limbs. A form of *marche à petit pas* that superficially may resemble the small-stepped gait usually associated with Parkinson's disease may be seen. It is widely based, however, and the patient often seems to be uncertain as to where he is going. A peculiar characteristic is the ability of some patients to step over lines and to climb stairs when they cannot walk on a flat, unmarked surface. Difficulty with the initiation of gait can be encountered in Parkinsonism as well as in gait apraxia, but this symptom of Parkinsonism can be treated successfully with L-DOPA whereas frontal gait apraxia does not respond to this medicine. Increased flexor tone caused by frontal lobe damage ultimately may lead to paraplegia in flexion.

Area 8 of the frontal lobes controls voluntary conjugate eye movements. Stimulation of area 8 causes the eyes to deviate conjugately to the opposite side. Destruction of area 8 leads to deviation of the eyes conjugately to the side of the lesion; but this is a temporary phenomenon, seen mainly in the first days and weeks following acute lesions. During convulsive seizures, the head and eyes characteristically turn away from the lesion, and during the postictal phase, they deviate back again toward the lesion.

Therapeutic Destruction of Frontal Lobe

After Moniz (1936) reported his results with frontal lobotomy for psychiatric illness, for which he received a Nobel prize, surgery on the frontal lobe became a widely practiced mode of therapy in psychiatry. Portions of the frontal lobes anterior to the motor strip were removed, but the areas and the amount of tissue removed varied widely. More conservative procedures isolated the frontal regions by sectioning the underlying white matter. Reports of success in treating psychiatric patients by lobectomy or lobotomy seemed to support a view of the frontal lobes as an intellectual "center" of the brain, the region in which disordered thinking arose. In this unsophisticated view, removing or disconnecting the frontal lobe from the rest of the brain would extirpate or quarantine the origin of the psychiatric symptoms.

It is surprising that, despite the large number of patients who underwent frontal lobotomy in the 1940s and 1950s before effective drugs were available, very little was learned about the efficacy of the procedure. Several basic medical questions have never been satisfactorily answered: What were the indications for the procedure? What were the complications and what was their incidence? What changes in the patients could be measured by pre- and postoperative psychological evaluation? What were the long-term results? One of the critical deficiencies has been the lack of a truly controlled study.

In many instances, the selection of patients for frontal lobotomy, the operation, and the postoperative evaluation were performed by the same individuals. Operations were often performed on patients who had been housed in public institutions for years—understimulated, undernourished, and all but forgotten. The beneficial effects attributed to the surgery cannot reliably be distinguished from the effects of resocialization, supportive treatment in an acute medical facility, postoperative care, better nutrition, and discharge to a family environment. The fundamental importance of these factors is suggested by a report on the late results of leucotomy in 84 "psychotic" patients that pointed up the correlation between good results and the presence of a relative responsible for the patient after the operation (Tucker, 1966).

Despite the weakness of the data, some lessons have been learned. There is a consensus among psychiatrists that frontal lobe surgery is inadvisable for chronic schizophrenia but may be useful in conditions in which anxiety is a prominent symptom; these include disabling phobias, obsessive-compulsive states, and agitated depression. It is also fairly clear that extensive surgery may have serious side effects. In a 10-year, follow-up study of 134 men who had undergone such surgery, Miller (1967) found that nearly half were disabled by seizures and a quarter by severe intellectual impairment; "less than 10% could be discharged from hospital." To be sure, these dreadful results have not been the experience of all groups performing psychosurgery, but they are very disturbing nevertheless.

Several surgeons have attempted to minimize the adverse effects of extensive frontal surgery by performing more limited operations, cutting only some of the frontal white fibers, or making stereotactic lesions in the inferior frontomedial region. Some have planted radioactive yttrium "seeds" or used cryoprobes to produce limited damage. Some have operated on the cingulate gyrus or its subcortical white matter. But the greater precision and sophistication of these surgical techniques, applied mainly in the 1960s, does not compensate for the continued imprecision of diagnosis, the ambiguous criteria by which success is measured, and especially, the lack of well-controlled studies. Though no published study of patients who have undergone limited frontal leucotomy fails to endorse its use, at least for intractable affective psychosis or disabling, intractable neurosis, in no series has uniform success been claimed for any group of patients (Valenstein and Heilman, 1979).

The symptomatic relief of anxiety that follows any destructive procedure could be a nonspecific result of brain damage, which can dull a person's response to stress. If so, according to the findings of Chapman and Wolff (1959), any supratentorial lesion in the nervous system would be likely to produce the same result, depending only on the size of the lesion. Thus, whatever the success of frontal lobe surgery, it does not necessarily derive from damage to a major center of intellectual functioning, the source of the emotional disturbance.

We find ourselves in agreement with Sweet (1973), who reviewed the subject thoroughly and concluded that a randomized study is badly needed to determine if limited surgery could help incapacitated psychiatric patients who have not benefited from medication or psychotherapy. Enough information is now available to indicate that psychosurgery may possibly help some patients, but not without substantial risk (Shevitz, 1976). For both ethical and scientific reasons, it seems to us that such surgery should no longer be performed unless it is part of a well-controlled study to determine under what circumstances, if any, it can be useful. For many reasons, it is very unlikely that such a study could be performed in this country now (Kolb, 1973).

Parietal Lobe Syndromes and Language Functions

Like frontal lobe dysfunction, parietal lobe disease gives rise to rather nonspecific symptoms. Many of the deficits seen with parietal injuries may also be the result of lesions elsewhere in the brain and of diseases that involve the brain diffusely. In general, patients with parietal disease are poor observers, have no awareness of their deficits, and perform variably on psychological tests from day to day. Lesions of the dominant hemisphere usually produce disturbances of speech, and lesions of the nondominant hemisphere produce gnostic deficits, faulty corporeal awareness, and defective visuospatial conceptualization. When such deficits are seen in patients who are not grossly disoriented, or dysmnesic, parietal lobe dysfunction should be suspected. The deficits produced by parietal lobe disease have been considered fully in Critchley's classic monograph (1953). His categorization of abnormality is summarized in Table 4-1. Table 4-2 indicates some of the variability in the location of single retro-Rolandic lesions that may give rise to "parietal" symptoms.

Table 4-1
Some Neurological Deficits
Seen with Parietal Lobe Damage

Tacticle Dysfunction
"Primary": Hemihypalgesia for touch, pain, heat, and cold
"Cortical": Astereognosis, agraphesthesia, extinction on simultaneous bilateral stimulation, two-point discrimination loss, position sense deficit with pseudoathetosis, sensory ataxia

Motility Disturbance
Apraxia for learned activities (following commands) or automatic acts (walking), *gegenhalten*, perseveration, echopraxia
Ataxia
Muscular wasting

Constructional Apraxia

Gerstmann Syndrome: Finger agnosia, dyscalculia, right-left disorientation, agraphia

Disordered Body Image
Unilateral neglect
Anosognosia
Denial

Visual Defects
Cortical blindness
Anton's syndrome (blindness with confabulation)
Hemianopia
Distortions: Macropsia, micropsia, obliquity, drifting, alexia

Source: Critchley, 1953

It is difficult to find evidence quantifying the prevalence of intellectual deficits in patients with parietal lesions. Clearly, the manifestations of injury, their severity and their duration are variable. A close reading of Hecaen (1962) and Hecaen and Angelergues (1962) does provide a basis (Tables 4-3, 4-4) for certain generalizations. Dysphasia and dyscalculia are characteristic of posterior left hemisphere lesions, but do not occur in all patients. The speech of sinistrals in general is less seriously and less permanently affected by single posterior lesions of either hemisphere. Ideomotor apraxia, when it is the result of a single posterior lesion, is seen only with lesions of the left hemisphere and only in a small minority of these

Table 4-2
Origin of Some "Parietal"-type
Deficits in Single Retrorolandic Lesions

Dysfunction	Hemisphere	Lobe(s) Mainly Involved
Apraxia		
Constructional	R > L 4:1	Parietal
Dressing	R > L 5:1	Parietal
Agnosia		
Somatognosia		
Denial of half of body opposite lesion	R	Parietal
Finger agnosia (bilateral)	L > R 6:1	Parietal, especially supramarginal and angular gyri
Visual Agnosia		
Neglect of space on side opposite lesion	R > L 10:1	Parietal
Nonrecognition of faces	R > L 3:1	Parietal
Nonrecognition of objects, pictures, colors	L	Occipital or post-temporal
Numbers not correctly placed	L > R 3:1	Parietal
Alexia	L	Temporal-occipital parietal
Agraphia	L	Temporal-parietal occipital
Acalculia	L > R 3:1	Temporal or parietal
Aphasia		
Fluent		
Wernicke (poor comprehension poor repetition)	L	Temporal-parietal
Conduction (good comprehension, poor repetition)	L	Parietal-temporal
Anomic-amnestic (good comprehension, good repetition)	(a) Widespread brain disease (b) Recovery from other forms of aphasia (c) Also L parietal (angular gyrus) L posterior temporal	
Nonfluent (motor)	L[a]	Frontal, temporal, parietal, rolandic

Source: Based on Hécaen (1962) and Geshwind (1971)
[a] R in a minority of sinistrals

Table 4-3
Frequency of Deficits in Patients
with Unilateral Retrorolandic Lesions

Deficit	Dextrals	
	Left Hemisphere Lesion (n = 206) (%)	Right Hemisphere Lesion (n = 151) (%)
Dysphasia	70	0
Dyscalculia	91	20
Ideatory apraxia	5	0
Ideomotor apraxia	19	0
Dressing apraxia	4	22
Constructional apraxia	40	62
Somatognosia		
Unilateral	4	29
Bilateral	20	3
Spatial agnosia	4	39
Metamorphopsia	8	16
Catastrophic reactions	26	13
Indifference to failure	17	33
Confusion—Dementia	20	36

Source: Hécaen, H. Clinical symptomatology in right and left hemispherical lesions in Interhemispheric Relations and Cerebral Dominance. V. B. Mountcastle (ed.) Johns Hopkins Press, Baltimore, 1962, pp. 215–243; Hécaen, H. & Angelerques, R. L'aphasie, l'apraxie, l'agnosie chez les gauchers: modalités et fréquence des troubles selon l'hémisphère atteint. *Rev. Neurol.* 106:510–516, 1962.

cases. Dressing apraxia and spatial agnosia are most characteristic of right hemisphere disease but affect only a minority of patients. Symptoms characteristic of dementia or "frontal" disease such as indifference to failure, catastrophic reactions, and confusion can be encountered in many patients with unilateral posterior lesions.

Language

Because language is a cortical function unequally represented between and within the hemispheres, its study promises to provide insights into how cortical functions are organized in the central nervous system. Yet the literature on this subject is complex, con-

Table 4-4
Frequency of Deficits in Patients
with Unilateral Retrorolandic Lesions

Deficit	Sinistrals	
	Left Hemisphere Lesion ($n = 37$) (%)	Right Hemisphere Lesion ($= 22$) (%)
Expressive dysphasia	64 (24 permanent)	50 (9 permanent)
Receptive dysphasia	14	9
Amnestic dysphasia	54 (28 permanent)	14
Dyscalculia	50	50
Ideomotor apraxia	8	0
Ideatory apraxia	8	0
Dressing apraxia	19	18
Constructional apraxia	51	53
Somatognosia	43	32
Spatial agnosia	9	7
Metamorphopsia	8	22

fusing, and often contradictory. Part of the problem is methodological, and part is conceptual; there has not yet been a complete resolution of the opposing views that cortical functions reside in certain anatomical centers and that the cortex is more or less equipotential.

Methodological Problems

Any student of aphasia immediately confronts at least two methodological problems. The first is how to define accurately the anatomical site of the lesion producing aphasia; the second is how to interpret tests for aphasia.

Language is generally considered a uniquely human trait, and humans are therefore the only proper subjects for experimentation and research. This means that anatomical correlations with functional deficits must depend in large part on the study of patients with neurological disease. A variety of lesions can give rise to language deficits in many different ways. Some conditions are progressive, and others are not; some tumors produce cerebral edema (causing dysfunction in brain regions far removed from the primary lesion), and others do not. A low-grade glioma and a metastatic lesion may have strikingly different effects even when they occur in the same anatomical location. Similarly, old scars from trauma or strokes may give rise to seizure activity, which can spread to distant brain regions and produce disorders of language that may be incorrectly attributed to the area of the primary lesion. Dominant or left hemispheric strokes sustained in early childhood produce disorders of language quite different from those that follow strokes in adults. Many studies of structure-function correlation in aphasia following traumatic injuries have been based on a presumed area of brain injury as calculated from a missile trajectory, though distant or contralateral effects of trauma cannot be ruled out before a full pathological investigation (Russell and Espir, 1961). Even when a full pathological examination has been performed, some investigators have concentrated on one aspect of a lesion and disregarded others. For example, Broca attributed aphasia to lesions of the frontal operculum and the immediately adjacent cortex. Yet when Marie (1906) restudied Broca's material several years later, he found that the lesions extended into temperoparietal regions. On other occasions, more than one infarct has been found, but functional deficits have been attributed to the largest one, and the small lesions in other regions have been regarded as "insignificant" (Nielsen, 1946). The "insignificance" of such small lesions has not been proven.

A major difficulty in studying aphasia is the variability of the tests used in different studies. The deficits revealed in patients by a specific examination are not necessarily their only deficits. In other words, the type and degree of deficit is a function of the type and completeness of testing, and in this respect, all studies are not comparable. It is not our purpose to discuss aphasia testing in detail. At a minimum, however, clinical evaluation should include tests of the ability to understand spoken and written material, to repeat and to write the names of objects and to identify objects correctly. Notations should be made on the fluency of speech, articulation, and correct use of words in sentences. Nonetheless, even the most thorough testing for aphasia has proven unsatisfactory, to some degree, in providing a reliable, reproducible method for investigating that complex of factors that determines one's ability to use language. Dissatisfaction with standard tests has provided a stimulus for the development of newer psychological and linguistic analyses of language disorders (Jakobson, 1964). No testing system has been devised, however, that provides a completely reliable basis for correlating anatomical findings with clinical observations.

Conceptual Barriers

Many of the notions commonly held about the organization of language are inaccurate, though they have been handed down from generation to generation and do bear some relation to the truth. Three such notions are: (1) that the left hemisphere is dominant for language in right-handed persons (dextrals) and the right hemisphere is language dominant in left-handed persons (sinistrals); (2) that speech is located in one hemisphere and the organization of language in that hemisphere can be studied by analyzing language deficits in patients who have sustained damage to it; (3) that motor (expressive, nonfluent, or Broca's) aphasia is caused by anterior lesions in the dominant hemisphere, whereas sensory (receptive, fluent, or Wernicke's) aphasia is caused by posterior lesions in the dominant hemisphere and anomic (nominal or amnestic) aphasia may result from temporal lobe lesions in the dominant hemisphere.

ASSUMPTION (1) *There is left speech dominance in dextrals and right speech dominance in sinistrals.* There is no question that speech is represented in the left hemisphere in virtually all dextrals. In countless instances, destruction of the left hemisphere in dextrals by tumors, strokes, trauma, or surgery has resulted in aphasia. Destruction of the right hemisphere, on the other hand, virtually never causes serious persistent speech problems in otherwise normal right-handed adults. Still, amytal injections of the right carotid by the Wada technique in epileptic dextrals have been reported to cause speech arrest in five of 48 cases (Milner et al.,

1964). Thus, right cerebral contributions to speech in some dextrals cannot be entirely discounted, though it is conceivable that in these cases some amytal entered the left circulation.

The situation in sinistrals is more complex. Ettlinger et al. (1956) found left cerebral speech dominance in 7 of 10 sinistrals. By using intracarotid amytal injections, Milner et al. (1964) found that roughly two-thirds of 44 sinistrals or ambidextrous patients had speech function localized in the left hemisphere. Only in sinistrals with a history of damage to the left hemisphere early in life was speech represented on the right side in the majority of patients (18 of 27). Nonetheless, a minority (20 to 30 percent) of normal left-handed individuals are right cerebral dominant for speech and, to this degree at least, handedness does correlate with hemispheric speech localization. Hécaen and Angelergues (1962) studied 59 sinistrals with unilateral, postrolandic lesions in either the right or the left hemisphere. They also found that left hemispheric lesions more often caused aphasia but noted that language disorders were less serious than they were in dextrals, that there was a better prognosis for recovery and that, despite the posterior location of the lesion, the disorder tended to be expressive rather than receptive in nature.

ASSUMPTION (2) *Speech is localized in one hemisphere.* There is evidence that the speech function potential of the two hemispheres is equal early in life though this has been questioned (Woods and Teuber, 1977). It seems that both hemispheres participate as speech develops in the second and third year of life and that lateralization develops afterward at more or less the same time that reading and writing skills are being acquired. Thus, destruction of the left or right hemisphere during the first years of life usually does not prevent the ultimate development of speech, unless there is severe retardation; nor does subsequent surgical removal of the damaged hemisphere cause deterioration of speech (Basser, 1962). Furthermore, damage to either hemisphere in young children who are beginning to speak when brain damage occurs may result in a temporary loss of speech. The bulk of the present evidence indicates that, at some time in the middle portion of the first decade, major speech functions become established in the left hemisphere in most individuals and that permanent aphasia is likely to result from left hemispheric damage thereafter.

The completeness and permanence of the lateralization of speech in normal adults has long been taken for granted, whereas the possibility of a contribution to speech by the right hemisphere in normal dextrals has commonly been overlooked. But the conclusion that the right hemisphere does not participate in speech has largely rested on an inadequate factual basis, that is, that destruction of the right hemisphere does not disturb speech. In fact, stimulation of the right hemisphere may cause vocalization or alter speech (Penfield and Roberts, 1959), and destruction of the right hemisphere may occasionally result in a certain hesitancy of speech or other temporary speech deficits.

The contribution of the minor hemisphere to speech has been investigated by Gazzaniga and Sperry (1967) in patients whose cerebral hemispheres were functionally separated by commissural section. Testing each hemisphere independently, they found that information perceived by the minor (right) hemisphere could not be communicated in speech or writing and that complex calculation likewise appeared to be solely a function of the major (left) hemisphere. Nonetheless, the minor hemisphere showed considerable ability to comprehend written and spoken language, though less than the major hemisphere. These experiments suggest that in individuals with intact left hemispheric speech function, the right hemisphere may make some contribution to the understanding of language but is incapable of producing language.

The most impressive evidence of right hemispheric participation in adult language function has been presented by Kinsbourne (1971); he studied three right-handed men who suffered left hemispheric strokes that caused aphasia and found that all three were able to speak a little at the time of testing and that one had shown considerable improvement. The speech in all three, however, was markedly impaired. Intracarotid injections of amytal caused complete speech arrest when the right carotid was injected but not when the left carotid was injected. It thus appears that whatever speech these patients retained or recovered after they sustained left hemispheric damage originated not in the remaining undamaged portion of the left hemisphere but in the right hemisphere. This is a remarkable demonstration, since it casts great doubt on the validity of some of our most cherished beliefs about language.

It is commonly implied that dysphasic language in adults with left hemispheric lesions originates in the remaining intact portions of the left hemisphere and that recovery from aphasia is a result of recovered function in partly damaged left hemispheric cells or of recruitment of other previously unused language circuits in the left hemisphere. On the basis of the Kinsbourne study, it appears likely that dysphasic language is largely right hemispheric and that recovery from aphasia depends largely on how completely the right hemisphere can redevelop language skills (i.e., understand and take over the motor language apparatus in the brain stem). The participation of the right hemisphere in dysphasic speech may well be the reason why various forms of aphasia correlate as incompletely as they do with the anatomical locus of the lesion. Clinical testing of aphasics, in other words, is at least as much a measure of right hemispheric adequacy as it is of left hemispheric damage. Kinsbourne's study provides a good reason for our relative inability to correlate aphasia with anatomical pathology.

ASSUMPTION (3) *The quality of aphasia is of value in localizing a cerebral lesion.* Neurologists, for over a century, have been intrigued by the possibility of localizing a cerebral lesion by psychological tests. Their goal has been elusive though, and for those who are trying to develop ever more sensitive tests, Monrad-Krohn's caveat still has force: "Nothing can be gained by an untimely anticipation of an anatomical-clinical correspondence, which no doubt exists, but the details of which still for the greater part remain unknown. Until the necessary knowledge has been gathered, all we can do is to avoid muddying the problem in question" (1958).

Most neurologists, nevertheless, agree that large anterior lesions are likely to produce disturbances of articulation, hemiparesis, and a form of aphasia in which the patient speaks slowly and with great effort, using single words in a telegraphic style. There is little speech, and sentence structure is poor. This form of expressive (motor) aphasia can be seen when the patient's understanding of written and spoken language is largely intact. Even in expressive aphasia, there is usually some receptive component to the deficit.

Large posterior lesions are less likely to produce hemiparesis and more likely to produce a disturbance in comprehension. Aphasic speech in these patients may be fairly well articulated, but often there is some defect of articulation. Speech is fluent in the sense that long phrases and sentences with some grammatical structure are used even when words are incorrect and disorganized.

Comprehension and articulation may be normal in amnestic (anomic) aphasia. Patients with amnestic aphasia cannot remember the names of objects. Though this may often be seen in patients with temporal lobe damage, it is quite nonspecific and is encountered in patients with dementia, metabolic encephalopathy, or lesions elsewhere in the brain.

Though many have tried, it is not clear that much more can be usefully said about anatomical-clinical correlation in aphasia. The inability of clinicians to establish an extensive and reliable anatomical-clinical correspondence is difficult to understand if the brain is organized into anatomical compartments or centers on which particular speech functions depend.

Two opposing theories about aphasia had arisen by the beginning of the twentieth century, and they are still maintained. According to one theory, language is a property of cortical centers that have a particular functional significance. Destruction of these centers, the association fibers between them, or the projection fibers from them, it is believed, will produce predictable forms of aphasia.

According to the other theory, the locus of the lesion is less important in determining the speech deficit than the adequacy of the remaining circuits. It seems to us that this theory is closer to the truth in view of the clinical facts and research data.

The classic work of Penfield and Roberts (1959) provides evidence that supports the second theory. During operations on epileptic patients whose seizures had been impossible to control with medication alone, they stimulated and excised virtually all areas of the cortex thought to have a role in speech. Stimulation in either hemisphere produced vocalization and arrest of speech. It never resulted in actual speech or even words, but only grunts or the enunciation of syllables. Despite the nonphysiological nature of the stimulus, one might have expected stimulation to produce some words or simple sentences if specialized, localized motor centers for speech exist.

In these and other studies that followed, such "speech areas" as the temporal and parietal regions, the supplementary motor area, and Broca's area have been removed. Excision of each area produced only temporary aphasic disturbances as long as the rest of the brain was intact. These studies indicate that the most sensitive area for language function is the left temporal-parietal region, followed by Broca's area. Other regions, such as the supplementary motor area, become indispensable only when the major speech areas are damaged.

Hécaen and Angelergues (1964) performed a systematic language study of 214 right-handed adult patients with left cerebral lesions in the frontal, rolandic parietal, temporal, and occipital regions. They confirmed the importance of the posterior temporal region (Wernicke's zone) in all language functions, even expressive ones, but emphasized that the effect upon language was devastating when more than one region was involved.

One is led to the conclusion that language depends on intact widespread, supple neuronal circuits in the left hemisphere and probably the right hemisphere, too. The functions of these circuits are not irrevocably set in a particular anatomical pattern. Though one or two areas in the left hemisphere may asume a leading role in the production of speech under normal conditions, other regions in the left and right hemispheres can take over these functions to a great extent. Destruction of particular brain regions will, according to this second theory, fail to produce predictable forms of aphasia, since the degree and type of speech deficit will depend on the potential ability of the remaining circuits in the left and right hemispheres to produce speech. This ability is realized chiefly in the presence of brain damage. Corollaries of this theory are that multiple or bilateral gray matter lesions will have a more devastating effect on particular aspects of speech than will single lesions; and single white matter lesions, by interrupting widespread circuits, will be more devastating than single gray matter lesions. These predictions conform to clinical experience.

What leads to the "dominance" of one hemisphere, how dominance is maintained, and how recovery from aphasia occurs are not known. Nor is it known whether the change in the language potential of the minor hemisphere that is thought to occur in childhood is the result of inactivity of that hemisphere or whether the dominant zone has some active role in the change. The mechanism of dominance may be analogous to the one demonstrated by Wiesel and Hubel (1965) for the visual cortex. If one eye of a newborn kitten is occluded for two to three months, the visual cortex becomes unresponsive to impulses from that eye permanently, but it is normally responsive to impulses from the unoccluded eye. When both eyes are occluded for two or three months and then tested, the visual cortical cells are still responsive to visual impulses from both eyes. Thus, it appears that the seeing eye of the monocularly occluded cat either preempts all the dendritic connections of the visual cortex or inhibits (suppresses) impulses that come from the occluded eye. This experiment, of course, is analogous to the condition amblyopia ex anopsia in humans (see Introduction).

In our view, the development of right-handedness is part of the process by which the left hemisphere becomes dominant for speech and other functions. The fact that major speech functions reside in the left hemisphere of most sinistrals indicates that the two functions—handedness and speech—are independent. Yet the state of left-handedness implies that the right hemisphere is not completely subordinate to the left, and in sinistrals, it appears that the speech dominance of the left hemisphere is not so well developed as it is in dextrals. This is manifested by the less serious and less permanent nature of speech deficits that result from left hemispheric lesions in sinistrals. From Kinsbourne's work, we suspect that the speech potential of the right hemisphere of sinistrals has not been permanently rendered ineffective by the dominant left hemisphere. We hypothesize that the right hemisphere of sinistrals is better able to produce speech after damage to the left hemisphere than that of dextrals.

Recovery from Aphasia

We also feel that the time-course of recovery from aphasia after a destructive lesion has been sustained reflects the time necessary for the reorganization of remaining circuits for the development of speech functions. This interval, however, may also represent a resumption of normal metabolism in cells damaged but not destroyed by anoxia, swelling, and other local abnormalities. Theoretically, it is conceivable that learning and practice can aid the redevelopment of language skills in previously underused circuits and that speech therapy could have a positive impact. Any improvement associated with speech therapy, of course, must be evaluated in the light of the natural history of recovery.

Some remission in the symptoms of acquired aphasia is typically seen in patients with nonprogressive brain diseases, such as cerebrovascular disorders. Significant spontaneous recovery is often thought to occur even three to six months after onset. Available data suggest that most spontaneous recovery occurs mainly in the first month after the onset of aphasia. Some improvement may continue for the next few months, but it usually is not significant (Culton, 1969). The most important factors in recovery are early age of onset, left-handedness, and lack of bilateral or widespread brain damage. It seems reasonable to suppose that recovery would be maximal in a supportive social milieu, but evidence of this is lacking. Similarly, no clear-cut statement can be made about the efficacy of aphasia therapy, since no studies have been performed with adequately matched control groups (Darley, 1975).

Other Cortical Functions

Like speech, there are other cortical functions that are unequally represented in various brain regions. Apraxia, agnosia, acalculia, agraphia, and alexia may result from retrorolandic lesions. The literature concerning aphasia is much more extensive than that concerning these deficits, but many of the caveats and principles that are relative to the study of the organization of speech seem to apply to these other cortical functions, too. Lesions in certain areas of the brain are apt to produce these deficits, and yet this does not prove that the lost functions "reside" in specific centers because lesions in these regions do not always produce the same constellation of symptoms, and recovery can occur even after destructive lesions have been sustained. The mechanism of recovery is not clear, and it is not yet known if one or both hemispheres participate. Like aphasia, apraxia, and agnosia in sinistrals are generally less severe and less permanent than in dextrals (Hécaen and Angelergues, 1962).

One's view concerning the efficacy of speech or physical therapy for any fixed deficit does imply an attitude toward the organization of central functions. Depending on one's view of the organization of the brain, it should be possible to predict the effect of active retraining on motor recovery or speech recovery after a given lesion. If one's view of the brain is that it is divided into centers that are irrevocably committed to performing particular skills, retraining would be ineffective if these skills were lost. If one's view is that the brain has considerable plasticity and that centers for higher skills and functions are not fixed, then redistribution of functions along other pathways could occur after a lesion, and retraining would be effective.

There is only one study of which we are aware that addresses this question quantitatively (Black et al., 1975). In this study, 27 rhesus monkeys were trained on two motor tasks. When a plateau of proficient performance was achieved in both hands (after six to eight months), the cortical precentral forclimb area was surgically ablated on one side. Each animal was then randomly assigned to

1

one of two experimental groups or to a sham-operative control group. To evaluate the contribution of spontaneous postoperative recovery independent of retraining, the training of one group was begun immediately after surgery; in the other experimental group, the weak forelimb remained idle for the first four postoperative months before retraining was started. Each of the groups was divided into subgroups, one of which received retraining directed toward both the weak and normal limbs and the other the weak limb alone.

They found that combined training of the weak and the normal limb, which resulted in an 85 percent recovery in the weak limb, did not differ significantly from training the weak limb alone. This suggests that the critical factor promoting recovery is the training of the weak part. The groups in whom training was begun immediately after the cortical ablation improved and reached a plateau at 82 percent of their preoperative performance after six months. The group in which training was delayed reached a plateau of 67 percent recovery six months after the start of training (10 months postoperatively). This difference in recovery between the immediate and delayed treatment groups was significant ($p > 0.05$).

Thus, it would appear from this study that active retraining facilitates recovery from fixed neurological deficits and that, to be most effective, training should begin as soon as possible after the insult to the brain. This study should encourage active early institution of physical and speech therapy in patients who have suffered neurological damage, since it lends support to the view of the brain as having considerable plasticity.

Apraxia can be defined as an inability to carry out a voluntary act which the patient should know how to do, the nature of which the patient understands, in the absence of paralysis, sensory loss, or ataxia. In dextrals, apraxia of both sides of the body is likely to result from lesions in the posterior left hemisphere, especially the supramarginal gyrus of the parietal lobe. Certain forms of apraxia are more likely to result from right parietal lesions; these include dressing apraxia and constructional apraxia (loss of the ability to copy an arrangement of matchsticks).

Agnosia is the failure to perceive the nature and meaning of a sensory stimulus when the sensory pathways conveying it are intact. Visual agnosia is present, for example, when a patient is unable to recognize an object he clearly sees. The inability to recognize objects, pictures, and colors is almost always the result of a lesion in the occipital or posterior temporal regions of the left hemisphere, but lesions in these regions do not always give rise to this form of agnosia. When present, these agnosias are usually associated with other deficits of mental and cognitive function including hemianopsia (Bender and Feldman, 1972; Benson and Greenberg, 1969; Rubens and Benson, 1971). The nonrecognition of faces (prosopagnosia) is likely to be associated with a right parietal lesion, though only a minority of patients with right parietal lesions manifest this sign (Hécaen, 1962; Meadows, 1974).

The Gerstmann syndrome—finger agnosia (the inability to name the fingers), agraphia, acalculia, and the inability to distinguish between right and left—was once thought to be specific for lesions of the angular gyrus of the left parietal lobe (Gerstmann, 1940). Though the observation that lesions in this region can produce this constellation of symptoms, as well as dyslexia, is correct, the left angular gyrus is not a "center" for these functions. Agraphia, acalculia, and alexia may result from left temporal lobe lesions, agraphia and alexia from left occipital lobe lesions, and acalculia from right hemispheric lesions (Hécaen, 1962). This information is summarized in Table 4-2.

Split Brains

The theory that supple widespread neuronal circuits exist for all the higher functions is supported by the innovative experiments on commissurotomized patients. The nature of the functional differences between the left and right hemispheres has been explored by psychological testing of epileptic patients in whom commissurotomy was performed as a reasonable measure of last resort to control their seizures.

In the initial postoperative period, such patients characteristically appear somewhat dull; there is temporal confusion, but orientation and speech are intact. Patients restrict their physical activity and have to be urged to perform the simplest body functions. As they begin to move about, a degree of spatial disorganization becomes apparent. The patient often settles into a repetitive pattern of behavior, such as closing a door with the right hand and opening it with the left, which stops only when they are distracted from the activity (Wilson et al., 1975).

It is remarkable that several weeks after section of the corpus callosum, there are no behavioral changes except those detectable by the most sophisticated testing. By flashing pictures, objects, written material, and numbers in a single visual field or by presenting objects for touch by one hand, the examiner can test each hemisphere independently. Material presented to the subject's right visual field or right hand registers in the left hemisphere and vice versa. Nonverbal responses derived from motor activity in one or the other arm by pointing, writing, and so on reflect activity in the opposite cerebral hemisphere.

In this general testing procedure a picture of an orange, for example, can be flashed to the left hemisphere. The patient can then correctly retrieve by touching with his right hand an orange from a series of test objects presented out of view. The subject would then say in a normal fashion that the stimulus had been an orange. If the patient had used his left hand, for which the major sensory projection is to the right hemisphere, and the orange were exclusively projected to the left hemisphere, this intermodal (visual to tactile) association would have failed. In order for such an association to succeed in a brain-bisected individual, the incoming visual and tactual information must be projected to the same hemisphere.

When a visual stimulus such as an orange is presented exclusively to the right hemisphere, the patient characteristically claims that he sees nothing (in other words, the left hemisphere "is talking"). Then, with the left hand, the patient can retrieve the orange from a series of objects. After each correct response, if the patient is asked what has been retrieved, he would reply that he didn't know. Once again, this represents the "left hemisphere talking." The left hemisphere neither "saw" the visual stimulus nor had direct access to the tactile information. Because the right hemisphere performs consistently and well in such tests over a longer period of time, one assumes that it "knows" and is "aware" of the test stimulus but isn't able to "talk" about it (Gazzaniga, 1970).

In many ways the right hemisphere is identical in function to the left; reaction times are the same, intermodal transfers from vision to touch and from touch to vision are as efficient in both, and the ability to respond emotionally to provocative stimuli is equal in both. The right hemisphere can "learn" any of a number of visual and tactile problems with the same rapidity as the left hemisphere. In short-term memory experiments, the right hemisphere functions as well as the left and its ability to control the left half of the body is equal to that of the left hemisphere in controlling the right. Stereognostic recognition for the left hand is present and intact in the right hemisphere as it is for the right hand in the left hemisphere.

The major differences between the right and left hemispheres are seen in the analysis of language, speech, and arithmetic. The left hemisphere is capable of speech but the adult right hemisphere is not; the left hemisphere has the capacity for complicated mathematical computations, but the right hemisphere is very poor at arithmetic.

In some tasks, mainly those involving spatial patterns, relations, and transformations, the right hemisphere is superior to the left. For example, the right hemisphere has a greater capacity than the left for drawing block designs and copying test figures. In addition, the right hemisphere apparently processes information ("reasons") by direct perceptual processing and does not depend on verbal reasoning processes for solving problems. It solves spatial problems directly and rapidly. In contrast, the left hemisphere solves similar problems slowly; the process is accompanied by a great deal of talking about the problem. It has been suggested that the left and right hemispheric modes of reasoning might interfere with each other if they were both located in the same hemisphere. If so, this would give some rationale for the development of cerebral dominance in human beings (Sperry, 1974).

In young patients who have had commissurotomies and in patients who were born with the congenital absence of the corpus callosum, the interhemispheric differences noted in commissurized adults have disappeared. The functions normally associated with either the left or the right hemisphere may become established in both hemispheres. In independent tests of each hemisphere in such patients, it has been determined that the right hemisphere can produce spoken language, writing, and calculations as well as the left, and the left can perform spatial tasks as well as the right. In both young commissurotomized patients and patients with congenital agenesis of the corpus callosum, there is a tendency for language facility to develop normally but for nonverbal functions to be somewhat impaired (Sperry, 1974). This indicates plasticity of the nervous system and argues against the identification of a cerebral structure, even a hemisphere, with a particular function. It supports the view that the higher intellectual functions, including language, calculation, and writing, can be subserved by neuronal circuits that are not irrevocably set in a particular pattern.

It has become a popular idea in recent years that the brain is a "dual processor" in which each hemisphere carries out specific tasks. The left hemisphere is thought to be specialized for language and to process information by sequential analysis; the right hemisphere, in most individuals, is thought to mediate spatial functions, emotional states, and complex nonverbal tasks in a synthetic mode of information processing. As indicated above, there is some evidence to support this though the view is oversimplified.

Much less evidence relating the hemispheres to psychiatric illness is available, despite what might be called a clinical renaissance of cerebral localization in psychiatry. There have been about 40 studies of schizophrenia alone, most of which advance the hypothesis that some form of left hemisphere hyper- or hypoactivity is present in schizophrenia.

These theories have little factual basis and often depend on unreliable or untested indicators of cerebral dominance and cerebral activity. For example, the lateralized amplitude of EEG activity or initial eye movements to the right or left are proposed as indicators of hemispheric dominance, but their correlation with other standards of dominance or with normal functioning is unknown (Marin and Tucker, 1981; Taylor and Abrams, 1984). Current evidence suggests that the major psychoses are characterized by widespread rather than by localized dysfunction and that they possibly involve certain amine pathways.

When lesions of the temporal lobes produce cognitive deficits, there may be concomitant psychosis, depression, sexual dysfunction, and rarely, episodic violence. These phenomena have been discussed under the limbic system and complex partial epilepsy. The language deficits that may occur with temporal lobe lesions have been presented above. The temporal lobe also plays a role in memory functions, though the mind's ability to record, store, and recall events cannot be regarded as localized in that region. Recent memory loss is the hallmark of all severe organic brain syndromes, whether they are induced by focal or diffuse disease, and it is usually associated with extensive cortical dysfunction. There is no doubt, however, that the medial temporal lobe and the rest of the limbic system play an especially important role in memory function.

In humans, limited bilateral lesions in regions of the limbic system can produce a severe, permanent disturbance of recent memory. This has been repeatedly noted after bilateral hippocampal destruction or after unilateral lesions in patients whose other hippocampus was impaired. That both of the hippocampuses are important for recent memory has been further emphasized by the observation that bilateral destruction of the amygdala, another limbic structure, does not cause any memory deficit. The fornix, however, must play some role in memory, since its bilateral destruction makes the mental recording of ongoing events and their subsequent recall difficult, but the extent of memory deficit after sectioning of the fornices is not as great as that caused by hippocampal lesions (Ojemann, 1966).

Lesions in other areas of the brain can also disrupt memory

function. Destruction of both the dorsomedian thalamic (DMT) and medial pulvinar nuclei produces severe recent memory deficits even when the hippocampus is intact. DMT lesions are now thought to be the major anatomical correlate of recent memory loss in Wernicke's encephalopathy. Lesions in the mamillary bodies had previously been regarded as the locus of dysmnesia in that condition (Victor et al., 1971). Stimulation of the lateral surface of the temporal lobes, especially the superior temporal gyrus, in neurosurgical patients under local anesthesia, evokes remote memories, chiefly auditory and visual, apparently of long forgotten events. Usually these events were trivial and not of obvious "psychodynamic significance" (Penfield and Perot, 1963). Removal of the stimulated regions has not obliterated such memories, however, so it would be incorrect to conceive of the temporal cortex as a unique memory storage center.

Delirium

In addition to the size and site of a lesion, the nature of the disease process is important in determining the character of an organic brain syndrome. The organic brain syndromes of acute onset, most of which have a toxic or metabolic etiology, are often characterized by delirium. Delirium is not a characteristic of chronic brain syndromes. In addition to disorientation and poor memory, delirium has other features. There is fluctuating awareness, with occasional lucid periods and somnolence. Often patients are fearful and irritable and suffer from visual hallucinations. Motor signs commonly encountered in delirium include myoclonus, asterixis, and tremulousness.

It must be emphasized that personality changes and thought disorders of a kind usually associated with schizophrenia or depression may be the prominent presenting symptoms of both the chronic and acute forms of an organic brain syndrome. This is frequently a source of diagnostic confusion; patients with structural neurological diseases or toxic and metabolic abnormalities are often misdiagnosed as schizophrenic, depressed, or hysterical on the basis of their most prominent symptoms. Careful attention to the history and physical examination, as well as detailed mental status-testing and appropriate laboratory tests, will minimize such errors. The most important point in avoiding a mistaken diagnosis is the awareness that a differential diagnosis exists and must be considered whenever a thought disorder develops (see p. 182).

The prognosis for organic brain syndromes in adults depends on their etiology. It is quite clear that the chronic, slowly developing syndromes generally have a poorer prognosis than acute cases, but this is not always so. Most of the diseases that cause brain syndromes are potentially reversible, either by medical or surgical means (Table 4-5). Unfortunately, most demented patients suffer from irreversible, progressive disease processes, such as arteriosclerosis or senility. Even in these cases, however, the physician can play a positive role by minimizing the discomfort of the patient and his family through wise counsel and judiciously administered medication. For an excellent discussion of the management of the organic brain syndromes, see Detre and Jarecki (1971).

Of the chronic conditions causing dementia, one of the most difficult to diagnose is occult hydrocephalus. Accuracy of diagnosis is important because this condition can be reversed by a relatively simple neurosurgical procedure, the placement of a ventriculoarterial shunt. Occult hydrocephalus is usually confused with one of the nontreatable causes of chronic dementia, such as senile or presenile dementia. The classical patient is a middle-aged or elderly person with gait disturbances, incontinence, and dementia, whose ventricles are large and whose cerebrospinal fluid pressure, measured at lumbar puncture, is normal (Adams et al., 1965). In some patients, a previous history of head trauma, subarachnoid hemorrhage, meningeal inflammation, or tumor suggests the possibility of a deficit in the absorption or circulation of cerebrospinal fluid; in most cases, however, in which the diagnosis of occult hydrocephalus is considered, the patient has become progressively demented over a period of months or years without any such history.

At an early stage these patients sometimes consult a psychiatrist for symptoms like apathy, psychomotor retardation, and forgetfulness, which may easily be mistaken for a depressive reaction (Price

Table 4-5
The Differential Diagnosis of Dementia

Degenerative	*Neoplastic*
Alzheimer	Gliomas[a]
Pick	Meningiomas[a]
Huntington's chorea	Secondary tumors[a]
Mechanical	*Infectious*
Trauma[a]	Lues[a]
Occult hydrocephalus[a]	Abscess[a]
Subdural hematoma[a]	Chronic meningitis[a]
	Subacute sclerosing panencephalitis
Metabolic	Creutzfeldt-Jacob disease
Hypothyroidism[a]	
Hyponatremia[a]	*Exogenous Poisoning*
Hypercalcemia[a]	Metals[a]
Hypoglycemia[a]	Bromides[a]
Porphyria[a]	Alcohol[a]
Hypoxia[a]	Barbiturates[a]
Wilson's disease[a]	Belladonna alkaloids[a]
Uremia[a]	Organic phosphates[a]
Hepatic coma[a]	Hallucinogens[a]
Carbon dioxide narcosis[a]	Psychotropics[a]
Vascular	*Vitamin Deficiency[a]*
Arteriosclerosis	especially:
Collagen disease[a]	B_1[a]
	B_6[a]
	B_{12}[a]
	Niacin[a]
	Folate[a]

[a] Potentially reversible by medical or surgical means

and Tucker, 1976). Following pneumoencephalography, they may appear catatonic. Characteristically, a gait disturbance (apraxia) appears first and is more severe than the accompanying mental changes. This contrasts with Alzheimer's disease, which begins with dementia and does not impair gait until a relatively late stage of illness.

Pneumoencephalography and CT scanning have not been very useful tools for distinguishing hydrocephalus ex vacuo (in which brain cell loss has resulted in large ventricles) from hydrocephalic dementia. Enlarged ventricles and atrophy of the cortical gyri may be seen in both conditions.

A more dynamic procedure, isotope cisternography, was devised. In this procedure, the pattern of radioisotope distribution is traced after the subarachnoid injection of radioactive material in the lumbar region. If the isotope travels normally, rather than passing "upstream" to reflux into the ventricles, and if it does not remain concentrated in the basal cisterns but passes over the convexities of the cerebral hemispheres (where it is absorbed), primary hydrocephalus can presumably be ruled out.

Unfortunately, this procedure has not been as valuable as one might have predicted, since the results are seldom unequivocal. Though few patients with completely normal isotope cisternograms have responded favorable to shunting procedures, some have. Many patients, perhaps the majority of those who do not benefit from shunting, have had abnormal cisternograms; in other words, ventricular reflux and slow absorption does not indicate that a favorable response to shunting procedures will be obtained (Wolinsky et al., 1973; Wood et al., 1974). The same failures have occurred with such other diagnostic techniques as constant infusion manometric testing.

Evidence of enlarged ventricles, when unassociated with widening of the cortical sulci, as demonstrated by computerized axial tomography and when the cerebrospinal fluid pressure is normal, may suggest occult hydrocephalus (Gawler, 1976). But this too is not likely to avoid misdiagnosis.

Direct continuous monitoring of the intraventricular pressure via a catheter placed in one of the lateral ventricles for periods of 24 to 72 hours in patients suspected of being hydrocephalic has revealed intermittent increases above the normal range in some patients, particularly during REM sleep when the cerebral blood flow is increased. Some of these patients have subsequently benefited dramatically from shunting. Transient improvement after removal of 15 to 20 ml of cerebrospinal fluid may predict improvement with shunting (Fisher, 1982), but this test has not been fully evaluated. The choice of patients for shunting relies on the art of medicine, which is to say that no firm criteria have been established. In general, the patients who have most consistently benefited from shunting have been those with demonstrable pathology whose symptoms have developed subacutely. Examples are patients with parasellar or posterior fossa tumors or malformations, and those who have had meningitis, subarachnoid hemorrhage, or head trauma.

Unfortunately, the most common cause of dementia is Alzheimer's disease or senile dementia of Alzheimer's type (SDAT), a progressive, untreatable condition of unknown etiology that is often fatal within seven years of diagnosis characterized by neurofibrillary tangles and neuritic plaques in the cerebral cortex. It is familial in about 10 percent of cases (Heston, 1979).

It is common knowledge that the brain shrinks in the course of aging and it is commonly assumed that the loss of cortical neurons is even greater in SDAT. Using a computerized method of image analysis that permits the high speed counting of large numbers of cells, Terry (1979) compared the brains of 20 clinically and histologically diagnosed cases of SDAT with 20 brains from normal individuals who died between the ages of 70 and 90. He found that the SDAT brains showed no significant loss of small neurons, no significant increase in glia, and no significant shrinking of neuronal or neuropil size. There was, however, a 40 percent decrease in the number of large neurons throughout the neocortex (Terry and Katzman, 1983).

Clearly, the qualitative changes in neurons are as significant as the quantitative loss of cells. The microscopic hallmarks of SDAT are neuritic plaques, masses of ring-shaped silver-staining material in the cortex and neurofibrillary tangles, and intraneuronal fibers that stain with silver. A correlation exists between the numbers of these lesions and the psychometric deficiency (Blessed et al., 1968). Some cases of SDAT, especially familial ones, show "lawless" secondary growth of dendrites with bizarre clusters of spine-rich dendrites (Scheibel, 1979). Other signs of dendritic abnormality in SDAT have been reported (Buell and Coleman, 1979).

Biochemical studies of SDAT have indicated that there are no major deficits in several neurotransmitters, including norepinephrine, 5-hydroxytryptamine, dopamine, and gamma-aminobutyric acid (GABA), but that acetylcholine is seriously impaired. The major enzymes responsible for acetylcholine synthesis and hydrolysis, choline acetyltransferase and acetylcholinesterase, are markedly reduced. A presynaptic acetylcholine deficiency in SDAT is thought to exist, as there is no loss of postsynaptic acetylcholine receptors in the brains of SDAT patients (Davies, 1979). The loss of cholinergic neurons is specific rather than generalized; those of the basal nucleus of Meynert are heavily affected whereas those of the caudate, putamen, and anterior horn cells are not.

Encouraged by the successful use of L-DOPA treatment in Parkinsonism, some have tried to treat SDAT with acetylcholine precursors (choline, lecithin), but the results have been disappointing. However, preliminary results with a centrally active acetylcholinesterase inhibitor, physostigmine, do indicate an improvement in memory test scores during a relatively brief period following the injection of the drug (Davies, 1983; Johns et al., 1983).

Often demented patients appear to be depressed. Depressed patients can also appear to be demented. Confusion, psychomotor retardation, and general apathy are commonly observed in depressed patients. While these symptoms often appear "organic," clinicians have been reluctant to regard them as symptoms of organicity because they are reversible. With the increasing use of neuropsychological tests in psychiatry, however, it has become clear that most psychiatric syndromes, particularly schizopherenia and affective disorders, have manifestations that are characteristic of neurological impairment. To explain these reversible symptoms of dementia in psychiatric patients, the term "pseudodementia" has been used. There are no validated diagnostic criteria for "pseudodementia," but Caine (1981) has stipulated the following characteristics: (1) A patient with a primary psychiatric diagnosis is intellectually impaired. (2) The features resemble, at least in part, a clear cognitive deficit. (3) The intellectual disorder is reversible. (4) The patient does not appear to have any significant neuropathology. Some have added various other discriminating features such as when the patient often acts as a caricature of a demented patient and frequently answers "I don't know" to many of the questions that one would think he should be able to answer (Wells, 1979).

Why should some elderly patients with depression appear demented? Perhaps they are not really demented but distracted. This is refuted by the failure to find "dementia" in equally distracted young depressed patients. If depression represents a failure in the activity of the ascending pathways of certain amines that influence cognitive functioning by focusing or sustaining the activity of cortical neurons, the effect of this failure on cognition might be most clear in individuals such as the elderly who, with aging, gradually lose cortical neurons (McHugh and Folstein, 1979). According to this hypothesis, the dementia syndrome in depression would be the result of the combination of cerebral neuronal loss with a potentially reversible disorder of a biogenic amine pathway (McAllister, 1981; McHugh and Folstein, 1979).

NEUROPSYCHOLOGICAL TESTING

When deficits are moderate or severe, psychological testing usually serves to confirm the physician's clinical impression, but in cases of mild or questionable brain damage, psychological tests can provide clinical information that is not readily apparent to a careful interviewer (Lezak, 1983). Many of these tests can give information about the lateral site of a lesion and, when repeated at intervals, can provide precise information as to the progression or regression of signs of intellectual dysfunction. Psychological testing is most valuable in the diagnosis of questionable cases, in which the question of referral of the patient to a neurologist or a psychiatrist is important for both diagnosis and treatment, as well as in longitudinal studies to document the changes in a disease process (Schreiber et al., 1976).

The major tests used to evaluate organic brain damage are performance tests. Projective tests and personality inventories have been of little use in the study of brain damage. The Wechsler Adult Intelligence Scale (WAIS) is divided into verbal and performance sections. Organic deficit usually manifests itself as the disparity between the verbal scales and the performance scales. One would expect patients with left cerebral lesions to do more poorly on the verbal scales than on the performance tasks (spatial and numerical abilities), while the converse would be true of patients with posterior right hemisphere lesions (Matarazzo, 1972). The performance scales for the WAIS, in terms of block design, picture arrangement, and the assessment of various memory functions, are similar to those for the more widely used Halstead-Reitan Battery. Batteries of tests like this one are useful in determining "organicity" and in assessing changes over time.

The Halstead-Reitan Battery consists primarily of the following tasks:

1. The *category test*. This is a test of concept formation or abstracting ability in which the patient is asked to apply an abstract principle in classifying a series of objects by size, shape, number, position, or brightness in color. This may be looked upon as a variation of the many object sorting tasks that were devised by Goldstein and Sheerer.

2. The *tactile performance test*. In this test a blindfolded patient is asked to place blocks of varying geometric shapes in the appropriate space on the board by touch alone. He does this with each hand separately and then with both hands. Then he is asked to draw a diagram of the board from memory. The patient is scored for total time to place the blocks with each hand, with both, and finally for the accuracy of his diagram (memory).

3. A *rhythm test*. The patient is asked to discriminate between rhythmic beats.

4. A *speech sounds perception test*. Here the patient compares spoken nonsense words with a printed form.

5. *Finger-tapping speed*. This is measured for each hand.
6. A *time sense test*. The patient is asked to estimate a period of time.
7. A *trial-making test*. This demonstrates the patient's ability to follow numbered sequences randomly distributed on paper.
8. A test for *aphasia*.
9. The *WAIS*.
10. The *Minnesota Multiphasic Personality Inventory* (MMPI).

Tests such as these lend themselves to statistical and computerized analysis. Diagnostic possibilities raised by the testing can be generated by the computer too. Qualitative, more individually tailored tests have been proposed by Luria (1973), though recently there has been an attempt to standardize his proposed neuropsychologic investigations (Christensen, 1975; Golden, 1980). What has emerged is a test battery of 269 tasks which takes about 2½ hours to administer. The areas tested include motor, rhythm, tactile and visual functions; receptive speech; expressive speech; writing, reading, and arithmetical skills; memory, and intellectual processes. The proponents of this battery claim that it is not only shorter than the Halstead-Reitan, which takes about six hours to administer, but also gives more information relevant to diagnosis and rehabilitation. The usefulness of this battery has been questioned because there have been few validation studies in relation to the neuropsychologic functions purportedly measured (Delis and Kaplan, 1983).

Differentiating organic brain syndromes from schizophrenia by psychological testing is quite difficult. The most pervasive disturbance of thinking evident in brain-damaged patients is their concreteness (inability to abstract). As mentioned before (p. 108), the concreteness manifested by organic patients differs somewhat from that of schizophrenic patients. In brain-damaged patients, concreteness is present consistently rather than intermittently. Intermittent concreteness is more characteristic of schizophrenia. The schizophrenic tends to be more bizarre and idiosyncratic, though "organics" can be quite bizarre. One is also more impressed by the "stimulus boundedness" of patients with organic brain syndromes. This psychological term refers to perseveration that is stimulated by and bound to the most recent verbal or visual cues. Schizophrenics tend to go off on wild tangents of loosely connected thoughts when given a particular cue. Often, however, differences between dementia and "dementia praecox" are subtle, and as yet there has not been enough research on the precise differences between the two conditions to be able to reliably distinguish between them on the basis of psychological tests. In fact, there seem to be more similarities than differences.

ORGANIC BRAIN SYNDROMES IN CHILDREN

Especially at an early age, children have a different response to brain damage than adults. Lateralization and dominance with regard to speech, reading, writing, praxis, and so on are not fully established until several years after birth. After early unilateral injury to either hemisphere, most of these functions become established on the healthy side and surgical removal of the damaged tissue produces no further deficit. Thus, unilateral brain damage in children is less likely to cause permanent loss of speech or the other "lateralized" functions. Large unilateral injuries in infants, however, tend to produce a more widespread deficit in intellectual abilities than do similar injuries in adults. It is not clear why this is so. The older a child at the time of injury, the more likely he is to suffer impairment resembling that of an adult with a similar lesion. The classical cortical dysfunction that may result from single lesions in adults are seen only in young children who have sustained bilateral cortical damage because these functions have not yet become lateralized. These dysfunctions include dyscalculia, right-left confusion, finger agnosia, constructional apraxia (Hansen, 1963), and aphasia (Landau et al., 1960).

EARLY CHILDHOOD AUTISM

Disorders of speech are the hallmark of early childhood autism, a behavioral syndrome first described by Kanner (1957) and often mislabeled "childhood schizophrenia." The syndrome includes speechlessness and an inability to make meaningful patterns out of auditory or visual stimuli. It begins in the first few years of life. Characteristically, the first year of life is marked by feeding difficulties and excessive screaming. Motor developmental milestones are usually somewhat delayed but within the normal range. Social withdrawal, odd behavior, and peculiar affect are usually quite noticeable by the second or third year of life. Autistic children have a marked inability to form human relationships and give a sharp impression of extreme solitariness. The severity of these symptoms varies, and those children who develop speech by five years of age have a fair chance of achieving independence in later life. Nearly all those who do not speak by this age require permanent care. Autism is often seen in children who also show strong evidence of neurological abnormality; it may be associated with phenylketonuria, tuberous sclerosis, and infantile spasms during the first year of life. Many autistic children have multiple cognitive deficits and perhaps half have electroencephalographic abnormalities or a history of seizures or both (Kolvin et al., V & VI, 1971; Rutter, 1966; Schain and Yannet, 1960). The symptoms of autism resemble those of congenital aphasia, and some neurologists feel it is often nothing more than that.

About the only feature that childhood autism shares with schizophrenia is the term "autism," which is one of Bleuler's fundamental symptoms. Otherwise, the two conditions are very different in age of onset, symptomatology, sex distribution (1 : 1 schizophrenia; 4 boys to 1 girl in childhood autism), and the social and intellectual status of the patient's family (high in autism and tending toward low in schizophrenia) (Kolvin et al., III, 1971). The most convincing evidence that the two conditions are not identical is genetic. There is no increase in the prevalence of schizophrenia in the parents or siblings of autistic children. Of 521 sibships of autistic children, only seven contained more than one affected member (Wing, 1966). As noted earlier, the prevalance of schizophrenia in first-degree relatives of schizophrenics is 10 to 15 percent.

Kanner (1957) and others have noted anecdotally that the

mothers of autistic children were emotionally frigid and gave their autistic children only mechanical care. This had been deemed of etiological significance until a controlled study of the attitudes of mothers toward childrearing failed to confirm the idea. In this study, carefully matched groups of the mothers of autistic, mongoloid, and normal children (100 mothers in each group) were compared. There was very little difference in such traits as overprotection, acceptance, and rejection (Pitfield and Oppenheim, 1964). Therefore, it seems likely that the cold parental handling of autistic children, when present, is a response to the child's behavior rather than the cause of it (Kolvin et al., IV, 1971).

The bulk of evidence seems to suggest that autism is not a disease entity itself but rather a behavioral syndrome of childhood that can result from many different disorders of the central nervous system that cause bilateral dysfunction and defective speech. In these terms, it is not difficult to understand why autistic children often have varying deficits in comprehension, symbolic thinking, and the formation of abstract concepts that reflect varying degrees of central nervous system dysfunction and the diseases that cause it. This could easily explain why the pattern of cognitive functioning is often uneven, with "islets of intelligence."

One strange aspect of autism is the occasional appearance of an isolated, unusual, and highly developed skill in an autistic child. Such is the case of the "idiot-savant," who can tell on what day of the week any date will fall, though he is otherwise incapable of doing simple arithmetic and generally functions at a grossly retarded level. Similarly isolated and abnormally developed skills relating to music, memory, or reading have been described in children who appear to be autistic and retarded (Scheerer et al., 1945). The abilities demonstrated by idiot-savants are especially striking because they contrast so vividly with the individuals' low intelligence. Such talents, however, are not seen exclusively in idiot-savants but may be encountered in persons of average or above-average intelligence.

Hardly any information on the neuropathological correlates of childhood autism has been published. It is a nonprogressive, non-fatal syndrome, and brain biopsies cannot usually be justified. Those few cases that have been autopsied in which some previously unsuspected progressive neurological disease was not revealed have shown no changes in the brain that could be detected by inspection or by light microscopy with standard staining techniques. Though no morphological correlates of autism and mental retardation have yet been defined, the severity of the functional disruption in these conditions stands in stark contrast to the lack of morphological findings. This demonstrates the inadequacy of neuropathological techniques, not the "functional" nature of the condition.

ATTENTION DEFICIT DISORDER (MINIMAL BRAIN DAMAGE)

The Term

The most outstanding impediment to understanding this subject in children is the vagueness and variability of the syndrome. Although many children show abnormalities in only one category, three broad categories of dysfunction are distinguishable in this syndrome: disturbed conduct, intellectual deficit measured by academic records or psychological scores (or both), and minor physical abnormalities demonstrated by neurological examination. None of the categories, not even the third, has been linked to histological evidence of brain damage. The justification of the older diagnostic term "minimal brain damage" therefore depended on observations of behavioral, intellectual, and/or neurological abnormalities in individuals who are known to have suffered brain damage. After an episode of viral encephalitis, for example, a previously normal, well-adjusted child may become impulsive, overactive, provocative, dull in his schoolwork, and clumsy in performing fine motor tasks. The role of brain damage in such behavioral changes is easy to accept, but in most cases to which the term MBD was applied, the situation was much less clear. Reading disability, for example, is sometimes considered to be a hallmark of brain damage. In many instances, this deficit may be relatively isolated. Genetic factors, which are clearly present in isolated reading disorders, may account for many kinds of intellectual deficit that are often unaccompanied by behavioral, neurological, or generalized intellectual abnormalities (Bakwin, 1973). Though it is evident that some dysfunction of the nervous system exists in such cases, "brain damage" seems an inappropriate designation and it has thus been generally discarded. Instead, the widespread recognition by clinical researchers that the deficit in attention span is critically important in developing hyperkinetic behavior and learning difficulties has led to the rechristening of the syndrome as "attention deficit disorder" (ADD). ADD has replaced MBD in common medical parlance (Nosology of disorders of higher cerebral functioning. Developmental Disabilities Committee, Child Neurology Society, 1981; DSM-III, American Psychiatric Association, 1980).

Though brain damage can cause subtle or pronounced changes in behavior and intellectual and body function, it does not necessarily follow that brain damage always produces such changes. Since virtually every minor abnormality ascribed to ADD can be seen in normal children in the preschool age group, many have questioned the significance of these phenomena when they are encountered in older children and have viewed the entire syndrome as resulting from delayed maturation of the central nervous system, psychological immaturity, or the response of a normal central nervous system to an abnormal environment at home or at school; that is, to a "functional" abnormality. A high rate of correspondence among the three categories of dysfunction and the persistence of problems in these areas into adult life would favor the organic view, but definitive information on this is lacking

The Syndrome

The most common symptoms of ADD may be described as inappropriate, poorly controlled behavior, a shortened attention span, and an intellectual deficit (Pincus and Glaser, 1966).

Inappropriate activity usually takes the form of hyperkinesis; the child, seemingly driven by some internal force, is constantly on the move, touching and handling objects, often quite briefly and to no discernible purpose. Such behavior is maximal in anxiety-provoking situations and unfamiliar surroundings. The distinction between a normally active child and a hyperactive child is largely a matter of clinical impression, and it may be made on the grounds of impulsive rather than excessive activity.

Attention span is characteristically altered, so that affected children cannot concentrate on anything for a sustained period. In severe cases, the child will respond in rapid succession and with equal intensity to any stimulus in his environment. This probably accounts for the frenetic activity so characteristic of the syndrome. Attention span is not only shortened but inappropriate and unpredictable; attention sometimes becomes riveted to trivia, and at other times the child is completely inattentive.

Impulsive, poorly controlled behavior may be destructive when the child rapidly touches and moves objects. It may also involve aggressive acts, tantrums, sexual displays, and verbal outbursts directed at others. Changes in accustomed routine or unfamiliar demands can provoke such outbursts. Some clinicians have observed a decreased capacity for spontaneous affectionate behavior and a failure to respond to reprimand or punishment.

The procedures most often used to assess the possibility of brain damage in ADD children are a carefully taken medical history that includes inquiries about events known to be associated with brain damage, such as prematurity, parental Rh incompatibility with neonatal jaundice, and epilepsy; complete physical and neurological examinations; and psychological tests.

School failure caused by intellectual deficits of many varieties is a regular occurrence among children with ADD. These deficits may be generalized or patchy. There is often a history of delayed developmental milestones. Specific difficulty with arithmetic and delayed acquisition of reading and writing skills are common. Learning disabilities may also reflect difficulties in hearing, language comprehension, memory, and speech and in the ability to generalize and classify. Such perceptual limitations may contribute to the difficulties these children have in controlling their activity. The IQ may be normal, and sophisticated psychological testing may be necessary to reveal areas of dysfunction and define them.

Intelligence, however, is generally low, being in the borderline or defective range in about half the cases.

Most children with this syndrome show no major sign of neurological deficit, such as hemiplegia, but many do have minor signs. These include clumsiness; impaired succession movements; excessive synkinesis; motor impersistence; mild involuntary movements of a choreiform nature; inability to perform tandem gait, to stand on either foot, to hop, or in children more than seven years of age, to skip. Stereognosis, graphesthesia, and two-point discrimination may also be impaired. There is no evidence af anatomical abnormalities using current computerized tomographic techniques (Shaywitz et al., 1983).

Correspondence of the Symptom Categories

To determine whether hyperactivity was correlated with neurological abnormality, Shaffer et al. (1974) divided 41 boys, five to eight years of age, into four groups: those with both neurological damage and a conduct disorder, those with the former, those with the latter, and those with neither (Shaffer et al., 1974). The subjects with no neurological disorders were chosen from the general and specialized pediatrics clinics of the Yale–New Haven Hospital and included children referred for behavioral problems at home or at school. Children with demonstrable neurological signs or an abnormal EEG were excluded and so were those who showed evidence of athetoidlike movements of the outstretched hands, dysdiadokokinesis, marked motor impersistence during the performance of rapid alternating movements of the wrists, or ataxia on tandem gait. In addition, any of the following conditions led to exclusion from the non-neurological groups: a history of abnormal pregnancy, birth weight below five pounds, a complicated delivery, a history of delayed motor and speech development, a history of seizures or trauma or infection of the central nervous system. The neurological groups were made up of boys attending the private and public clinics of the pediatric neurology unit of the Yale–New Haven Hospital. Subjects diagnosed as suffering from epilepsy or from a nonprogressive lesion above the level of the brainstem were considered for inclusion; but, progressive, malignant, or chronically debilitating conditions; conditions associated with deafness or blindness; a markedly disabling motor handicap; or an IQ below 70 were excluded. The criterion for conduct disorder was a high score on the conduct disorder dimension of the Peterson-Quay behavior problem checklist, which was filled out by parents and teachers. Differences in family background, race, social class, and IQ were controlled.

Attentional behavior was measured by automated techniques in a free play situation and during a continuous attention test. The findings indicated that the two most important features of the "hyperactivity syndrome"—overactivity and impulsivity—were also the major components of "conduct disorder." There was, however, no obligatory relation between these behaviors and brain damage or neurological dysfunction. The group of children with neurological but with no conduct disorders failed to differ in behavior from the normal control group, and children with both a neurological and a conduct disorder were no more active, impulsive, or inattentive than the children with a conduct disorder alone.

The neurological cases in the Yale study comprised virtually all of the five- to eight-year-old boys registered in the pediatric neurology service of the Yale–New Haven Hospital. Of the group, 66 percent showed conduct disorder on the basis of the Peterson-Quay questionnaires. Even when the possibility that this is an overestimate is allowed for, the incidence of ADD among the brain-damaged children must still be very high. This may reflect inadvertent selection—epileptic children who attend a hospital or clinic are more likely to be psychiatrically disturbed than epileptic children who are treated by their family doctors (Pond and Bidwell, 1960). Nevertheless, the high incidence of conduct disturbance among neurologically abnormal boys strongly suggests that brain damage in children does result in an increased *vulnerability* to a conduct disturbance (Shaffer et al., 1974).

Psychological test results and neurological findings seem to correlate fairly well in assessments of the presence or absence of a brain disorder. In a study by Klatskin et al. (1972), fifty children aged seven to twelve were studied independently by two neurologists and a psychologist to determine whether minor neurological signs would correlate with abnormalities on the Wechsler Intelligence Scale for Children (WISC) and the Bender Visual-Motor Gestalt Test. All children had full-scale WISC scores above 85, no history of seizures, and a normal head circumference. Twenty-five showed minor abnormalities on neurological examination. These children did not differ in age, sex, or full-scale IQ from the 25 who were normal. Agreement between the psychological and neurological examinations was found in 43 cases. In their WISC performances, children identified as damaged on neurological examination did less well than the normal children on the decoding subtest and on a perceptual organization test. Mental age on the Bender Test was one year or more below chronological age in 21 of 25, as compared with 7 out of 25 in the normal group ($p < 0.001$).

Thus, intellectual problems appear to correlate with neurological findings and both are likely to be present with brain dysfunction. The conduct disturbance is not a direct manifestation of brain damage, but brain damage seems in some way to predispose a child toward such behavior.

Natural History

Any accurate picture of the natural history of a behavioral syndrome like ADD must take into account its many etiological facets. Prognosis always depends to some degree on etiology, and there is no substitute for prospective studies to establish this pattern. Since etiology is so often in doubt, and there have been few convincing longitudinal studies, a really clear picture of ADD cannot be drawn.

Baumann et al. (1962) reported a five-year, follow-up study of 19 children, 5 to 12 years of age, in whom the original diagnosis was brain damage. In general, acute symptoms were found to decrease with age. Though the children matured socially, problems in academic work continued, showing only slight improvement in five years. Impulsivity and aggressiveness, which had at first been characteristic, gradually diminished with time but were replaced by withdrawn behavior. Peer group relations continued to be disturbed. A short attention span remained a problem but was associated more with daydreaming and withdrawal from social contact than with the restlessness seen initially. These findings are in general agreement with the impressions of others who claim that the hyperkinetic behavior syndrome tends to be replaced by other symptoms by the time the children have grown up (Laufer and Denhoff, 1957).

O'Neal and Robins (1958) correlated childhood problems with adult psychiatric status in a retrospective study of 150 subjects who had been evaluated in childhood, but not treated, at the St. Louis Municipal Psychiatric Clinic. This group was compared with a control group of 150 individuals of similar age and background who had been seen in nonpsychiatric clinics. No further selection was imposed on this study; it was necessary only to have been seen for any cause in either the psychiatric clinic or the pediatric clinic. A very high rate of sociopathy and psychosis was found in the group that had been evaluated in the psychiatry clinic compared with the control group. How many of the disturbed children might have had ADD was not indicated; but, since a very high proportion (perhaps 80 to 90%) of children referred to psychiatric clinics and child guidance clinics do have academic problems and behavior disorders, it is probably safe to assume that many of the individuals in O'Neal and Robins's study did have the syndrome as children. From this, it might be further assumed that ADD in childhood increases the risk of psychosis or sociopathy later in life.

Indeed, the work of Pollin and Stabenau (1968) with identical twins discordant for schizophrenia indicated conduct, behavioral, intellectual, and neurological impairment in the twin who became schizophrenic. The high incidence of neurological impairment among sociopaths lends support to the view that ADD increases the risk of sociopathy or psychosis. Whether this is actually so, however, can be determined only by prospective studies.

In the past, though there was not much published evidence, most physicians believed that the symptoms of ADD disappeared as the child or central nervous system matured. Indeed, the behavioral constellation does change over the years, but not necessarily for the better. Long-term follow-up studies have now begun to delineate a relationship between childhood ADD and adult conditions such as alcoholism and drug abuse (Schuckit, 1978; Goodwin, 1975), chronic delinquency (Satterfield et al., 1982), psychiatric symptoms (Gomes, 1981; Morrison, 1979), and continued symptoms of ADD or hyperkinesis (Wood, 1976; Bellak, 1973). Conversely, Reider (1979) found a much higher incidence of hyperactive symptoms in the offspring of schizophrenics than one would expect by chance.

One suspects that the disruption of the nervous system that gives rise to ADD is often not "minor" or "minimal." In combination with genetic propensities toward serious psychiatric illness and possibly as a manifestation of such vulnerabilities, ADD can have a devastating impact upon the life of an individual and his family.

Treatment

It is widely believed that hyperkinetic behavior can be controlled by drugs. Alerting drugs, such as the amphetamines and methylphenidate, paradoxically seem to calm hyperkinetic children and help them organize their behavior, perhaps by reducing fluctuations in alertness and improving attention span. Controlled, short-term studies using ratings by parents, teachers, and medical professionals have consistently shown that stimulant drugs improve behavior at home and at school as well as performance in the classroom and on standard psychological tests (Conners, 1971; Knights and Hinton, 1969).

Despite these impressive results, there is no reason to believe that there are long-term advantages for children who receive amphetamines chronically. Conrad et al. (1971) did not find any significant improvement on a large number of clinical and cognitive measurements and rating data after several months of drug treatment. Eight- to eleven-year-old children treated with stimulants for several years still had trouble at home and in school and often showed antisocial behavior (Weiss et al., 1971; Mendelson et al., 1971). The potentially negative effects of chronic stimulant therapy have been summarized by Sroufe and Stewart (1973). Drugs may be substituted for contact with a physician and render children more prone to drug abuse in adolescence.

In contrast to the effects of stimulants, sedating drugs, and one excellent anticonvulsant (phenobarbital) often exacerbate hyperkinetic behavior. Anticonvulsants usually do not alleviate behavioral disorders in children, even children with abnormal EEG's.

An interesting experimental model of hyperactivity in animals was presented by Shaywitz et al. (1976). These investigators correlated hyperactivity with selective depletion of brain dopamine in young rats in which a favorable response to amphetamine and behavior (temporary hyperkinesis and permanent learning disabilities) called to mind the response of hyperkinetic children. There is also some evidence of a brain dopamine deficiency in children with hyperactivity and ADD; Shaywitz et al. (1975) found a significantly reduced turnover of homovanillic acid, the major metabolite of dopamine, in the cerebrospinal fluid of these children (Shaywitz et al., 1978).

NUTRITION AND THE BRAIN

In the past several years, there has been more and more evidence that malnutrition, and environmental isolation, particularly during early life, can impair the biochemical and functional development of the brain. Some of this evidence also suggests that the observed impairment may be permanent and that it can persist as ADD, which appears to be a major contributing factor to school failure and to impulsive behavior, particularly repeated acts of violence; it may also play an important role in determining the expression of genetic potential for psychosis and epilepsy.

Many animal experiments have demonstrated that malnutrition, prenatally and neonatally, leads to physiological and biochemical alterations in the central nervous system. These are expressed as decreases in brain weight; in cell number, size and organization; in myelin formation; and in RNA, DNA, protein, glycoside, lipid, and enzyme levels (Winick, 1976). Animals malnourished prenatally show deficits in several problem solving situations later in life. Behavioral changes have also been described in neonatally malnourished animals. These include decreased motivation, decreased drive, and evidence of increased frustration and fright. But most of these behavioral and learning changes could be reversed by adequate diet and/or other environmental manipulations. In such experiments, it is difficult to separate the effects of non-nutritional environmental deprivation and nutritional deprivation in producing behavioral and learning deficits in later life.

Behavioral and learning deficits very similar to those just described can be produced by early social isolation with proper nutrition. Winick has reported that, as in malnourished rats, in socially isolated rats the rate of myelination will be reduced; in socially stimulated rats, the rate increases. Other disturbances in brain development that are associated with early social isolation resemble those found in the brains of animals subjected to early malnutrition. This underlines the need for strict environmental control in experiments on the effects of malnutrition and suggests the possibility that environmental deprivation and malnutrition may interact during the early postnatal period.

The difficulties in distinguishing the effects of malnutrition from those of environmental deprivation in animals can be illustrated by considering an experimental procedure in which early malnutrition in the rat was produced by increasing the litter size during lactation. By increasing litter size, the amount of milk available to each pup is reduced, resulting in malnutrition and subsequent behavioral changes. This method, however, also decreases the amount of attention paid by the mother to each pup. Are the resulting changes in behavior attributable to diet or to social factors?

One way of answering this question has been to introduce a trained virgin female as an "aunt" into the cage with the mother and pups for 8 hours a day. The "aunt" assists the mother in caring for the pups: she retrieves them, grooms them, and generally provides a heightened level of stimulation. The result is an increased interaction between individual pups and more interaction between the pups and their mother when the "aunt" is present.

This form of stimulation improves the pups' behavior. The improvement is quite marked in malnourished animals but not so marked in well-fed ones. Such studies have provided the first clear-cut evidence that environmental and nutritional states interact in determining behavior in the adult animal (Frankova, 1974).

In general, it can be said that animal experiments have not demonstrated an association between early malnutrition and the ability to learn. Rather, they have shown that animals malnourished in a variety of ways, both prenatally and postnatally, develop behavioral abnormalities. An abnormal behavioral pattern persists to some degree even after rehabilitation. Similar behavioral abnormalities, however, have been induced in young animals by isolating them socially, and partial reversal of the effects of either malnutrition or social deprivation is possible if the environment alone is enriched. Very much the same situation exists in humans.

Many investigators have tired to link the effects of malnutrition in early life to subsequent abnormalities in human behavior. Most of these studies have focused on intelligence tests because these tests are readily available and often standardized. But the interpretation of results is often difficult because malnourished populations also suffer from the effects of limited education, poor sanitation, recurrent infection, and a possibly higher incidence of accidents, including head trauma, as well as from malnutrition. Thus, non-nutritional environmental factors have contaminated most studies.

Prospective and retrospective studies have usually shown that mental deficiencies occur in malnourished humans. Malnourished children tend to come from more deprived classes than nonmalnourished controls and from even more deprived families when the controls are of a similar class. There is also a problem in using intelligence tests standardized in industrial nations in cultures where malnutrition is common. Despite these shortcomings, it may be worth while to review some of these studies.

In India, 19 children who suffered from kwashiorkor between the ages of 1½ and 3 years were followed and studied when they reached 8 to 11 years of age. The controls chosen for this study included three children for each of the 19 who had recovered from kwashiorkor. These controls were matched for age, sex, religion, caste, socioeconomic status, family size, parental education, school class, and locality. The IQ tests used had been standardized in India. The previously malnourished children were found to be retarded in perceptual and abstracting abilities as compared with the controls. Smaller differences were found between the malnourished children and the controls in tests of memory and verbal ability (Champakam et al., 1968).

This study emphasizes that kwashiorkor is associated with subsequent mental deficiency, but should we conclude that malnutrition caused the retardation? It would appear that we should, and yet the purist could insist that the prolonged inactivity caused by malnutrition and the prolonged hospitalization for the treatment of kwashiorkor led to a loss of learning time and to a functional separation from the family. Uncontrolled variables still persist, however, even in this careful study, and to these must be added such other possibilities for variation as the motivation of the parents in caring for children with kwashiorkor, child spacing, and the presence of infectious disease.

The major methodological problem in these studies is the selection of controls. Nonmalnourished children, even when they come from the same socioeconomic background are not necessarily as exposed to poor sanitation, poverty, lack of food, neglect, or parental indifference as malnourished children. We cannot assume that all children in one family have equal access to food and parental attention. But there have been studies using "nonmalnourished" siblings as controls, and in some of these studies no difference in IQ between the malnourished and the nonmalnourished siblings was found. These studies demonstrate the opposite problem in the selection of controls; for the so-called nonmalnourised siblings may well have been malnourished too, subclinically perhaps, but in some studies the "nonmalnourished" sibling was below national standards in height and weight, parameters that serve as indices of nutrition. In less developed countries, there is a positive correlation between height and weight and intelligence. In populations in which malnutrition is not prevalent, there is no such correlation (Winick, 1976).

In populations of uniform socioeconomic backgrounds in Mexico and Guatemala, Cravioto (1965, 1966, 1967) found that performance on psychological tests could be related to dietary practice, but not to differences in personal hygiene, housing, cash income, crop income, percentage of family income spent on food, or parental education. In these studies, it was found that the earlier the malnutrition the more profound the psychological retardation. The most severe retardation occurred in children admitted to the hospital for malnutrition at less than 6 months of age; on serial testing, the degree of developmental retardation in these children did not improve after 220 days of therapy. Children who were admitted to the hospital with malnutrition later in life did improve within this time span.

The exact age at which a child is most at risk for brain damage from malnutrition or its associated social factors is not clear from these studies. A Jamaican study (Hertzigetal, 1972) suggested that the first two years were the most important; Cravioto suggested that the first six months were critical. The exact nature of the depprivation is also unclear; if solely nutritional is it purely a caloric deficiency? a protein deficiency? a vitamin deficiency? or are exogenous factors, such as alcohol, drugs, tobacco, food additives in the forms of crop sprays, and so on at work?

Several interesting studies in nondeprived environments in industrialized countries have been made. One of the best known of these took advantage of the Dutch "hunger winter" at the end of World War II. In 1944–1945, there was severe famine in some parts of the Netherlands, and malnutrition was well documented. For six months in the famine areas of western Holland, 750 calories or less per person per day were consumed on average. In nonfamine areas, 1300 calories or more per person per day were consumed. The death rates from starvation were high in the famine areas, as was edema, and the average weight loss was 25 percent. The average birth weights of children in the famine areas were significantly lower than those in the nonfamine areas.

Many years later, a retrospective cohort study of male inductees to the army from both areas of Holland was performed (Stein et al., 1972). The subjects were divided into separate groups depending on whether they were conceived before, during, or after the famine. The frequency of severe or mild mental retardation was *not* found to be related to conception, pregnancy, or birth during the famine. The test scores of several thousand young men on the Raven matrices showed no differences between those coming from famine or nonfamine areas. Nonetheless, the tests were sensitive enough to detect differences between manual and nonmanual workers. Thus, no effect of prenatal malnutrition on mental development could be documented, but there was a very significant association between the social class of the father and the IQ of the son.

There are several possible interpretations of this study, which apparently shows that a certain degree of prenatal malnutrition has no effect on mental development. On one hand, all infants who would have been retarded may have died. This seems very unlikely; it is much more likely that whatever impairment of mental development occurred as a result of maternal starvation was of a degree that could be overcome by standard Dutch childrearing practices, including good nutrition. The diet of infants during the famine was not inadequate, being assessed as over 100 percent adequacy in both calories and protein. Thus, it may be that pathological effects of prenatal malnutrition can be overcome by postnatal nutritional adequacy.

Another group studied was a series of middle-class children with cystic fibrosis (Lloyd-Still et al., 1972). Although pregnancy is normal, the infant suffers from malnutrition induced by a malabsorption syndrome in this disease. The disease is also associated with frequent infections, chronic pancreatic insufficiency, and chronic lung disease. The study group suffered from malnutrition, in at least four of the first six months of life, which was severe enough to produce symptoms of kwashiorkor or marasmus. Twenty-nine normal siblings were used as controls; IQ tests were given to most of the parents as well. Both the normal and the malnourished children were divided into two groups at the time of testing: those under five years of age and those over five years of age. The malnourished children under five years of age showed lower scores on the Merrill-Palmer tests than their control siblings; but in the group over five years of age, there was no significant difference between the scores of the malnourished children and the control children on the WISC, Vineland, and WAIS tests. Thus, early malnutrition may slow development temporarily, but subsequent recovery is possible in an adequate environment; by environment, of course, one means both the nutritional and the social environment.

Several studies have shown a dramatic and critical effect of social factors on mental development. In one such study performed in the 1960s, a group of socially deprived children was tested and then some were given special care and instruction through home visits and daycare center experiences. In these children, the IQ improved dramatically as compared with controls from the same environment. But the children in the experimental group experienced a drop in IQ to control levels after the study was discontinued, when they returned to their "normal environment" (Schaeffer, 1967).

Another study concerned 141 Korean girls who came to medical attention at under one year of age. Of these, 42 were severely malnourished and were below the third percentile in height and wight by Korean standards, 52 were marginally nourished and were between the 3rd and 25th percentile, and 47 were well-nourished and were above the 50th percentile. All were adopted before their second birthdays by American families on a first-come, fiirst-served basis. All families had been screened for the adequacy of their home environment. These children were followed up at 7 to 16 years of age.

By age 7, there was no difference in average weight among the three groups. All were normal by Korean standards, although they were somewhat small by American standards. In height, the severely malnourished group was significantly smaller than the other two groups. The mean IQ of the malnourished group was 102; the mean IQ of the marginally nourished group was 105.9. This was not a significant difference. The previously well-nourished group had a mean IQ of 111.7, which was significantly greater than the severely malnourished group. Performances on achievement tests showed similar differences (Winick, 1976).

Similar results were reported in a prospective study (Klein et al., 1975). Four Guatemalan villages of comparable population were studied. In the first village, pregnant women and young chlidren received a high protein supplement; in the second, they received a nonprotein caloric supplement; in the third, they received the same medical care as was provided in the supplemented villages, and in the fourth, they received neither supplements nor medical care. In general, mothers from villages receiving food supplements (protein or caloric), had fewer low birth-weight infants, and the infants showed a significantly smaller percentage of growth and developmental retardation at 36 months. Piaget-based tests indicated an advantage in the supplemented groups at 48 months, but at that time the nonsupplemented groups were closing the gap. Prenatal supplementation provided a greater advantage than postnatal supplementation.

These studies show that environmental stimulation and a good diet will reverse many, if not all, the adverse effects on IQ and achievement of early malnutrition, but that neither psychosocial environment nor diet is sufficient to allow the full mental potential to develop if either one is seriously inadequate. One of the critical points made by these studies is that the adverse effects of nutritional or social deprivation or both are potentially reversible.

Severe malnutrition seldom occurs in the United States, but milder or chronic forms of undernutrition resulting from long-term deficits in diet are seen. Unfortunately, it is not yet possible to predict the effects of mild undernutrition on learning and behavior; there is good reason, however, to think that such deficits constitute a significant problem. In some of our cities, 15 percent of the population is on welfare. Most welfare recipients are women of childbearing age and children. Surveys have shown that a majority of welfare mothers (more than 80%) run out of food money before their next check arrives, and in some surveys, more than one-half experience hunger from time to time as a result.

Primrose and Higgins (1970) studied 1544 pregnant women seen in 1963–1967. Their children were born at 28 or more weeks of gestation. The mothers were from the lowest socioeconomic groups in Montreal; 62 percent were unwed and under 19 years of age. The pregnant girls were placed in one of two groups on the basis of family income. If the family income was below a certain minimum level, the girls were given instruction and food supplements; if their income was above this level, they were given instruction only, since it was assumed that they had enough money to buy food. Dietary adequacy, in terms of calories and protein, was calculated by means of careful dietary histories before and after supplementation. It was assumed that an adequate diet for someone 13 to 15 years of age would be 2600 calories per day, including 80 gm of protein plus an additional 25 gm for each infant in utero; for girls 16 to 19 years of age, 2400 calories per day with 75 gm of protein was considered adequate, although the diet was adjusted for underweight mothers.

On the average, the supplemented group had an average *deficit of 43 gm of protein per day* when first seen; this dropped to a deficit of 4 gm of protein per day during the study. The nonsupplemented group had an average *daily deficit of 26 gm of protein* when first seen, and this was reduced to 10 gm during the study.

This treatment had a significant impact on the rate of low birthweight children. This rate was 9.6 percent for girls who had less than 12 weeks of instruction and food supplements. For girls who received supplements and instruction for more than 20 weeks, the rate was only 4.7 percent. The lowest average birthweights were found among infants of mothers who had been underweight and had received no supplements. The length of clinic service had more impact on the birthweight of the child than did illegitimacy.

Other studies support these findings. In 1975, mothers who began prenatal care in the first trimester of pregnancy had a 6.6 percent incidence of low birthweight. Mothers who received prenatal care in the second and third trimesters had an incidence of 8.7 percent. The incidence of low birthweight among infants whose mothers received no prenatal care was 21.1 percent (Ma and Russell, 1975).

Interestingly in the Montreal study, mothers who smoked had children with significantly lower birthweights than those who did not smoke, even though the average caloric intake of smokers was higher than that of nonsmokers.

We can draw several important conclusions from this study. Dietary protein deficiency in pregnant lower-class women is widespread in North America. This, perhaps in addition to other adverse environmental factors, results in a rate of low birthweight of approximately 20 percent in women who do not receive prenatal medical care, 10 percent in women who receive prenatal medical care for only three months, and 5 percent in women who receive prenatal medical care for over three months. Medical intervention in the form of instruction and food supplementation can thus reduce the rate of low birthweight by 75 percent if it occurs early in the pregnancy and continues to term. Also, exogenous toxic factors, such as smoking, can have a significant impact on the birthweight of infants.

It is well known that low birthweight is among the most important risk factors in the development of cerebral palsy and mental retardation. Lesser degrees of neurological damage can also be attributed to low birthweight. In a study at Johns Hopkins University (Wiener, 1965), 500 low birthweight infants and 492 full-term infants were matched for race, season of birth, parity of mother, hospital of birth, and socioeconomic level of parents. All were examined at 40 weeks of age and followed up at six to seven years of age. At this time, 442 of the low birthweight children and 415 of the full-term children were given a battery of six psychological tests.

The tests showed that many of the premature children were psychologically impaired. The degree of impairment increased with decreasing birthweight. Low birthweight children could be identified by perceptual motor disturbances, as measured by the Bender-Gestalt test; by flaws in comprehension and abstract reasoning; by perseveration trends; by poor gross motor development; by immature speech; and by lower IQ.

If 20 percent of infants born to unserviced lower class mothers have a low birthweight, and if one-third of these infants show brain damage as a result, a significant public health problem exists.

One of the most controversial nutritional issues today is the possibility that food additives (artificial colorings, flavorings, and preservatives) cause conduct disturbance in children. Several groups have claimed that hyperactive behavior disturbances in some children can be eliminated by removing food additives from the diet (the "Feingold hypothesis"). As yet, there have been no conclusive studies to prove this point, and no convincing papers on the subject have been published in reputable journals. Preliminary data do not offer strong support in favor of the Feingold hypothesis (Harley et al., 1978).

Another important exogenous factor to consider is alcohol. The fetal alcohol syndrome, characterized by microcephaly, pre- and postnatal growth retardation, multiple congenital anomalies, and significant degrees of mental retardation, is well recognized. It is reasonable to suppose that since maternal alcoholism can severely damage the developing fetus, an entire spectrum of disorders should be apparent, ranging in severity from the fully developed syndrome to minimal toxic effects. Evidence accumulating from several lines of investigation suggests a relationship between maternal alcohol use and minimal brain damage in the offspring (Ouellette et al., 1977).

REFERENCES

Adams, R. D., et al. Symptomatic occult hydrocephalus with normal cerebrospinal fluid pressure. *New Eng. J. Med.* 273:117, 1965.

Anthony, J., L. Resche, V. Niaz, M. Van Korff, and M. Folstein. Limits of the "Mini Mental State" as a screening test for dementia and delirium among hospital patients. *Psychol. Med.* 12:397, 1982.

Bakwin, J. Reading disability in twins. *Devel. Med. Child Neurol.* 15:184, 1973.

Basser, L. S. Hemiplegia of early onset and the faculty of speech with special reference to the effects of hemispherectomy. *Brain* 85:427, 1962.

Baumann, M. L., F. A. Ludwig, R. H. Alexander, et al. *A Five Year Study of Brain Damaged Children.* Springfield Mental Health Center, 1962.

Bellak, L.   Psychiatric states in adults with minimal brain dysfunction. *Psychiat. Ann.* 7:575, 1977.

Bender, M. B. and M. Feldman.   The so-called "visual agnosias." *Brain* 95: 173, 1972.

Benson, D. F. and J. P. Greenberg.   Visual form agnosia: A specific defect in visual discrimination. *Arch. Neurol.* 20:82, 1969.

Black, P., R. S. Markowitz, and S. N. Cianci.   Recovery of motor functions after lesions in motor cortex of monkeys. In: *The Outcome of Severe Damage to the Central Nervous System.* CIBA Foundation Symposium. 34. Elsevier, Amsterdam, 1975, p. 65.

Blessed, G., B. E. Tomlinson, and M. Roth.   The association between quantitative measures of dementia and of senile changes in the cerebral gray matter of elderly subjects. *Brit. J. Psychiat.* 114:797, 1968.

Buell, S. J. and P. D. Coleman.   Dendritic growth in the aged human brain and failure of growth in senile dementia. *Science* 206:854, 1979.

Caine, E.   Pseudodementia. *Arch. Gen. Psychiat.* 38:1359, 1981.

Caroff, S. N.   The neuroleptic malignant syndrome. *J. Clin. Psychiat.* 41:79, 1980.

Champakam, S., S. G. Srikantia, and C. Gopalan.   Kwashiorkor and mental development. *Amer. J. Clin. Nutr.* 21:844, 1968.

Chapman, L. F. and H. G. Wolff.   The cerebral hemispheres and the highest integrative functions of man. *Arch. Neurol.* 1:357, 1959.

Christensen, A. L.   Luria's Neurophychological Investigation. *Spectrum,* New York, 1975.

Connors, C. K.   Recent drug studies with hyperkinetic children. *J. Learn. Disab.* 4:476, 1971.

Conrad, W. G., E. S. Dworkin, A. Shai, et al.   Effects of amphetamine therapy and prescriptive tutoring on the behavior and achievement of lower class hyperactive children. *J. Learn. Disab.* 4:509, 1971.

Cravioto, J. and B. Robles.   Evolution of adaptive and motor behavior during rehabilitation from kwashiorkor. *Amer. J. Orthopsychiat.* 35:449, 1965.

———, E. R. DeLicarde, and H. G. Birch.   Nutrition, growth and neurointegrative development: An experimental ecological study. *Pediatrics* 38:319, 1966.

———, H. G. Birch, and E. R. DeLicarde.   Influencia de la desnutrición en la capacidad de apprendizaja del niño escolar. *Bol. Med. Hosp. Infantil Mexico* 24:217, 1967.

Critchley, M.   *The Parietal Lobes.* Edward Arnold, London, 1953.

Cruickshank, W. M., F. A. Bentzen, F. H. Ratzburg, and M. T. Tannhauser. *A Teaching Method for Brain-Injured and Hyperactive Children: A Demonstration Pilot Study.* Syracuse University Press, Syracuse, 1961 (Series 6, Syracuse University Special Education & Rehabilitation Monograph).

Culton, G. L.   Spontaneous recovery from aphasia. *J. Speech Hear. Res.* 12:825, 1969.

Darley, F. L.   Treatment of acquired aphasia. In: *Advances in Neurology,* vol. 7, W. J. Friedlander, ed. Raven Press, New York, 1975, p. 111.

Davies, P.   Biochemical changes in Alzheimer's disease-senile dementia. In: *Congenital and Acquired Cognitive Disorders*, R. Katzman, ed. Raven Press, New York, 1979.

————.   An update on the neurochemistry of Alzheimer's disease. *Advances in Neurology*. Raven Press, New York, 1983.

Delis, D. and E. Kaplan.   Hazards of a standardized neuropsychological test with low content validity. *J. Consult. Clin. Psychol.* 51:396, 1983.

Detre, T. P. and H. G. Jarecki.   *Modern Psychiatric Treatment*. J. B. Lippincott, Philadelphia, 1971.

Ettlinger, G., C. V. Jackson, and O. L. Zangwill.   Cerebral dominance in sinistrals. *Brain* 79:569, 1956.

Fisher, C. M.   Hydrocephalus as a cause of disturbances of gait in the elderly. *Neurology* 32:1358, 1982.

Frankova, S.   In: *Symposia of the Swedish Nutritional Foundation* 12: *Early Malnutrition and Mental Development*. Almquist and Wiksell, 1974.

Galin, D.   Implications for psychiatry of left and right cerebral specialization. *Arch. Gen. Psychiat.* 31:572, 1974.

Gazzaniga, M. S. and R. W. Sperry.   Language after section of the cerebral commissures. *Brain* 90:131, 1967.

Gelenberg, A. J. and M. R. Mandel.   Catatonic reactions to high-potency neuroleptic drugs. *Arch. Gen. Psychiat.* 34:947, 1977.

Gerstmann, J.   Syndrome of finger agnosia, disorientation for right and left, agraphia, and acalculia. *Arch. Neurol. Psychiat.* 44:398, 1940.

Golden, C. J.   A standardized "version of Luria's neuropsychological tests." In: *Handbook of Clinical Neuropsychology*, S. Filskov and T. Ball, eds. John Wiley, New York, 1981, p. 608.

Goldstein, K.   *After-Effects of Brain Injuries in War: Their Evaluation and Treatment*. Grune & Stratton, New York, 1948.

Gomez, R., D. Janowsky, M. Zetin, L. Huey, and P. Clopton.   Adult psychiatric diagnosis and symptoms compatible with hyperactive child syndrome. *J. Clin. Psychiat.* 42:389, 1981.

Goodwin, D. and F. Schulsinger.   Alcoholism and the hyperactive child syndrome. *J. Nerv. Ment. Dis.* 160:349, 1975.

Hansen, E.   Reading and writing difficulties in children with cerebral palsy. In: *Minimal Cerebral Dysfunction*, R. C. MacKeith and M. Bax, eds. 1963 (No. 10, Little Club Clinics in Developmental Medicine), p. 58.

Harley, J. P., R. S. Ray, L. Tomasi, et al.   Hyperkinesis and food additives: Testing the Feingold hypothesis. *Pediat.* 61:818, 1978.

Hécaen, H.   Clinical symptomatology in right and left hemisphere lesions. In: *Interhemispheric Relations and Cerebral Dominance*, V. B. Mountcastle, ed. Johns Hopkins University Press, Baltimore, 1962, p. 215.

———— and P. Angelergues.   L'aphasie, l'agnosie chez les gauchers: modalités et fréquence des trouble selon l'hémisphère atteint. *Rev. Neurol.* 106: 510, 1962.

———— and ————.   Localization of symptoms in aphasia. In: *Disorders of Language*. Little, Brown, Boston, 1964 (CIBA Foundation Symposium), p. 223.

Hertzig, M. E., H. G. Birch, et al. Intellectual levels of school children severely malnourished during the first two years of life. *Pediatrics* 49:814, 1972.

Heston, L. L. Genetic relationships to Down's syndrome and hematologic cancer. In: *Congenital and Acquired Cognitive Disorders*, R. Katzman, ed. Raven Press, New York, 1979.

Jakobson, R. Towards a linguistic typology of aphasic impairments. In: *Disorders of Language*, H. Hécaen and P. Angelergues, eds. Little, Brown, Boston, 1964, p. 21.

Johns, C., B. Greenwald, R. Mohs, and K. Davis. The cholinergic treatment strategy in aging and senile dementia. *Psychopharm. Bull.* 19:185, 1983.

Kanner, L. *Child Psychiatry*, 3rd ed. C C Thomas, Springfield, Ill., 1957.

Kaufman, P., J. Nemberger, J. Strain, and J. Jacobs. Detection of cognitive deficits by a brief mental status examination. *Gen. Hosp. Psychiat.* 247, 1979.

Kiloh, L. G. Pseudodementia. *Acta Psychiat. Scand.* 37:336, 1961.

Kinsbourne, M. The minor cerebral hemisphere as a source of aphasic speech. *Arch. Neurol.* 25:302, 1971.

Klatskin, E. H., N. E. McNamara, D. Shaffer, and J. H. Pincus. Minimal organicity in children of normal intelligence: Correspondence between psychological test results and neurological findings. *J. Learn. Dis.* 5:213, 1972.

Klein, R., B. Lester, C. Yarbrough, et al. On malnutrition and mental development: Some preliminary findings. In: *International Conference on Nutrition*, A. Chavez, ed. Karger, New York, 1975.

Knights, R. M. and G. Hinton. The effects of methylphenidate (Ritalin) on the motor skills and behavior of children with learning problems. *J. Nerv. Ment. Dis.* 148:643, 1969.

Kolb, L. C. Psychosurgery—justifiable? *New Eng. J. Med.* 289:1141, 1973.

Kolvin, I., C. Ounsted, L. M. Richardson, and R. F. Garside. III. The family and social background in childhood psychoses. *Brit. J. Psychiat.* 118:396, 1971.

———, R. F. Garside, and J. S. H. Kidd. IV. Parental personality and attitude and childhood psychoses. *Brit. J. Psychiat.* 118:403, 1971.

———, C. Ounsted, and M. Roth. V. Cerebral dysfunction and childhood psychoses. *Brit. J. Psychiat.* 118:407, 1971.

———, M. Humphrey, and A. McNay. VI. Cognitive factors in childhood psychoses. *Brit. J. Psychiat.* 118:451, 1971.

Landau, W. M., R. Goldstein, and F. R. Kleffner. Congenital aphasia: A clinicopathologic study. *Neurology* 10:915, 1960.

Lashley, K. S. *Brain Mechanisms and Intelligence.* University of Chicago Press, Chicago, 1929.

Laufer, M. W. and E. Denhoff. Hyperkinetic behavior syndrome in children. *J. Pediat.* 50:463, 1957.

Lloyd-Still, J. D., P. H. Wolff, et al. Studies in intellectual development after severe malnutrition in infancy in cystic fibrosis and other intestinal lesions. Presented at IX International Congress of Nutrition, Mexico, 1972.

Ma, P. and W. R. Russell. Memorandum to Chairmen of Medical and Other Professional Advisory Committees. The National Foundation, White Plains, New York, November 13, 1975.

Marie, P. Revision de la question de l'aphasie: la troisième circonvolution frontale gauche ne joue aucun rôle spécial dans la fonction du language. *Sem. Med.* 26:241, 1906.

Marin, R. and G. J. Tucker. Psychopathology and hemispheric dysfunction. *J. Nerv. Ment. Dis.* 169:546, 1981.

Matrazzo, J. D. In: *Wechsler's Measurement and Appraisal of Adult Intelligence*, 5th ed. Williams & Wilkins, Baltimore, 1972.

McAllister, T. Pseudodementia. *Amer. J. Psychiat.* 140:528, 1983.

———. Cognitive functioning in the affective disorders. *Compr. Psychiat.* 22: 572, 1981.

Meadows, J. C. The anatomical basis of prosopagnosia. *J. Neurol. Neurosurg. Psychiat.* 37:489, 1974.

Mendelson, W., N. Johnson, and M. A. Steward. Hyperactive children as teenagers: A follow-up study. *J. Nerv. Ment. Dis.* 153:273, 1971.

Miller, A. The lobotomy project—a decade later: A follow-up study of a research project started in 1948. *Can. Med. Assoc. J.* 96:1095, 1967.

Milner, B., C. Branch, and T. Rasmussen. Observations on cerebral dominance. In: *Disorders of Language*, H. Hécaen and P. Angelergues, eds. Little, Brown, Boston, 1964, p. 200.

Moniz, E. Les premières tentatives opératoires dans le traitement de certaines psychoses. *Encéphale* 31:1, 1936.

Monrad-Krohn, G. H. *The Clinical Examination of the Nervous System.* Lewis, London, 1958.

Morrison, J. Diagnosis of adult psychiatric patients with childhood hyperactivity. *Amer. J. Psychiat.* 136:955, 1979.

Nielsen, J. M. *Agnosia, Apraxia, Aphasia: Their Value in Cerebral Localization.* 2nd ed. P. B. Hoeber, New York, 1946.

Ojemann, R. G. Correlations between specific human brain lesions and memory changes: A critical study of the literature. *Neurosci. Res. Prog. Bull.* 4:1, 1966.

O'Neal, P. and L. N. Robins. The relationship of childhood behavior problems to adult psychiatric status: A 30 year followup study of 150 subjects. *Amer. J. Psychiat.* 114:961, 1958.

Ouellette, E. M., H. L. Rosett, N. P. Rosman, et al. Adverse effects on offspring of maternal alcohol abuse during pregnancy. *New Eng. J. Med.* 297:528, 1977.

Penfield, W. and P. Perot. The brain's record of auditory and visual experience. *Brain* 86:595, 1963.

——— and L. Roberts. *Speech and Brain Mechanisms.* Princeton University Press, Princeton, 1959.

Pincus, J. H. and G. H. Glaser. The syndrome of "minimal brain damage" in childhood. *New Eng. J. Med.* 275:27, 1966.

Pitfield, M. and A. N. Oppenheim. Child rearing attitudes of mothers of psychotic children. *J. Child Psychol. Psychiat.* 5:51, 1964.
Pollin, W. and J. Stabenau. Biological, psychological and historical differences in a series of monozygotic twins discordant for schizophrenia. In: *Transmission of Schizophrenia*, D. Rosenthal and S. Kety, eds. Pergamon, London, 1968.
Pond, D. A. and B. H. Bidwell. A survey of epilepsy in 14 general practices. *Epilepsia* 1:285, 1960.
Price, T. R. and G. J. Tucker. Psychiatric and behavioral manifestations of normal pressure hydrocephalus. *J. Nerv. Ment. Dis.* 164:51, 1977.
Primrose, T. and A. Higgins. A study in human antepartum care. *J. Reprod. Med.* 7:257, 1971.
Reitan, R. M. Research program on psychological effects of brain lesions in human beings. In: *International Review of Research in Mental Retardation*, N. R. Ellis, ed. Vol. 1. Academic Press, New York, 1966, p. 153.
Rieder, R. and P. Nichols. Offspring of schizophrenics III. *Arch. Gen. Psychiat.* 36:665, 1979.
Rubens, A. B. and D. F. Benson. Associative visual agnosia. *Arch. Neurol.* 24:305, 1971.
Russell, W. and M. L. E. Espir. *Traumatic Aphasia.* Oxford University Press, London, 1961.
Rutter, M. Behavioural and cognitive characteristics of a series of psychotic children. In: *Early Childhood Autism: Clinical, Educational and Social Aspects.* J. K. Wing, ed. Pergamon, London, 1966, p. 51.
Satterfield, J. H., C. M. Hoppe, and A. M. Schell. A prospective study of delinquency in 110 adolescent boys with attention deficit disorder and 88 normal adolescent boys. *Amer. J. Psychiat.* 139:795, 1982.
Schaeffer, E. S. Infant education research project: Implementation and implication of a home tutoring program. In: *The Preschool in Action—Exploring Early Childhood Programs.* Allyn and Bacon, Boston, 1971.
——— and E. C. Griffieth. Hyperactivity and cognitive deficits in developing rat pups born to alcoholic mothers. Presented at Fetal Alcohol Syndrome Workshop, San Diego, CA, February 14, 1977.
Schain, R. J. and H. Yannet. Infantile autism: An analysis of 50 cases and a consideration of relevant neurophysiologic concepts. *J. Pediat.* 57:560, 1960.
Scheerer, M., E. Rothman, and K. Goldstein. A case of "idiot savant": An experimental study of personality organization. *Psychol. Monogr.* 58, No. 4, 1945.
Scheibel, A. Dendritic changes in senile and presenile dementias. In: *Congenital and Acquired Cognitive Disorders*, R. Katzman, ed. Raven Press, New York, 1979.
Schuckit, M., J. Petrich and J. Chiles. Hyperactivity: Diagnostic confusion. *J. Nerv. Ment. Dis.* 166:79, 1978.
Shaffer, D., N. McNamara, and J. H. Pincus. Controlled observations on patterns of activity, attention, and impulsivity in brain damaged and psychiatrically disturbed boys. *J. Psychol. Med.* 4:4, 1974.

Shaywitz, B. A., D. J. Cohen, and M. B. Bowers, Jr.   CSF amine metabolites in children with minimal brain damage evidence for alteration of brain dopamine. *Ped. Res.* 9:385, 1975.

———, R. D. Yager, and J. H. Klopper.   Selective brain dopamine depletion in developing rates: An experimental model of minimal brain dysfunction. *Science* 191:305, 1976.

———, S. E. Shaywitz, T. Byrne, et al.   Atttention deficit disorder: Quantitative analysis of CT. *Neurology* 33:1500, 1983.

Shaywitz, S. E., D. J. Cohen, and B. A. Shaywitz.   The biochemical basis of minimal brain dysfunction. *J. Pediat.* 92:179, 1978.

Shevitz, S. A.   Psychosurgery: Some current observations. *Amer. J. Psychiat.* 133:266, 1976.

Sperry, R. W.   Lateral specialization in the surgically separated hemispheres. In: *The Neurosciences, Third Study Program,* F. O. Schmitt and F. G. Warden, eds. M.I.T. Press, Cambridge, Mass., 1974, p. 5.

Sroufe, L. A. and M. A. Stewart.   Treating problem children with stimulant drugs. *New Eng. J. Med.* 289:407, 1973.

Stein, Z., M. Susser, et al.   Nutrition and mental performance. *Science* 178: 708, 1972.

Sweet, W. H.   Treatment of medically intractable mental disease by limited frontal leucotomy—justifiable? *New Eng. J. Med.* 289:1117, 1973.

Taylor, M. A.   *The Neuropsychiatric Mental Status Examination.* S. P. Medical and Scientific Books, New York, 1981.

——— and Abrams, R.   Cognitive impairment in schizophrenia. *Amer. J. Psychiat.* 141:196, 1984.

Terry, R.   Ultrastructural changes in Alzheimer's disease and quantitative studies. In: *Congenital and Acquired Mental Disorders,* R. Katzman, ed. Raven Press, New York, 1979.

Tucker, W. I.   Indications for modified leukotomy. *Lahey Clin. Found. Bull.* 15:131, 1966.

Valenstein, E., and K. M. Heilman.   Emotional disorders resulting from lesions of the central nervous system. In: *Clinical Neuropsychology,* K. M. Heilman and E. Valenstein, eds. Oxford University Press, New York, 1979.

Van Putten, T. and P. R. A. May.   "Akinestic depression" in schizophrenia. *Arch. Gen. Psychiat.* 35:1101, 1978.

Wells, C. E.   Pseudodementia. *Amer. J. Psychiat.* 136:895, 1979.

Wood, D., F. Reimherr, P. Wender, and G. Johnson.   Diagnosis and treatment of minimal brain dysfunction in adults. *Arch. Gen. Psychiat.* 33: 1453, 1976.

Zubenko, G. and Pope, H.   Management of a case of neuroleptic malignant syndrome with bromocriptine. *Amer. J. Psychiat.* 140:1619, 1983.

Chapter 5

MOVEMENT DISORDERS, DEPRESSION, PSYCHOSIS, AND SLEEP

Recent advances in the study of the catecholamines have led to a greater understanding of Parkinson's disease and the biochemical mechanisms of action of drugs that modify its symptoms. Many of the drugs used to relieve or induce Parkinsonism are known to be effective in treating other neurological and psychiatric conditions, especially chorea, depression, and thought disorders. Combined with clinical experience in using these drugs, the insight into their mechanisms of action provided by basic research has made it possible to advance a hypothesis concerning the biochemical abnormalities that may underlie depression, some movement disorders, and some psychoses.

PARKINSON'S DISEASE

Clinical Features

There are three major clinical features of Parkinson's disease: tremor, rigidity, and bradykinesia. The *tremor* of Parkinsonism is apparent mainly when the patient is resting or holding sustained postures and is diminished during voluntary movements. For this reason, of the three cardinal symptoms, tremor interferes least with willed body movements. *Rigidity* is a manifestation of increased muscle tone, and it is maximal in flexor muscles. This results in the stooped posture with slight flexion of the knees, hips, neck, and elbows so characteristic of Parkinsonism. In practical terms, rigidity means that the patient with Parkinsonism must overcome increased tone in antagonistic muscles in order to move and that extensor functions are especially limited. The extra effort needed to move is often interpreted by the patient as weakness, but individual muscle testing frequently provides little evidence of loss of strength. The *bradykinesia* of Parkinsonism is best defined as a disability in initiating and sometimes arresting movement. Patients with Parkinson's disease may have great difficulty carrying out associated or spontaneous movements, such as swinging the arms while walking, and it often takes them a few seconds to begin walking. Not infrequently, they will run into a wall or a door in order to stop. An inability to adjust rapidly to postural changes may result in frequent falling.

Other clinical features of Parkinsonism that relate to the three cardinal symptoms are: expressionless features, a feeling of weakness and of being slowed down, flattening and weakness of the voice, micrographia, *marche à petit pas*, festinating gait, and cogwheel rigidity. Oily seborrheic skin, excessive salivation, constipation, difficulty in focusing the eyes, and sleep disturbances suggested autonomic dysfunction, namely parasympathetic overactivity, in Parkinsonism many years before much was known about its pathogenesis.

Parkinson's disease has many causes. The most common one today is probably the use of tranquilizing medications, such as the phenothiazines, and other major tranquilizers, or *Rauwolfia* alkaloids. The idiopathic, postencephalitic, and arteriosclerotic causes of Parkinson's disease are also fairly common. In these forms, the disease affects people over 50 years of age and is seldom familial. The etiology of idiopathic Parkinsonism is in doubt, but the idea that a slow virus could be responsible has gained wide currency. Other rare causes of Parkinson's disease are carbon monoxide poisoning, manganese intoxication, hypocalcemia, and degenerative diseases of the nervous system in which Parkinsonian features are seen. In this discussion, we will be concerned mostly with drug-induced and idiopathic syndromes.

It is not usually difficult to distinguish Parkinsonism from other neurological disorders. The condition most easily confused with

Parkinsonism is depression. In depression, generalized weakness, slowing down of movement, expressionless features, a weakened voice, small steps, diminution of spontaneous movements, constipation, and sleep disturbances are seen. All these symptoms are similar to features of Parkinsonism. Many clinicians have claimed that depression to some degree is virtually always seen in patients with Parkinson's disease. This has been disputed, but it is true that most patients with Parkinson's disease do look depressed, especially when they are at rest.

The histopathology of idiopathic and postencephalitic Parkinson's disease appears minor, giving one little indication of the clinical severity of the disorder. Though a person may be virtually imprisoned in his body, almost unable to move, the neuropathology of Parkinsonism may not be very dramatic. The substantia nigra is the primary site of lesions. Though other regions may be affected, this is the only part of the nervous system in which lesions always occur. There is a disappearance of neurons and a displacement into extracellular space of the pigment ordinarily present in the neurons of this region. In addition, some reactive gliosis is seen. Peculiar cytoplasmic inclusion bodies, called Lewy bodies, occasionally appear in the neurons of the substantia nigra.

Physiology

The neurophysiological defects in Parkinson's disease have been difficult to define, but a sensible theory has been put forward by Carmen (1968). Lesions of the substantia nigra, according to his theory, produce movement problems because of a loss of nigrostriatal influence. The substantia nigra is conceived as having an inhibitory effect on the globus pallidus, which, when unopposed, has an excitatory effect upon motor movements that results in tremor. This excitation is mediated mainly by pathways that travel from the globus pallidus to the ventral anterior and ventral lateral nuclei of the thalamus. These nuclei, in turn, project to the motor cortex and influence movement. In other words, Carmen has suggested an ascending pathway: the substantia nigra inhibits the globus pallidus; the globus pallidus sends messages to the thalamus; the thalamus transmits these messages to the motor cortex. In Parkinson's disease the messages are incorrect because of the change in the substantia nigra. Destruction of the globus pallidus was long ago shown by Cooper (1968) to relieve the tremor of Parkinsonism. A modification of the operation, which has been more effective, involves destruction of portions of the thalamus, the way station in the transmission of incorrect afferent information to the motor cortex. Many movement disorders that may result from dysfunction of the basal ganglia can be relieved by placing lesions in this region of the thalamus. Intention tremor, which presumably arises from a disorder of the dentate nucleus of the cerebellum; hemiballismus, which is caused by lesions in the subthalamic nucleus; and dystonia, which sometimes results from abnormalities of the putamen, may be abolished by thalamic lesions. The advantage of thalamotomy over operations that destroy the corticospinal pathways is that though poor procedures abolish excessive abnormal movement, the former does not produce paralysis; the latter always does.

This operation is not the ultimate "cure" for Parkinson's disease because beyond the obvious risks of operating on elderly people, and the fact that unilateral lesions are not sufficient to treat an essentially bilateral disease, thalamotomy does not abolish bradykinesia and has a disappointingly mild effect upon rigidity. It has been very effective in abolishing tremor, but tremor is the least disabling of the three major symptoms of Parkinson's disease. The failure of thalamic lesions to ameliorate all the symptoms of Parkinson's disease suggests that Carmen's theoretical model of the pathophysiology underlying the condition is oversimplified and possibly incorrect.

Biochemistry

Biochemical studies in the last decade offer a promising approach to a fuller understanding of Parkinson's disease and other related conditions. One of the initial breakthroughs was the demonstration that certain neurons in the central nervous system contain catecholamines (dopamine, norepinephrine) and serotonin. It was further demonstrated that these amine-containing neurons are not uniformly distributed. Serotonin is found primarily in the cells of the median raphe and, via their projections in the hippocampus and hypothalamus. Norepinephrine is widely distributed throughout the cerebral cortex, cerebellum, and spinal cord in terminals of neurons that often originate in the locus ceruleus. Norepinephrine reaches its highest concentrations in the hypothalamus. Higher concentrations of dopamine are found in the caudate nucleus and putamen than the globus pallidus and substantia nigra. Presynaptic nerve terminals contain 10 to 100 times more transmitter than the cell bodies in which transmitter-containing vesicles are synthesized, and it has been estimated that each cell has about 10^5 nerve terminals. Thus, adrenergic cells in the substantia nigra that terminate in the caudate, putamen, and globus pallidus produce higher concentrations of dopamine than the cells in the substantia nigra (Cooper et al., 1974). In postmortem studies of the brains of patients with Parkinson's disease, dopamine and its principal metabolite, homovanillic acid (HVA), were found to be reduced to one-tenth their normal concentration in the basal ganglia (Hornykiewicz, 1966). These findings have led to the development of a rational and highly effective drug treatment for this condition.

Other biochemical findings in Parkinsonism are a 50 percent diminution of brain norepinephine and serotonin. These changes may be important in understanding the emotional concomitants of this disease.

Catecholamine Metabolism

The catecholamines dopamine and norepinephrine are synthesized from the amino acid tyrosine by a series of steps (see Fig. 5-1). Tyrosine is taken into neurons and hydroxylated through the action of the enzyme tyrosine hydroxylase to DOPA. DOPA, by means of the enzyme DOPA-decarboxylase, is converted to dopamine. Dopamine is stored in some neurons (called dopaminergic) in which it is thought to be a neurotransmitter. Dopaminergic neurons are concentrated in the basal ganglia. In those neurons that store norepinephrine ("noradrenergic"), the presumed transmitter

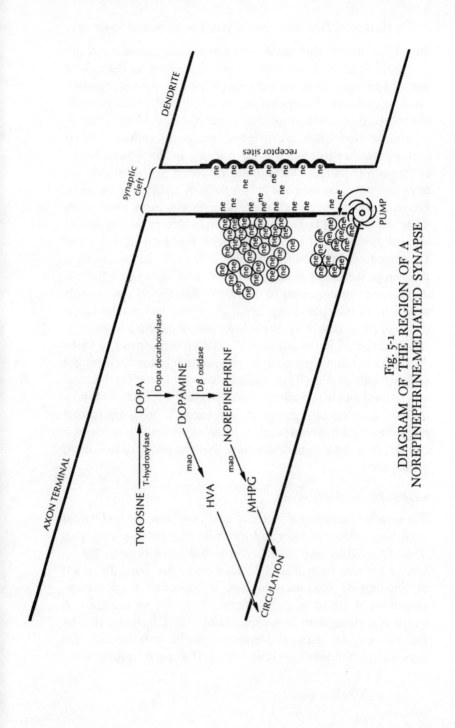

Fig. 5-1
DIAGRAM OF THE REGION OF A
NOREPINEPHRINE-MEDIATED SYNAPSE

substance is norepinephrine. In noradrenergic neurons, dopamine is a precursor of norepinephrine. By the action of dopamine beta oxidase, norepinephrine is synthesized from dopamine. Though widely distributed, noradrenergic neurons are highly concentrated in the hypothalamus.

In the conversion of tyrosine to dopamine or norepinephrine, it has been established that the step catalyzed by tyrosine hydroxylase is the rate-limiting step. This means that a reduction in the activity of this enzyme reduces the production of both dopamine and norepinephrine proportionally. Inactivation of other enzymes in this pathway does not lead to proportional decreases in the production of the catecholamines. That tyrosine hydroxylase activity is inhibited by the catecholamines suggests a negative feedback mechanism, whereby the production of norepinephrine and dopamine provokes a decline in their production. Direct nerve stimulation has been shown to accelerate norepinephrine biosynthesis, presumably by release of the transmitter; it thus depletes the pool of norepinephrine within the neuron, which reduces enzyme activity.

An analogous set of reactions occurs in the formation of the indoleamines. Thus, tryptophan is taken up by serotonergic neurons and converted to 5-hydroxytryptophan and then to 5-hydroxytryptamine (5-HT or serotonin). The rate-limiting step in this series is the one catalyzed by tryptophan hydroxylase. In all tissues in which catecholamines and indoleamines are found, they are located within highly specialized subcellular particles. In the central nervous system, these particles are called synaptic vesicles, and they are concentrated at axon terminals (see Fig. 5-1). Stimulation of the axon releases the contents of these vesicles into the synaptic cleft, where they then activate receptor sites on the dendritic membrane and thus impulse transmission from cell to cell is accomplished.

Catecholamines undergo a rather complex fate. One moiety is metabolized by catechol-O-methyl transferase (COMT) and another by monoamine oxidase (MAO), which also degrades 5-HT. Enzymatic degradation, however, plays a relatively minor role in the inactivation of these transmitter amines. Most of the released neurotransmitter is taken up again by the neuron. This process, called reuptake, depends upon an active pumping mechanism, which rapidly and economically terminates the action of the released transmitter. Reuptake is the major mechanism by which indoleamines, as well as catecholamines, are removed from the receptor sites. At cholinergic sites, on the other hand, the major mechanism for the inactivation of acetylcholine is enzymatic.

Once the released amine is taken up by the axon, it is stored again in vesicles. Only a minority of the amine-containing vesicles release their contents during nerve stimulation; thus, most of the amine within the axon terminals is essentially in an inactive form. This allows us to roughly equate "reuptake" with "inactivation" in speaking of transmitter amines.

Monoamine oxidase, which is present within the amine-containing axons, serves to inactivate any excess catecholamines that may leak out of the storage vesicles. As a result of MAO action, by-products of the amines are formed and then excreted via the blood and spinal fluid and finally the kidneys. These by-products include 3-methoxy, 5-hydroxy phenylethylene glycol (MHPG), a breakdown product of norepinephrine, and homovanillic acid (HVA) and dihydroxyphenylacetic acid (DOPAC), breakdown products of dopamine. Five-hydroxy indoleacetic acid (5-HIAA) is the major breakdown product of serotonin. These by-products can be measured in the spinal fluid and urine to provide information concerning the role of catecholamines in neurological and psychiatric diseases. It is difficult to correlate urine concentrations of HVA and 5-HIAA to changes in the central nervous system, since the source of nearly all these catabolites in the urine is peripheral. Of the urinary MHPG, however, 30 percent is derived from norepinephrine in the brain and spinal cord.

Several groups of drugs are effective in treating Parkinson's disease. The most effective, in order of their chronological introduction into the pharmacopoeia for treatment of Parkinson's disease, are: (1) belladonna alkaloids (anticholinergics), (2) levo-dihydroxyphenylalanine (L-DOPA), (3) amantadine, and (4) bromocriptine (Calne et al., 1974). Other drugs that have some beneficial effect in patients with Parkinsonism are the amphetamines, the

MAO inhibitors, and the tricyclic mood elevators. Other commonly used medications may induce or exacerbate Parkinson's disease. The *Rauwolfia* alkaloids (reserpine), the phenothiazines, and the major tranquilizers (haloperidol, etc.), administered in high doses to neurologically normal individuals, can produce all the symptoms of Parkinsonism.

Treatment of Parkinson's Disease and the Biochemical Basis
of Drug Action: Anticholinergics

Because of the apparent parasympathetic overactivity in patients with Parkinson's disease, anticholinergic drugs, such as scopolamine (Hyoscine) and stramonium, were used. These drugs have been supplanted by synthetic compounds, such as trihexyphenidyl (Artane) and benztropine (Cogentin), which are slightly effective in reducing salivation and rigidity. Bradykinesia is occasionally alleviated by these drugs, but tremor is largely unaffected. In idiopathic Parkinson's disease, the best result one can expect is a 20 to 30 percent improvement in 60 to 70 percent of patients (Goodman and Gilman, 1970). The phenothiazine-induced Parkinsonism responds very differently, however. Immediate remission of symptoms occurs after intravenous injection of an anticholinergic drug or even after injection of certain anticholinergic antihistamines, such as diphenhydramine (Benadryl). Total remission of Parkinsonian symptoms is the rule when anticholinergics are administered orally to psychiatric patients who are receiving high doses of phenothiazines or related major tranquilizers.

The demonstration of low dopamine levels in postmortem studies of the brains of Parkinsonian patients has led to the "balance" theory of Parkinsonism and its treatment (Van Woert et al., 1972; Weintraub and Van Woert, 1971). According to this theory, cholinergic and adrenergic brain mechanisms must be in balance. In Parkinsonism, the adrenergic mechanisms are weakened by loss of dopamine. The anticholinergic drugs reduce cholinergic activity and thus restore a balance that leads to clinical improvement. Support for this theory comes from experiments that demonstrate a worsening of Parkinsonism when the centrally acting antiacetylcholinesterase medication physostigmine (Eserine) is injected. This deterioration is conceived as the result of an increased cholinergic activity induced by physostigmine. Though attractive, the balance theory does not offer a ready explanation for the difference in the effectiveness of anticholinergic drugs with idiopathic and phenothiazine-induced Parkinsonism.

It has been found that the anticholinergic drugs are potent inhibitors of dopamine reuptake into synaptosomes isolated from rat corpus striatum (Coyle and Snyder, 1969). This may well be a major site of action of the anticholinergic drugs used to treat Parkinsonism. By reducing reuptake, these drugs may lead to an accumulation of dopamine in the extracellular region, thus prolonging the time it can act at receptor sites on the dendritic membrane. In idiopathic Parkinson's disease, however, since there is little dopamine in the brain and therefore little to be released into the synaptic cleft, the anticholinergic drugs would be expected to have little effect.

The phenothiazines are thought to act primarily by competitively blocking the postsynaptic receptor sites of the transmitter amines. In animals treated with large doses of phenothiazines, total brain dopamine levels are not reduced and, in fact, may be elevated. Thus, the amount of dopamine that is released from the axon by nerve stimulation is much greater in phenothiazine-induced Parkinsonism than it is in idiopathic Parkinson's disease. Inactivation of the reuptake mechanism in phenothiazine-induced Parknsonism would lead to a marked elevation in the concentration of dopamine in the synaptic cleft and would be expected to overcome the competitive block formed by phenothiazines. Thus, it is possible that the anticholinergics may modify Parkinsonism primarily through their effect on the catecholamine inactivation system; this theory offers a reasonable explanation of the differential efficacy of anticholinergics in the treatment of idiopathic and phenothiazine-induced Parkinsonism.

Though anticholinergic drugs are infrequently used in neurology and psychiatry beyond the treatment of Parkinsonism, some of their other effects should be noted. In toxic doses, they may produce nightmares, agitation, and delirium. The mental state that can be produced by the anticholinergic compounds may strikingly resemble that seen in schizophrenia. The drugs may give rise to loose associations, auditory hallucinations, and inappropriate affect in people who have normal orientation and memory. The dose of an anticholinergic drug does not have to be unusually high to induce psychosis, since there seems to be a large element of individual sensitivity to these drugs. For this reason, it is wise to start anticholinergic medication with very small doses to be sure that the patient can tolerate the drug. The delirium caused by these drugs is usually associated with tachycardia, fever, dilated pupils, flushing of the skin, visual hallucinations, and disorientation, but these signs may not be prominent. When high doses of anticholinergic compounds are used in combination with phenothiazines for the treatment of schizophrenia, they occasionally exacerbate psychosis.

Theoretically, the belladonna compounds might have some antidepressant action (cf. p. 235), since they reduce reuptake of dopamine. They are not known, however, to have any antidepressant effect. Yet, their effect upon depression apparently does not differ from that of an effective antidepressant, imipramine. In a study of the treatment of depression performed in 1965, in which imipramine was compared with an active placebo (atropine), no difference between imipramine and the placebo was found (Tucker, unpublished). Atropine was chosen for this study because such cholinergic side effects as dry mouth, constipation, and visual blurring are the same as those produced by imipramine. In the light of many subsequent studies indicating the great usefulness of imipramine in the treatment of depression, the question can be raised whether belladonna compounds might, in fact, have an antidepressant effect. There is some evidence that this is so. Scopolamine has long been known to have a tranquilizing effect when used preoperatively, and it often relieves a patient's agitation. In therapeutic doses, it normally causes drowsiness and euphoria. Its major drawback is that it may occasionally produce excitement and delirium in doses in the usual therapeutic range (Goodman and Gilman, 1970).

L-DOPA

The suspicion and final demonstration that dopamine deficiency in the basal ganglia is the basic chemical defect in Parkinson's disease led to clinical trials with agents with the ability to replenish the deficient amine. Because dopamine itself does not cross the blood-brain barrier, the precursor, DOPA, first in the racemic form and now in the levo form, has been used. This compound is unquestionably the most effective therapy that has yet been devised for Parkinson's disease. The drug markedly reduces rigidity and bradykinesia and though less effective for treating tremor, it helps this symptom also. Roughly 80 percent of all patients on L-DOPA experience 60 to 70 percent improvement. In order to be effective in Parkinson's disease, large doses of L-DOPA must be used; most patients do not experience a significant beneficial effect unless they are taking between 3 and 8 gm/day by mouth. As a result, side effects are extremely common. Some of these, like nausea, can be reduced or eliminated by the use of a DOPA decarboxylase inhibitor, which does not enter the brain. This type of drug allows much lower oral doses of L-DOPA to enter the central nervous system in effective concentrations by preventing its peripheral metabolism. The lower dose results in fewer peripheral side-effects but the central nervous system side-effects are not changed, and these are the most relevant to our discussion. They consist of movement disorders and emotional changes.

In about half the patients treated with L-DOPA, involuntary movements, ranging from mild and fleeting to severe and prolonged, develop. Choreiform movements of the legs, arms, and face are often seen, and these involuntary movements can become so severe that they may resemble hemiballismus. The development of such movements is definitely linked to the improved control of Parkinsonism. In some cases, it is impossible to relieve the major symptoms of Parkinson's disease without inducing choreiform movements (Cotzias et al., 1969).

Many treated patients alternate between Parkinsonism and chorea several times daily—the "on-off" effect. Others have sudden episodes of akinesia that last for varying periods of time, usually from seconds to minutes ("sudden transient freezing"). It has been suggested that akinesia and the on-off effect may be the result of the accumulation of such condensation products as tetrahydropapaveroline, which is formed by the joining of two molecules of dopamine. These substances can be taken up by peripheral adrenergic terminals and possibly by central ones. If central terminals take them up, their temporary accumulation could cause a buildup of false transmitter in the dopaminergic terminals, and this could explain the sudden development of Parkinson-like symptoms in patients who are taking high doses of L-DOPA. Sometimes these symptoms are alleviated by lowering the dose.

About 10 percent of all patients being treated for Parkinson's disease with L-DOPA experience changes in their mental state that are occasionally severe enough to warrant stopping the medication. These changes include confusion, with paranoid features; frank psychotic breaks; hypomania; agitation; and aggressive-impulsive behavior. The drug also aggravates psychosis in schizophrenics (Yaryura-Tobias et al., 1970). The mechanism by which L-DOPA induces such mental aberrations is not clear.

Analyzing the brains of L-DOPA-treated Parkinsonian patients at autopsy, Hornykiewicz (1970, 1973) found that there was increased dopamine formation in the nervous system wherever DOPA decarboxylase was found, but that the dopamine accumulated only in the basal ganglia. Homovanillic acid levels are very high throughout the brain, which suggests a rapid turnover and a high rate of activity in the conversion of DOPA to dopamine and then to the breakdown product HVA. The HVA/DOPA ratio is higher in the basal ganglia than in the temporal cortex, indicating a higher dopamine turnover rate in the basal ganglia than in the cerebral cortex.

All the changes induced by L-DOPA may not be related to dopamine only, since exogenous L-DOPA affects other brain amines as well. The drug is known to augment the release of serotonin, and dopamine is taken up into serotonergic neurons during L-DOPA therapy. Thus, dopamine derived from exogenous DOPA may, to some degree, act as a false transmitter at serotonin receptor sites, and some of its clinical effects in Parkinsonian patients may be the result of a relative deficiency of serotonin. As noted earlier, brain levels of serotonin (and norepinephrine) are reduced by 50 percent in untreated Parkinsonian patients, and serotonin turnover in Parkinsonian patients is markedly reduced, as 5-HIAA cerebrospinal fluid studies have shown (Chase, 1972). If dopamine, or one of its condensation products, acts as a false transmitter at serotonergic synapses, a deficiency of serotonin could occur. According to the catecholamine hypothesis of depression (see p. 260), this might be expected to induce depression. It is our impression that the development of depression in L-DOPA-treated patients whose Parkinsonian symptoms have been largely relieved is a frequent and unsettling phenomenon, though as yet it is incompletely documented.

L-DOPA does not significantly increase the amount of norepinephrine in the brain, though MHPG levels are elevated diffusely in the central nervous system after treatment with L-DOPA. This indicates an increase in norepinephrine turnover. Exogenous L-DOPA in cats decreases norepinephrine levels in the hypothalamus. This may be the result of a dopamine-induced increase in norepinephrine release. L-DOPA has been shown to induce manic episodes in manic-depressive patients (Murphy et al., 1971). The catecholamine hypothesis of depression is consistent with the concept that increased norepinephrine release could cause a manic episode. Thus, the interaction between the indoleamines and catecholamines is highly complex. An excess of one is likely to lead to increased release and possibly to depletion of the others. This complexity renders tentative any simple theory of the mechanism by which L-DOPA and other drugs used to treat Parkinsonism produce behavioral and neurological changes.

Amantadine

Amantadine, which was first introduced as an antiviral agent, was accidentally found to be active against Parkinsonism. Until recently, its mechanism of action was unknown. Many of its side-effects are similar to those of the anticholinergic drugs. These include dryness of the mouth, difficulty in focusing, insomnia, and psychosis. Nonetheless, the drug has been shown to have no anticholinergic activity. There is good evidence, however, that amantadine increases the release of both dopamine and norepinephrine in the peripheral and central nervous systems. It is similar in this regard to amphetamines but much less potent (Farnebo et al., 1971). The range of its therapeutic efficacy is similar to that of the anticholinergic compounds. The drug appears to be most effective when it is added to an existing treatment regimen consisting of anticholinergic agents or L-DOPA or both (Yahr and Du-Voisin, 1973). Its effects upon depression have not been studied but it can cause a toxic psychosis.

Bromocriptine

Several drugs that are effective in treating Parkinson's disease are thought to stimulate postsynaptic dopaminergic receptors directly. Apomorphine, bromocriptine, and piribedil are three such drugs. Their development came about as the result of a search for agents that can act directly at dopaminergic receptor sites without having to undergo chemical transformation in the brain. Such drugs would not require that presynaptic dopaminergic cells be intact, since they would mimic the action of dopamine at the postsynaptic receptor site. This class of drugs would be of potentially great importance to patients whose Parkinson's disease had progressed to the point at which presynaptic cells were markedly diminished in number. In such patients, the chemical network necessary to convert DOPA to dopamine would not exist, and L-DOPA would be relatively ineffective. Indeed, it has been well established that the anti-Parkinsonian response to L-DOPA diminishes over the course of years and that this agent does not prevent progression of the disease.

The first dopamine agonist ever to be used in clinical practice was apomorphine. In early trials with subcutaneous administration, all the cardinal features of Parkinsonism were alleviated in most patients. The effects of the drug were short-lasting, however, and repeated injections were required. Side-effects, including severe nausea and vomiting as well as hypotension, proved to be a major impediment to the use of apomorphine.

In 1971, Corrodi co-workers introduced piribedil. A double-blind study failed to demonstrate that the drug had a statistically significant action, though tremor seemed to be lessened in a small number of patients. The major dose-limiting factor was the development of involuntary movements (Claveria et al., 1975).

Of the dopamine agonists thus far investigated, bromocriptine appears to be the most effective. It has been reported that some severely disabled patients who could not tolerate L-DOPA or who had failed to experience significant benefit from its use showed significant improvement with bromocriptine (Calne et al., 1974).

The evidence that dopamine agonists actually stimulate post-synaptic dopamine receptors is rather indirect. It is true that all such compounds, in both animals and humans, produce similar effects to those of L-DOPA, and they can reverse the biochemical and behavioral effects of phenothiazines. But detailed studies of the pharmacological properties of dopamine receptors in the central nervous system have proven difficult, due to the absence of a simple model for such receptor sites in the peripheral nervous system. Nonetheless, a biochemical test system that is considered a valid model for testing agonist and antagonist drug interactions with dopamine receptor sites in the central nervous system has been developed. This test is based on the finding that dopamine in low concentrations stimulates the production of cyclic AMP in bovine superior cervical ganglia and other neural tissues. The effects of dopamine on some of these animal tissues are mimicked by drugs thought to be dopamine-receptor stimulators, such as apomorphine, and are antagonized by such neuroleptic drugs as chlor-promazine and haloperidol (Iversen et al., 1975).

Another line of indirect evidence that "dopamine receptor stim-ulators" deserve this label derives from the theory that there is a neuronal feedback loop from cells receiving dopamine input back to the cell body or dendrites of the presynaptic, dopamine-contain-ing neurons. This theory proposes that drugs that block the post-synaptic dopamine receptors increase the firing rate of the presyn-aptic dopamine neurons by "turning off" this negative neuronal feedback loop. Conversely, in such a system, drugs that facilitate the release of dopamine or mimic its postsynaptic action would, by "turning on" the negative feedback loop, decrease the firing rate in the presynaptic dopaminergic cells. Piribedil, bromocriptine, and apomorphine have been shown to stop the firing of dopamine-containing neurons temporarily. This is the effect that would be predicted if a negative neuronal feedback loop existed and if these drugs did directly stimulate postsynaptic dopamine receptors (Wal-ters et al., 1975).

Amphetamines

Of the drugs with minor effects upon Parkinsonism, the amphet-amines have the longest history. Dextro-amphetamine (D-ampheta-mine; Dexedrine) is of mild benefit to patients with Parkinson's disease, but its use for this purpose has been limited by its side-effects and by the development of tolerance. The worst side-effects are cardiovascular, which are particularly dangerous in the aged. More significantly for our discussion, however, is the euphoria in-duced by amphetamines as well as the insomnia, loss of appetite, and occasional toxic psychosis, which closely resembles schizo-phrenia. Levo-amphetamine (L-amphetamine) has very little effect on mood, thought, appetite, or sleep and consequently has not been used much in medical practice.

Amphetamines accelerate the release of catecholamines and in-hibit their reuptake. D-Amphetamine is about ten times more po-tent than L-amphetamine in potentiating the release and inhibiting the uptake of norepinephrine. Both isomers are equally active in facilitating the release and inhibiting the uptake of dopamine (Coyle and Snyder, 1969; Taylor and Snyder, 1970).

When rats are treated with either D- or L-amphetamine, some locomotor stimulation results, D-amphetamine again being ten times more potent than L-amphetamine in producing this effect. The amphetamines also elicit stereotyped compulsive behavior in rats, and both isomers of amphetamine are equally effective here. The locomotor stimulation produced by D-amphetamine has been related to its effect on norepinephrine. The stereotyped behavior elicited by both amphetamines has been related to their effects on dopamine release and reuptake. It is very interesting that inhibition of the rate-limiting enzyme tyrosine hydroxylase by the drug alphamethylparatyrosine, which prevents the synthesis of both dopamine and norepinephrine, also prevents all the behavioral effects of both D- and L-amphetamine (Taylor and Snyder, 1971).

As noted, D-amphetamine is at least ten times more potent than L-amphetamine in eliciting euphoria, anorexia, insomnia, and psychomotor activity in humans. For this reason, the theory has been advanced that D-amphetamine produces these behavioral changes in humans by virtue of its more potent effect on norepinephrine release and reuptake. Both L- and D-amphetamine are equally active in inducing paranoid psychosis in human beings (Snyder, 1972) and in improving the hyperkinetic behavior of children diagnosed as having minimal brain dysfunction (Arnold et al., 1976). These findings have been interpreted as suggestive evidence that both paranoid psychosis and hyperkinetic behavior may be mediated by central dopaminergic mechanisms.

The similar range of their dopaminergic effectiveness suggests that L-amphetamine might be at least as useful as D-amphetamine in Parkinson's disease and would be relatively free of the unpleasant side-effects of D-amphetamine. If this hypothesis were correct, it would also lend credence to the theory that central noradrenergic systems are more involved than dopaminergic systems in the mood, thought, appetite, and sleep changes induced by D-amphetamine. It could be taken as evidence that dopamine is more in-

Table 5-1
Comparison of D-Amphetamine and L-Amphetamine

D-Amphetamine Roughly Equal to L-Amphetamine in:
1. increasing release of dopamine
2. decreasing uptake (inactivation) of dopamine
3. causing stereotyped behavior in rats
4. inducing paranoid psychosis in man

D-Amphetamine Ten Times More Potent than L-Amphetamine in:
1. increasing release of norepinephrine
2. decreasing uptake (inactivation) of norepinephrine
3. causing locomotor stimulation in rats
4. inducing euphoria, insomnia, anorexia, and psychomotor stimulation in man

---

volved in the movement disorder than in the emotional and thought changes induced by D-amphetamine. This hypothesis has been incompletely tested in human beings, but L-amphetamine appears to be quite effective in overcoming the drug-induced side effects in animals that resemble Parkinsonism (Snyder, 1970). D-Amphetamine and L-amphetamine are compared in Table 5-1.

MAO Inhibitors

Monamine oxidase inhibitors, especially tranylcypromine (Parnate) and isocarboxazid (Marplan), have proven useful in treating Parkinson's disease. These drugs probably produce their mild beneficial effect by partially alleviating the cerebral dopamine deficit. Since overactivity of MAO is not a factor in the pathogenesis of Parkinsonism, the MAO inhibitors would not be expected to have a major effect.

Tricyclics

The tricyclic antidepressants (imipramine and amitriptyline) are minimally effective in treating Parkinson's disease when used alone. In combination with other anti-Parkinsonian agents, they may be very beneficial. These drugs act by inhibiting the uptake of norepinephrine and serotonin in peripheral and central neurons (Himwich and Alpers, 1970). Their minor efficacy in relieving the symptoms of Parkinson's disease may reflect the fact that they have very little effect on dopamine reuptake and may derive primarily from their antidepressant effect. Though they are similar to the belladonna drugs in anticholinergic potency, their relative inefficacy in Parkinson's disease makes less tenable the hypothesis that belladonna compounds ameliorate Parkinsonism chiefly by their anticholinergic action.

Parkinsonism-inducing Drugs: Reserpine and Phenothiazines

Reserpine and its related natural and semisynthetic analogues are potent depleters of catecholamines and indoleamines because they interfere with the intraneuronal storage of amines. This marked depletion of dopamine, norepinephrine, and serotonin is the basis for its clinical effects, which are tranquilizing and antipsychotic, though the drug may induce Parkinsonism or depression or both. The other drugs that can induce Parkinsonism, the phenothiazines, haloperidol, and others, have their primary biochemical action at the amine receptor sites where they competitively block receptors. Both dopamine and norepinephrine synthesis is faster after administration of these drugs. This has been interpreted as compensation for the blockade of catecholamine receptor sites. Though the use of phenothiazines is associated with an increase in the total brain-level of catecholamines, the opposite of the reserpine effect, these drugs share with reserpine the crucial action of reducing catecholamine concentration at the postsynaptic receptor site. Like reserpine, they are antipsychotic and tranquilizing but may exacerbate depression and induce Parkinsonism. Pronounced dystonia and other movement disorders are also side-effects of these drugs. If these movement disorders appear soon after medication is started, they can almost always be overcome by the injection of anticholinergic compounds. If phenothiazines must be administered on a long-term basis, control of these drug-induced movement disorders can usually be maintained by the use of an anticholinergic compound.

After months to years of treatment with dopamine receptor

blockers, however, a form of movement disorder known as tardive dyskinesia can develop. This is a socially disabling disorder involving grimacing, chewing, and unsightly movements.

The major symptoms of tardive dyskinesia are abnormal movements of the cheek, face, and tongue, such as lip smacking, chewing, tongue "thrusting," lateral jaw movements, or sucking. Choreaathetoid movements of the extremities and dystonias have also been observed. Most of these symptoms are worsened under emotional stress or during other body movements (Klawans and Barr, 1982; Koller, 1983).

Tardive dyskinesia associated with drug use is most often encountered in elderly women and is often accompanied by evidence of brain damage. The reported incidence in patients receiving phenothiazines chronically varies from 2.9 to 41 percent, probably because of variation in the criteria for diagnosis. Drug use is not the only factor in the development of tardive dyskinesia. A review by Kane and Smith (1982) revealed an average 5 percent prevalence of spontaneous dyskinesias in 19 different samples of untreated psychiatric patients of all diagnoses as compared with a 20 percent incidence in populations treated with neuroleptics. Many of the buccal-lingual movements of tardive dyskinesia can be seen in old people, and particularly in those who are toothless, who have no special history of drug exposure. And many of the characteristic facial movements of tardive dyskinesia were noted in schizophrenics before the advent of phenothiazines (Stevens, 1974). It is possible that tardive dyskinesia could be related to the "soft" neurological signs found in untreated schizophrenics. These signs include choreiform movements and reflect neurological dysfunction in schizophrenics. Furthermore, Granacher (1981) cautions against hastily attributing abnormal movements in a patient on neuroleptics to tardive dyskinesia, as one may overlook the onset or occurrence of other movement disorders.

Regardless of the precise etiology, which is not known, there are many biochemical possibilities. Tardive dyskinesia often becomes worse upon discontinuation of the drugs that are thought to have caused it; the condition will then persist or diminish slowly. Klawans (1970) has postulated that, due to the dopamine blockade produced by phenothiazines and the other major antipsychotic agents, a "denervation" hypersensitivity develops, which especially affects the facilitatory dopamine receptors in the caudate nucleus. This postulate draws its support from the similar response of patients with Huntington's chorea and tardive dyskinesia to certain drugs: both these movement disorders tend to improve with major antipsychotic medication and both can be exacerbated by anticholinergic drugs. It has been hypothesized that the cholinergic system has a counterbalancing effect in the dopamine system with regard to these movement disorders. Antipsychotic drugs that have the least extrapyramidal effect (thioridazine and clozapine) have the greatest muscarinic-cholinergic blocking effect, whereas haloperidol, which has the lowest muscarinic-cholinergic blocking effect, is perhaps the most effective of all these drugs in the treatment of Huntington's chorea, but with the highest incidence of extrapyramidal side-effects (Snyder et al., 1974). This complex dopaminergic-cholinergic balance may explain the varying extrapyramidal side-effects of antipsychotic drugs as well as the efficacy of the drugs that have been used to treat tardive dyskinesia and Huntington's chorea. Drugs that increase dopaminergic activity, such as L-DOPA, amphetamine, apomorphine, and amantadine, increase the abnormal movements in both conditions; drugs that block or deplete dopamine, such as phenothiazines, haloperidol, and reserpine, all have been variably reported to ameliorate these movements in both conditions. There is some evidence that tardive dyskinesia is associated with a neuroleptic-induced increase in dopamine receptors and in their binding of dopamine (Bacopoulos, 1984). Conversely, drugs that decrease cholinergic activity, such as atropine and benztropine, increase the hyperkinetic movement disorders; drugs that increase cholinergic activity, such as physostigmine, ameliorate these movements. It has been suggested that these differences in drug response are related to cellular hypersensitivity to dopamine in tardive dyskinesia and Huntington's chorea and to a decrease in the number of presynaptic dopaminergic cells that leads to a relative dopamine depletion in Parkinson's disease.

Alphamethylparatyrosine

Alphamethylparatyrosine (α-MPT) inhibits tyrosine hydroxylase and thus blocks the synthesis of both norepinephrine and dopamine. It has also been shown to induce Parkinsonism (Birkmayer, 1969) and ameliorate chorea (Chase, 1973) and the manic phase of manic-depressive illness (Bunney et al., 1971); it potentiates the effect of phenothiazines in schizophrenia.

Intellectual and Emotional Changes in Parkinson's Disease

In his original description of the disease, James Parkinson excluded intellectual change as one of the discriminating symptoms. In light of the clinical and biochemical similarity between Parkinsonism and depression (see p. 218), one might expect depressive symptoms to be more prominent in Parkinsonian patients. In this regard, Schwab and others (1951) reported on the incidence of psychiatric symptoms in 200 patients who had Parkinson's disease for over five years. They noted four types of psychiatric complications in these patients: (1) psychiatric disease, which was assumed to be unrelated to Parkinson's disease, because it existed before the onset of the Parkinsonian symptoms; (2) "reactive" depression; (3) syndromes secondary to medication, especially psychotomimetic symptoms with anticholinergic drugs; (4) paroxysmal disorders that he felt were specifically related to Parkinson's disease.

Paroxysmal disorders were most often noted in patients who also had oculogyric crises. These patients had depressive feelings and anxiety attacks, even when there was no prior history or clear precipitating event. The anxiety attacks were terrifying to the patients, particularly when accompanied by feelings of imminent death. They were usually relieved by anti-Parkinsonian medication rather than by antianxiety drugs. Schwab also described attacks of compulsive thinking, counting, and word use; paranoid feelings; "strange feelings" in the limbs; and states of agitation, tension, and chronic fatigue. What was perhaps most noteworthy about these symptoms was their brevity and "attacklike" quality.

Mindham (1970) studied 89 patients with Parkinson's disease

admitted to a psychiatric hospital and noted that 90 percent of these patients showed a depressive mood disorder.

Though it is clear there are mood changes in Parkinson's disease, it is not clear if there are intellectual changes. Garron and co-workers (1972) found that patients with marked akinesia beginning late in life suffered more intellectual deterioration than a group with less pronounced akinesia and earlier onset. Donnelly and Chase (1973) did not confirm the finding of intellectual deterioration but noted that after L-DOPA treatment, full-scale IQ and memory function as measured by the WAIS increased. The improvement was evident both at 1 month and 17 months after the initiation of treatment. They found no relation between intellectual dysfunction and any motor difficulty.

In dealing with supposed mental changes in Parkinsonian patients, one of the major problems is that the etiology of the disease varies and some of the diseases that cause Parkinsonism, such as arteriosclerosis, also cause dementia. Another problem is that the older patient with Parkinsonism is likely to be senile or to have suffered intellectual deterioration caused by some process independent of that causing Parkinsonism (Mayeux, 1981). Indeed, there has been increased awareness of organic brain syndromes in patients with Parkinson's disease. Sorka and others (1981) noted that patients with both Parkinson's disease and organic brain syndromes had a 90 percent incidence of cortical atrophy on CT scanning, while only 15 percent of the Parkinson patients with only extrapyramidal symptoms had such cerebral atrophy. The etiology of the dementia is unclear; patients with Parkinson's disease share certain neuropathological features with patients suffering from senile dementia of the Alzheimer type including a selective loss of cells in the nucleus basalis of Meynert (Baller et al., 1980; Whitehouse et al., 1983; Nakaro and Hirano, 1983), but there are subtle differences in the neurofibrillary tangles of the two conditions (Yenchl, 1983). These do not seem to be related to lesions of the basal ganglia as there is no significant loss of neurons from the nucleus basilis of Meynert in Huntington's disease (Clark et al., 1983).

Rikland and Levita (1969) studied a large group of patients in whom neurosurgical ablations of various portions of the extrapyramidal tract for movement disorders had been performed. The patients who showed the greatest intellectual changes after destruction of these areas were those who had bilateral rather than unilateral operations. In the immediate postoperative period, there was a general decline in intellectual functioning, diminished drive and productivity, and loss of perceptual motor integration; in other words, the nonspecific organic brain syndrome that results from lesions anywhere in the cerebral hemispheres (see Ch. 4). Patients with ablations in the left hemisphere showed greater loss of verbal functioning than those with ablations in the right hemisphere. The right hemisphere group showed more changes in emotional reactivity. At six month follow-up, however, all the patients seemed to return to their preoperative level of functioning. The patients with bilateral lesions, however, not only took longer to recover at follow-up but seemed to have decreased initiative and motivation.

CHOREA

Clinical Features and Physiological Considerations

Chorea consists of involuntary jerky movements of the face, tongue, extremities, especially the distal portions, and even the trunk and respiratory muscles in some patients. Choreatic movements are rapid and irregular, and they become more pronounced during voluntary movement and attempts to maintain a posture. Patients with chorea tend to "cover up" their disability by blending the pseudopurposeful choreatic movements with normal voluntary movements. Sometimes, while walking, a patient may show a slight lilt to his gait and will appear to be dancing. Choreatic movements can sometimes be revealed by having a patient squeeze the examiner's fingers. The choreatic movements of the patient's fingers that this accentuates gives the examiner the sensation of being milked, hence the term "milkmaid's sign." Patients with chorea are often unable to maintain protrusion of the tongue, and when they put their arms above their heads, choreatic movements of the upper extremities are maximized and the hands tend to pronate (pronator's sign). Choreatic movements superimposed on deep tendon reflexes cause the relaxation phase of the reflex to be discontinuous (hung-up reflexes).

Chorea and the slower writhing movements of athetosis (with which it is often associated and from which it cannot always be clearly distinguished) may be manifestations of one of several diseases: perinatal brain injury, encephalitis, vascular disease, hypoparathydroidism, Wilson's disease, and rarely, brain tumor.

Huntington's chorea is a degenerative disease of the brain involving the cortical mantle as well as the basal ganglia. Because of the prominent involvement of the caudate nucleus and putamen in this disease, it has been suggested that chorea may be related to pathology of the striatum. It would, however, be a mistake to identify chorea with pathology of the striatum solely, because of the extensive striatal connections to the caudate, globus pallidus, and thalamus. Chorea may be the result of an interruption of or imbalance between other neural systems, for example, inhibitory and excitatory motor pathways, in the striatal-pallidal-thalamic circuit. Carrea and Mettler (1955) produced transitory choreatic activity in monkeys by placing bilateral lesions in the superior cerebellar peduncles. Unilateral lesions of the ventral-lateral thalamus and subthalamic nuclei in man and in monkeys sometimes produce choreatic movements. Chorea in such cases is believed to be the result of a loss of inhibiting influences on the globus pallidus. Lesions in the dorsal caudate and putamen have been described in oral-facial dyskinesia, a kind of localized chorea (Altrocchi and Forno, 1983).

Virtually all the diseases in which chorea occurs may be associated with severe emotional disturbance. Roughly half of the patients with Huntington's chorea present with psychiatric symptoms and half develop psychosis at some point in the illness. Of these patients, 25 percent are indistinguishable from schizophrenics (Heathfield, 1967). Emotional disturbances frequently accompany Sydenham's chorea and may persist for many years (Freeman et al.,

1965). Action tremor and residual chorea also persist for years, but half such patients who have no sequelae have the onset of adverse choreic reactions to drugs such as stimulants and anorectics. Such patients also show significant elevations in the psychotic tetrad of the MMPI, suggesting persistent dopaminergic sensitivity in Sydenham survivors (Nanseida et al., 1983). Psychosis and signs of dementia may be prominent in Wilson's disease; and in encephalitis, of course, emotional changes are common. All the conditions that cause chorea involve the brain diffusely, and emotional changes are not always present. These changes derive from involvement of parts of the nervous system that have little or no relation to those which give rise to chorea. Psychosis is thus a frequent, though not a constant, concomitant of chorea.

Effect of Medications

The drugs that help alleviate chorea can induce Parkinsonism, that is, reserpine, phenothiazines, and the other major tranquilizers and α-MPT. As noted above, all these drugs reduce catecholamine concentrations at their rector sites; reserpine by lowering catecholamine concentrations throughout the nervous system, phenothiazines and related compounds by competitively blocking catecholamine at receptor sites, and α-MPT by blocking catecholamine synthesis.

Drugs that potentiate catecholamine activity increase the choreatic activity. These include belladonna compounds (Aquilonius and Sjöström, 1971; Kalawans and Rubovits, 1972); and imipramine (Whittier et al., 1961). Of the drugs that make chorea worse, L-DOPA is by far the most important. About half of all patients receiving L-DOPA in therapeutic doses for Parkinson's disease develop a choreatic movement disorder. L-DOPA has been shown to make the movement disorder in patients with Huntington's chorea worse, and this has led to the suggestion that it might be useful in the detection of presymptomatic Huntington's chorea. Klawans et al. (1972) gave low to moderate doses of L-DOPA to the asymptomatic offspring of patients with Huntington's chorea. Roughly one-third developed chorea, and it was assumed that these individuals were carriers of a gene for the disease and would develop it in time. Follow-up studies have not been completed.

Though the effects of amphetamines upon chorea have not been systematically studied, patients who have taken overdoses of amphetamines, either acutely or chronically, may develop symptoms of restlessness, tremor, motor impersistence, and "jumpiness," which strongly resemble choreiform movements. Motor signs of amphetamine overdosage are minor in comparison with the abnormal mental state produced by amphetamine intoxication, however.

Since chorea is improved by drugs that have an antidopaminergic effect and made worse or induced by drugs that augment catecholamine activity, it has been hypothesized that chorea is the result of excessive dopaminergic activity or sensitivity. The pharmacological evidence that suggests that the extrapyramidal signs and symptoms of Huntington's chorea may be related to a hypersensitivity of dopamine receptors in the striatum to endogenous dopamine has ben summarized by Klawans (1970). When the brains of patients with Huntington's chorea are examined at autopsy, the basal ganglia, and especially the caudate and putamen, are characteristically depleted of neurons. Despite this serious loss of neurons, the dopamine content of the putamen and globus pallidus per gram of remaining tissue has been found to be normal and that of the caudate reduced to approximately 60 percent of normal. Since the number of neurons per gram is greatly reduced in Huntington's chorea in these regions, it has been hypothesized that each remaining striatal neuron in this disease may be exposed to a relative excess of dopamine. Alternatively, it has been suggested that a change of dopaminergic balance in the basal ganglia occurs, in which the pallidum and putamen are favored over the caudate, and that a relative dopaminergic excess in the putamen-pallidum system causes chorea (Bernheimer and Hornykiewicz,, 1973). In summary, there is pharmacological and some biochemical evidence that chorea is the result of excess dopamine or excessive sensitivity to dopamine. According to this view, chorea is pathophysiologically and biochemically the opposite of Parkinsonism (Klawans, 1970).

Although the basic defect that gives rise to Huntigton's chorea is not known, Gusella and co-workers (1983), by using recominant DNA techniques, have isolated fragments on choromosome 4 (near a single autosomal dominant allele) that transmit Huntington's disease. This work involved only two families, but it holds promise of developing a test for presymptomatic individuals at risk for Huntington's disease (Gumby, 1984).

Though an absolute or a relative dopamine excess may be responsible for the symptom of chorea so prominently seen in Huntington's chorea, this genetic disease is almost certainly the result of a primary inborn error of metabolism that is not related to any of the enzymes involved in the synthesis or degradation of dopamine. The diffuse degeneration of neurons that are not dopaminergic supports this conclusion. Investigators interested in Huntingtion's chorea have recently concentrated on other transmitter substances, chiefly the powerful inhibitory substance gamma-aminobutyric acid (GABA). This compound is synthesized from glutamic acid by glutamic acid decarboxylase. Tissue levels of this enzyme have been measured in several areas of choreic brain tissue; and a deficiency has been found only in the basal ganglia. In contrast, tyrosine hydroxylase was not found to be deficient in the brain tissue of patients with Huntington's chorea examined postmortem. This confers some degree of specificity on the reduction of glutamic acid decarboxylase, since the structural changes induced by Huntington's chorea are maximal in the caudate nucleus; but this finding is of uncertain significance in the pathogenesis of the movement disorder. Consistent with these findings is the report by Glaeser and others (1975) of low GABA levels in the cerebrospinal fluid of patients with Huntington's chorea, compared with controls.

In recent years, drug therapy of several disparate movement disorders has become possible. Insights into the mechanism of action of these drugs may ultimately provide clues to the pathogenesis of the disorders. Some of this information is summarized in Table 5.2.

Table 5-2

Movement Disorder	Medication	Presumed Mechanism of Action
Dystonia	Belladonna (Fahn, 1979)	Anticholinergic
Myoclonus (nonepileptic)	Valproic acid (Sotaniemi, 1982)	GABA agonist
Essential tremor	Propanalol (Calzetti et al., 1983)	Adrenergic blocker
Oral facial dyskinesia (Meige's syndrome)	Baclofen (Gollomps et al., 1983)	GABA-mimetic
	Tetrabenezine ⎫	Dopamine depletion
	Trihexyphenidyl ⎬ (Jankovic and Ford, 1983)	Anticholinergic
	Lithium ⎭	Norepinephrine uptake stimulator
Tardive dyskinesia	Tetrabenazine (Fahn, 1983)	Dopamine depletion

DEPRESSION

The fact that many drugs and neurotransmitters that improve or worsen Parkinson's disease are also effective in treating or inducing depression suggests that the two disorders may have a similar biochemical background. Though this is an inadequate basis for conclusions about the etiology of depression, there is good clinical and pharmacological evidence for the existence of biochemical disturbance in affective disorders. In recent years, research has been more fruitful in elucidating biochemical aspects of depression than of any other psychiatric disorder.

Clinical Features and Nosology

The major phenomenology of affective illness (depression or mania) is mood disturbance. Depressed feelings are usually described as sadness, feeling "blue," "low," or gloomy. Because of the ubiquity of these feelings, it is not clear when they should be considered pathological. Usually, this judgment is made on clinical grounds by weighing such factors as the severity of the symptoms, the amount of interference with the functioning of the individual, the duration of the symptoms, the age at which they occur, the number of similar episodes previously experienced by the patient, and the presence of a family history of similar disturbances. Because it is so difficult to quantify most of these factors diagnostic confusion often occurs, and this has resulted in an impressive diversity of classications used for depressive disorders. In the literature one finds such adjectives for depression as psychotic, neurotic, endogenous, reactive, agitated, retarded, involutional, and postpartum. These distinctions are descriptive, deriving primarily from the etiological theory the author espouses.

Most classifications that impute etiological differences to different states of depression must be tentative in our present state of knowledge (Blumenthal et al., 1971). Even the common distinction between reactive (psychological) and endogenous (biological) depression seems arbitrary, for every depressive state must have both a psychological and a biological component. Findings that usually lead to the classification of depression as reactive are the presence of precipitating factors, a history of previous neurotic traits, good insight, early night sleep disturbance, and emotional lability. The factors invoked to support the diagnosis of endogenous depression are delusions, psychomotor retardation, diurnal variation, and a family history of depression. This distinction between reactive and endogenous depression creates some problems. (1) The significance of a particular life event to which an individual is supposed to be reacting is determined only after he becomes depressed. Thus, the causal relationship between the depression and the event presumed to have caused it is a matter a of post hoc reasoning. It is seldom possible to predict whether an individual will become significantly depressed after a particular event. Since depressed patients frequently distort life events or overemphasize their unfavorable side, these allegedly causal events may actually be a product of the depressive feelings themselves. Fogarty and Hensley (1983) have demonstrated that mood influences the retrieval of memories that were encoded during similar mood states; thus, the depressed patient is more likely to recall events from periods of depression. A number of life events inventories, developed from discussions with depressed patients, aim to identify and weigh (with a point score) the type of experience that is likely to cause reactive depression (Cochrane and Robertson, 1973). Such distressing events as job loss, divorce, death of a loved one, and physical illness, however, are so common that one might think the majority of the population would be suffering from depression as a reaction to them. (2) The diversity in individuals' reactions to events that might be expected to evoke depression indicates that preexisting constitutional factors determine the timing and severity of "reactive" depression, and these constitutional factors are, of course, endogenous. (3) The use of the terms reactive and endogenous by clinicians frequently depends more on the severity of the symptoms than on the precipitating factors. If a patient's symptomatology is only moderate, not psychotic, and his functioning is not markedly impaired, the clinician frequently and arbitrarily will classify the depression as reactive. The severity of illness is not always a logical basis for this distinction because many patients suffering episodes of psychotic depression also experience episodes of milder depression, and both the mild and severe forms respond to antidepressant medications. Consequently, it is not likely that the distinction between "reactive" and "endogenous" depressions reflects a different biochemical pathogenesis. They are not necessarily different conditions, but different points on a spectrum of severity. Kendell (1968) has shown in longitudinal and cross-sectional studies of depressed patients that use of the labels "reactive" and "endogenous" or "neurotic" and "psychotic" often emphasizes the extremes of a symptomatic continuum and ignores the middle ground.

There are three types of depressive symptoms: (1) disturbance of mood; (2) alteration in the person's perception of himself and the environment surrounding him; and (3) biological disturbances. Patients with altered mood are aware that their mood has changed. In moderate or severe depressions, patients perceive themselves as being worthless, hopeless, helpless, guilty, even at times "evil." Frequently they view their accomplishments as meaningless and neither persuasion nor confrontation with reality can change their attitude. If they are delusional, the delusions usually relate to ideas of bodily illness, decay, or other dismal eventualities. Severe depression can be accompanied by paranoid delusions and even hallucinations. Differentiation from schizophrenia in such cases depends on the presence of depression, a relatively normal premorbid adjustment, and a family history of affective disorder. In manic conditions, we see the obverse of depressive feelings: euphoria, grandiosity, and a heightened sense of one's abilities. Among the body functions that may be disrupted are sleep, appetite, digestion, sexual activity, and psychomotor activity. Sleep disturbances are often manifested as hyposomnia, difficulty in falling asleep, awakening frequently throughout the night, early morning awakening, or any combination of these. Many depressed patients sleep excessively (hypersomnia). Anorexia and weight loss or hyperphagia and weight gain are common. Decreased sexual interest and activity are the rule. Changes in psychomotor function, either agitation or retardation, are frequently evident. Agitated patients seem anxious, wring their hands, pace about, and frequently sleep poorly. Psychomotor retardation is characterized by reduced physical and mental activity and often by hypersomnia. The slowing of thought processes in retarded depressions may suggest dementia (McAllister, 1983). Suicidal ideation is usually prominent in severe depression.

If the symptoms of depression are *present in mild form and transiently* (not lasting more than one to, at most, six months) and closely follow emotionally charged events (usually loss of job, health, or a loved one), the reaction may be considered to be grief (Parkes, 1970). If the symptoms are severe, regardless of the presence of precipitating factors, if they persist, and if they interfere with the patient's functioning from day to day, the condition should be regarded as depressive illness and should be treated. The severity of a depressive syndrome is best characterized by summing up the symptoms rather than weighing individual symptoms. Scales for quantitating the severity and variety of affective symptoms have been devised (Hamilton, 1969; Beck et al., 1961; Zung, 1965). We have found such a phenomenological classification to be quite useful. It is a relatively reliable method of judging the severity of depression, following the course of the disorder, and evaluating therapy.

The duration and tendency of depression to recur as well as the severity of symptoms vary from patient to patient. In some patients, depression occurs as a single episode in an otherwise normal life. Most patients having their first depression have no family history of depression. When the family history is negative, there is no way of predicting the course of illness. The chances are that a remission will occur and that the symptoms will respond to antidepressant medication. There is probably a greater likelihood that such a patient will again become depressed in the future than someone of the same age and sex who has never been clinically depressed, but information on this point is sketchy.

Other patients have repeated episodes of affective disorder and their illnesses may be divided into two groups:

1. UNIPOLAR—manifested by repeated depressive (or rarely manic) episodes.
2. BIPOLAR—characterized by repeated episodes of both mania and depression. In some bipolar patients, mania is more prevalent, almost to the exclusion of depression, though the opposite may occur. In such cases, the diagnosis of bipolarity rests on other clinical characteristics and genetic data. Family studies indicate that whereas both unipolar and bipolar depressions are familial, there is no genetic overlap between the two; that is, bipolar illness does not occur in the families of monopolar probands and vice versa. The parents and siblings of bipolar patients have a 20 percent risk of bipolar illness, and the parents and siblings of unipolar patients (defined in these studies as patients with more than three episodes of depression) have a 12 to 14 percent risk of unipolar illness (Slater and Cowie, 1971).

The mode by which recurrent depressive disorders are inherited is not clear, but the fact that they are inherited is virtually indisputable. Twin studies of the affective disorders have been limited to bipolar illness, which affects less than 1 percent of the general population. A review of these studies indicates that the all-over concordance rate for bipolar disease is 72 percent in monozygotic pairs and 19 percent in same-sex dizygotic pairs (not age corrected). In Kallman's series, concordance rates for monozygotic pairs reached 96 percent (Kallman 1950, 1954).

Other differences distinguish unipolar and bipolar depression. The sex ratio in bipolar illness is one to one, but unipolar depression is twice as common in females as in males. Color blindness and the Xg blood group have been linked with bipolar but not unipolar illness (Winokur et al., 1971); however, there are as many studies now that report no link (Gershon, 1983). Recently there have been reports of HLA association with depressive illness (Weitkamp, 1981), but others have not found this association (Crowe, 1981). The entire area of genetic and genetically transmitted marker research has become so statistical and based so heavily on complex probability models that it almost defies simple statements about relationships (Gershon, 1983). Unless the association is so overwhelming most of these studies have equal numbers of positive and negative studies and adherents. The average age at the time of occurrence of the first episode of unipolar depression severe enough to require hospitalization is 45; bipolar depressions of such severity first occur on the average at age 30 (Detre and Jarecki, 1971). In a review of follow-up studies of unipolar and bipolar affective disorders, Robins and Guze (1972) noted that the median duration of the first attack of a depressive illness varied. In unipolar depression, it was 13 months; in bipolar depressions, 6½ months. The mean duration of manic attacks was 3½ months. Individual unipolar depressions last longer than bipolar ones, but relapse is less likely. Between episodes of illness, unipolar patients tend to be insecure, sensitive, or obsessional, whereas bipolar patients tend to be more active and sociable. Beigel and Murphy (1971) compared the clinical characteristics of the depressive state in 25 patients with bipolar illness and in 25 patients with unipolar illness. Patients were observed for a 14-day, drug-free period in a research ward during which time mania was absent. Greater physical activity, more overt expressions of anger, and more somatic complaints distinguished the unipolar from the bipolar patients, who tended to be less active and more socially withdrawn. The difference was statistically significant. Some authors have emphasized the tendency of unipolar depressives to be agitated with hyposomnia and bipolar depressives to be retarded with hypersomnia (Detre et al., 1972).

In summary, we believe that depression falls into the following general categories: (1) grief reactions; (2) nonrecurrent depression, which may or may not occur in relation to environmental stresses; and (3) hereditary, recurrent affective disorder, either bipolar (manic-depressive) or unipolar; (4) longstanding dysphoric states (Akiskal, 1983). This categorization is arbitrary and does not conform precisely to DSM-III, but it does have clinical value.

Biological Changes in Depression

It is often difficult to interpret biological studies of depression because of the varied diagnostic categories. Only recently have such clear phenomenological distinctions as unipolar and bipolar depression been made. Therefore, earlier studies and studies lacking clear, clinical descriptions must be interpreted with caution. Recently, the soft signs of diffuse neurological dysfunction and the electroencephalographic abnormalities, so often present in schizophrenic patients, are now also being reported in patients with affective disorder (McAllister, 1983). Previously, patients with such features were diagnosed as having "pseudodementia" (see Ch. 4, p. 185). However, it is clear that many of these signs of central nervous system dysfunction are present in affective disorders and that most of them remit as the depressive illness abates. There is little or no EEG change in bipolar patients when they go from depression to mania or vice versa.

Since Sacher (1967) found that depressed patients have elevated blood and urine levels of corticosteroids, there has been a flood of investigations of neuroendocrine factors in affective illness. After many years of study, Carroll and colleagues (1981) published a paper with the firm title "A Specific Laboratory Test for the Diagnosis of Melancholia." This paper demonstrated that patients with affective disorders fail to suppress cortisol excretion as would a normal person when given dexamethasone. Thus, it not only confirmed Sacher's original findings but also pointed to some defect in the hypothalamic-pituitary-end-organ interaction. As with many studies of psychopathologic conditions, when the control group was extended to other types of psychiatric patients rather than just normals, the positive findings became less definitive. Cortisol nonsuppression after dexamethasone has now been noted in a wide range of conditions, including normal health, old age, dementia, obsessive-compulsive disorders, alcoholism, and weight loss (Spar, 1982; Amsterdam, 1982; Insel, 1982; American College of Physicians, 1984). There does seem to be evidence that the test may correlate with therapeutic outcome in that patients with affective disorder who still fail to suppress after treatment have a poorer prognosis (Nemeroff and Evans, 1984). While it is clear that the dexamethasone suppression test (DST) is not a specific biologic test of depression, it is also clear that in affective illness there is sometimes a disturbance of cortisol metabolism. This metabolic disturbance often responds to treatment in tandem with remission of the affective symptoms.

Though disturbance of cortisol metabolism may be a secondary effect related to the stress of a depressive illness, it is noteworthy that elevated steroid levels may affect the metabolism of biogenic amines (Curzon, 1971). Coppen (1967) has documented increased intracellular sodium concentration in both depressed and manic states. It has also been shown that lithium, which is interchangeable with sodium, decreases the intracellular exchange of sodium and normalizes the corticosteroid disturbance. This may be related to the effect of lithium in alleviating mania and depression. In depressed states, it has been shown that there is, in general, diminished secretion of gastric juice and saliva, reduced peristalsis, and a lower basal metabolic rate.

The possibility of another kind of neuroendocrine disturbance in affective disorders is raised by extensive studies of serum thyrotropin response (TSH) to a dose of thyrotropin-releasing hormone

(TRH), which have consistently shown aberrant responses in depressed patients. Many depressed patients who have normal T_3 and T_4 blood levels will have diminished or blunted TSH response to TRH stimulation (Loosen and Prange, 1982). Other neuroendocrine correlations have been found between major depressive illness and growth hormone, prolactin, gonadol hormones, CRH, melatonin, all of which have been shown to have diminished responses to usual stimulations in sub groups of affective disorders (Lewey et al., 1982; Rubin and Marder, 1983; Gold et al., 1984; Kupfer and Thase, 1983).

Hypothalamic dysfunction in depression is further suggested by sleep disturbances, slowed heart rate, lowered body temperature, loss of weight and appetite, disturbances of the menstrual cycle, and impotence and frigidity (Hill, 1968; Pollitt, 1965). A general state of hyperarousal has been demonstrated in the depressed patient. Some studies (Whatmore and Ellis, 1962) in depressed patients have shown both elevated galvanic skin responses and muscle tension (Whybrow and Mendels, 1969). Buchsbaum and colleagues (1971) noted that depressed patients tended to augment the intensity of incoming stimuli.

Sleep disturbance is one of the most consistent features of depressive illness. In general, it parallels depression in severity. Conventional wisdom in the past, supported mainly by clinical impressions, identified early morning awakening with depressive psychosis (Noyes and Kolb, 1963), involutional melancholia (English and Finch, 1954), and endogenous depression (Kiloh and Garside, 1963) as opposed to neurotic or reactive depression in which a difficulty in falling asleep was supposed to be characteristic. In more recent, quantitative, EEG-controlled studies, the clinical impression of early morning awakening as a distinguishing feature of these "different types" of depression was not borne out (Hawkins and Mendels, 1966), though hyposomnia was found to be a characteristic of most depressive illness. This is manifested as early-morning wakefulness, a longer latency of sleep onset, and a decrease in nonrapid-eye-movement sleep, both absolute and relative to total sleep. In contrast to other forms of depressive illness, the depressive phase of bipolar depressive illness is often characterized by increased total sleep and increased relative and total time spent in the rapid-eye-movement (REM) stage of sleep. During the manic phase, total sleep time is always lower as is the percentage in the REM phase (E. Hartmann, 1968; Detre et al., 1972). Recent studies seem to confirm the diagnostic utility of shortened latency (appearance) of the first REM sleep period in 60 to 90 percent of moderately to severely depressed patients. While conditions such as narcolepsy, drug and alcohol withdrawal, and dementia show a similar pattern, this shortened REM latency may be emerging as a consistent finding in major affective disorders (Kupfer, 1983).

An interesting hypothesis stimulated in part by sleep studies of affective disorders is that some depressive illness may reflect a disturbance of circadian rhythms. Wehr and Goodwin (1981) found diurnal variation in severity of symptoms, seasonal fluctuation of symptoms, and—in some patients—distinct patterns of REM sleep, body temperature, and cortisol excretion. They postulated that in these patients the normal phases of such biologic functions have been advanced and that depressive symptoms can be ameliorated when the biological clocks are corrected (Rosenthal et al., 1984). Other studies, however, indicate that these circadian changes may represent a blunted diurnal response rather than a phase advance (Avery, 1982).

Biochemical studies of depression have attempted to show that the level of brain amines, especially norepinephrine, is low. Five different groups of researchers have investigated the urinary excretion of 3-methoxy,5-hydroxyphenylethylene glycol (MHPG) in bipolar (manic-depressive) patients. Four found that these patients excreted less MHPG during periods of depression than they did during periods of either normal mood or hypomania. In two of these studies, it was noted that the increments in urinary MHPG preceded the shift in the behavioral status of patients from depression to mania (Maas, 1975). Further evidence was provided by Post et al. (1973), who measured MHPG in the spinal fluid of patients with moderately severe depression, comparing them with normal and neurological controls, including patients with Parkinson's disease. All the factors known to influence MHPG levels in the spinal fluid, such as diet, sleep, medication, and physical activity, were controlled. Depressed patients were found to have a significantly lower MHPG in the spinal fluid. These findings, however, were not reproduced by another group performing a similar study (Shopsin et al., 1973). Furthermore, the value of MHPG as a marker or a guide to treatment has been questioned on the grounds that the supposedly low MHPG levels found in depressed patients actually fall within the normal range (Kewala et al., 1983; Hollister, 1981); it has only been through the use of complex statistical methods that some minimal utility for MHPG as a diagnostic or treatment guide has been maintained (Schildkraut, 1983).

The possible influence of affective disorders on immune responses is receiving increasing attention (Rogers, Dubey, and Reich, 1979; Ader, 1983), and one hears the term "psychoneuroimmunology" more often nowadays. Schleifer and colleagues (1983) reported suppression of lymphocyte response in bereaved males. The possibility of a relationship between disturbed immune function and affective disorder is also suggested by the increasing number of reports of major affective and cognitive symptoms in patients with multiple sclerosis (Whittock and Sisking, 1980; Schiffer et al., 1983). While these are mostly anecdotal, the depression seems so profound as to be more than a reaction to the disease. In some instances the affective symptoms have preceded the occurrence of neurological symptoms (Dalos, 1983).

In summary, then, depressed patients commonly undergo a decrease in many physiological functions in their responsiveness to a wide range of stimuli. This is accompanied by a heightened state of arousal, which may be experienced by the patient as anxiety or tension.

Although DSM-III has made the diagnosis of affective disorders more reliable, the validity of the DSM-III categorization of affective disorders (bipolar, unipolar, psychotic and nonpsychotic, chronic [dysthymic], etc.) is still tentative. Affective illnesses are probably very heterogeneous with regard to etiology. For example, a unipolar depression and the depressive phase of bipolar illness are phenomenologically indistinguishable, but their chains of causation are probably quite different, a phenomenon that may represent the limited number of responses of the central nervous system to different stresses. With DSM-III and the increased interest in nosology, we are probably on the threshold of studies of more homogeneous subtypes of depression and with this homogeneity should come more consistent biologic findings.

Treatment

In any evaluation of the treatment of depression, there are two prevailing difficulties: the above-mentioned absence of a definitive classification of depression and the fact that even chronic, recurrent depressive illnesses usually have time-limited episodes. Nevertheless, the therapeutic efficacy of the tricyclic antidepressants imipramine and amitriptyline) is well substantiated. Sixty to 70 percent of depressed patients benefit from the use of these drugs (Paykel and Coppen, 1979; Jacobson and McKinney, 1980; Davis, 1985), whether they are older patients with endogenous psychotic depressions or young patients with "reactive" depressions (Wittenborn et al., 1962; Abraham et al., 1963).

The major untoward reactions associated with the use of tricyclic antidepressants (dry mouth, blurred vision, and urinary retention) can be attributed to their anticholinergiclike effect. Occasionally, a full-blown encephalopathy with thought disorder and seizures has been reported (Davies et al., 1971). Imipramine, though sometimes helpful in relieving the rigidity of patients with Parkinson's disease, has been known to aggravate the tremor. Imipramine has also been reported to aggravate chorea in depressed patients with Huntington's chorea (Whittier et al., 1961).

The tricyclic antidepressants were originally hypothesized as exerting their effects through inhibition of norepinephrine reuptake in the peripheral and central noradrenergic neurons. It has been demonstrated, however, that the reuptake of serotonin can also be blocked by the tricyclic antidepressants (Sulser and Sanders-Bush, 1971). The question arises whether the clinical antidepressant activity of this class of drugs is more closely related to their effects on serotonin or norepinephrine neurons. It has been suggested that tricyclic inhibition of norepinephrine reuptake may produce the psychomotor effect, whereas the drugs' inhibition of serotonin reuptake may be responsible for the brightening of mood in depressed patients (Carlsson et al., 1969). It has also been suggested that the therapeutic response depends on the relationship between norepinephrine and serotonin content on the brain (Schildkraut, 1970, 1973).

Not all depressed patients respond to tricyclic drugs, and some respond to imipramine but not amitriptyline or vice versa. This has led to a theory that depressed patients can be divided on the basis of biochemical and pharmacological criteria into two subgroups: those who respond favorably to imipramine but not to amitriptyline; and those who respond favorably to amitriptyline. The first group, it is claimed, suffer from depression of the central norepinephrine system. The second group is presumed to suffer from a depression of the serotonergic system (Maas, 1975).

In our view, any attempt to classify depression by the patients' response to drugs is premature unless blood levels of the drugs being used are determined (Risch et al., 1979). No such study has been performed to date. Such "mundane" issues as uncertain administration, poor absorption, and rapid metabolism or excretion of antidepressant drugs must be ruled out before a therapeutic failure can be ascribed to a specific limitation in the drug's spectrum of brain amine interactions. In the absence of blood drug levels, no conclusions concerning the etiology of depression can be securely based on therapeutic results.

There is general agreement that episodes of mania can be brought to an end within 10 days by the administration of lithium carbonate and that chronic lithium therapy prevents the recurrence of manic episodes in most individuals suffering from bipolar disease. Of the manic patients, 80 percent show distinct improvement after the initial lag period. The more certain the diagnosis of mania, the more likely the therapeutic response (Davis et al., 1973). Longitudinal studies of a large group of manic-depressive patients (Baastrup and Schou, 1967) showed that the average relapse rate was once every eight months. After the institution of lithium treatment, the relapse rate dropped to once every 60 months. When lithium treatment was stopped, almost all the patients had relapses within three to four months (Baastrup and Schou, 1967). Studies by Angst et al. (1970), Small et al. (1971), and a carefully controlled double-blind study by Baastrup et al. (1970) confirmed the above findings, indicating that lithium is an effective prophylactic in preventing relapses of a manic nature.

Whether lithium is effective as a prophylactic drug against depression is not yet known. The studies cited above indicate that lithium helps prevent relapses of depression in bipolar patients. Another study, performed in double-blind fashion over a 16-month period, showed no reduction in the frequency of depressive attacks in bipolar patients taking lithium (Dunner et al., 1976). It has also been reported that lithium reduces the frequency of recurrent unipolar depressions (Fieve et al., 1975; Quitkin et al., 1976). These studies, though double-blind, should be repeated before lithium can be accepted as an effective prophylactic agent in unipolar depression.

The use of lithium in treating schizoaffective disorders and other periodic behavioral disturbances is under investigation, but preliminary results indicate that it is much less effective in these disorders than in mania. Though the mechanism of action of lithium is not yet established, there are some indications that it accelerates presynaptic catabolism of norepinephrine, inhibits the release of norepinephrine and serotonin, and stimulates the norepinephrine uptake process (Davis and Fann, 1971).

Murphy et al. (1971) have shown that L-DOPA in therapeutic doses can regularly induce manic episodes in some bipolar patients. Patients with unipolar depression fail to benefit from L-DOPA but do not develop mania while taking the drug. When depressed patients are divided into retarded and agitated groups, the retarded group seems to benefit somewhat from L-DOPA. Agitated depression, if anything, tends to become worse (Murphy et al., 1971).

As mentioned above, the amphetamines produce euphoria in in-

dividuals who take them in large doses. At one time, the amphetamines were the only drugs used for depression. They were not
especially effective in treating depression, and their use had to be
curtailed because of side-effects and the development of tolerance.
With the spread of drug abuse, many physicians have become ac-
quainted with the effects of amphetamine overdose and withdrawal.

Amphetamines, as we have noted, are known to have several
biochemical effects. They reduce the reuptake of norepinephrine
and dopamine and facilitate their release. There is some evidence
that D-amphetamine has a direct effect upon noradrenergic receptors. Both effects potentiate the action of these catecholamines.
The drugs also inhibit the synthesis of dopamine and norepinephrine. With continued use, amphetamines deplete norepinephrine
in the nervous system. This could explain the tolerance that develops with the chronic use of D-amphetamine (Cooper et al., 1974).

When amphetamine is withdrawn, there should presumably be
a lag before depleted catecholamine stores return to normal. This
lag period would correspond to the depression ("crash") that is
regularly seen in Dexedrine users who have suddenly stopped taking
the drug.

Amine Hypothesis

The results of these clinical trials led to the catecholamine hypothesis of depression. According to this theory, a certain level of
amines and of receptor sensitivity to these neurotransmitters is
necessary for a normal mood. If the amine receptors are insensi-
tive, or if there is a deficiency in amine synthesis, storage, release,
or ability to reach the receptor, there will be depression. If the receptors are hypersensitive, or if there is an excess of active amines,
mania and/or psychosis will develop. The results of the drug studies reviewed above are in general consistent with this interpretation.

The MAO inhibitors and tricyclic compounds alleviate depression and induce mania or make it worse. They also increase catecholamine and indoleamine concentrations at postsynaptic receptors.
The same is true of amphetamines in relation to catecholamines.

Although L-DOPA, the catecholamine precursor, does not primarily relieve depression, high doses may induce mania. Conversely, reserpine and the phenothiazines, which reduce the amount of transmitter available at the dendritic receptor sites, induce or increase depression and are occasionally effective in treating mania. Lithium, which is effective in blocking episodes of mania, may act by decreasing release and increasing reuptake and catabolism of norepinephrine and thus may have exactly the opposite effect from that of tricyclic mood elevators.

Janowsky et al. (1972) demonstrated that manic symptoms could be suppressed, at least transiently, by the administration of an acetylcholinesterase inhibitor, physostigmine. The suppression occurred only with physostigmine and not with a placebo or a noncentrally acting cholinesterase inhibitor, neostigmine. They hypothesized that mania may be a disease of "relative adrenergic predominance" and depression a disease of "relative cholinergic predominance." They also noted that schizophrenic and manic patients receiving methylphenidate manifested increased talkativeness and activity and that this effect was antagonized by physostigmine. This is an interesting theory, since it raises the possibility that the biochemical basis of both mania and depression is related to the proper balance of neurotransmitters rather than just to a deficiency of any single substance. The conceptualization of depression as a state of inhibition and mania as a state of activation is consistent with the physiological findings of central nervous system hyperexcitability in both mania and depression. Mania would reflect this hyperexcitability when it "breaks through" the state of inhibition, depression.

This is really the same "balance" theory of cholinergic and adrenergic mechanisms that has been put forward to explain movement disorders. Physostigmine makes Parkinsonism worse and alleviates chorea. The mechanism by which these changes are produced is assumed to be the result of the drug's antiacetylcholinesterase activity.

In enthusiastic discussions of the catecholamine hypothesis of depression, contradictory data have often been ignored. The evidence that supports this theory is derived mainly from the clinical results of drug treatment and from animal experiments. As pointed out by Mendels and Frazer (1974), most of the evidence that reserpine causes depression in human beings comes from retrospective studies in which endogenous factors were not adequately ruled out. In their review of studies on brain biogenic amine depletion and mood, Mendels and Frazer also found that selective inhibitors of central biogenic amine synthesis, such as alphamethylparatyrosine (α-MPT) or parachlorophenylalanine (PCPA), do not regularly cause depression in humans. DeMuth and Ackerman (1983) recently observed that in 42 hypertensive patients treated with methyldopa (a potent inhibitor of DOPA decarboxylase, which lowers levels of CNS catecholamines and indoleamines) there was no greater incidence of depressive symptoms than in a control group of hypertensives treated with other antihypertensives agents. The absence of marked depressive symptoms when these drugs are used, even though they produce a more consistent and greater reduction in amine metabolic concentration in the urine and spinal fluid than reportedly occurs in depressed patients, is an important observation. Also important is the fact that new, equally effective antidepressants (Table 5-3) have different modes of action than earlier drugs. Nevertheless, the catecholamine hypothesis of depression must be more fully refuted before it is abandoned. So far there is no other theory to replace it.

Studies of the newer drugs and molecular studies of central nervous system receptors have shifted the theoretical focus from the presynaptic aminergic neuron to inhibition of MAO activity and/or neuronal uptake of either catecholamines or indoleamines. The picture has become much more complex as evidence has accumulated that antidepressants affect many receptor systems (α_2-adrenergic dopamine, serotonin, adenylate cyclase, histamine$_1$ and histamine$_2$) and that their main action is on the receptor (often decreasing its sensitivity) rather than exclusively on either accumulation or turnover of neurotransmitters, as previously hypothesized (Sulser, 1983).

Sulser (1983) has outlined other factors that complicate any biochemical hypothesis of depression based on drug effects: (1) The biologic effects of antidepressants occur in minutes whereas the therapeutic effects usually take place only after 10 to 14 days. (2) There is marked variation in individual clinical responses despite uniform biochemical actions. (3) Some drugs, as noted above, are effective antidepressants but have no major effect on catecholamines and serotonin, while some drugs that do have marked actions on these neurotransmitters, such as amphetamines, L-DOPA, cocaine, and tryptophan, are not effective antidepressant agents.

"Kindling" is another interesting theory that posits a possible biologic factor in affective disorders and also stems from effective pharmacologic treatment. Ballenger and Post (1980) noted that certain patients with bipolar affective disorder responded to treatment with carbamazepine. To explain why this anticonvulsant could be effective in bipolar disorders, they postulated that these patients suffered from subthreshold cerebral seizure activity, which led to their aberrant behavior. They equated this to the concept of "kindling" in animals, where stimulation of the amygdala with currents inadequate to evoke seizures eventually leads to behavioral changes. That these behavioral changes may occur after a few stimulations spread over many months probably reflects long-term changes in neural excitability. Similar behavioral changes in animals can be produced with drugs (Post et al., 1982). In support of the kindling theory, Post (1983) reported a marked decrease in the number of manic and depressive episodes in a group of rapid-cycling bipolar patients who were treated with carbamazepine.

PSYCHOSIS

The symptoms of psychosis have been discussed in Chapter 3, along with some of the clinical considerations by means of which one can distinguish idiopathic (familial) schizophrenia from the schizophrenialike psychosis of epilepsy and the psychoses associated with neurological disease and drug effects. The similarities between drug-induced psychosis and schizophrenia are, on balance, more striking than the differences, and this has been the basis for speculation on the etiology of psychosis.

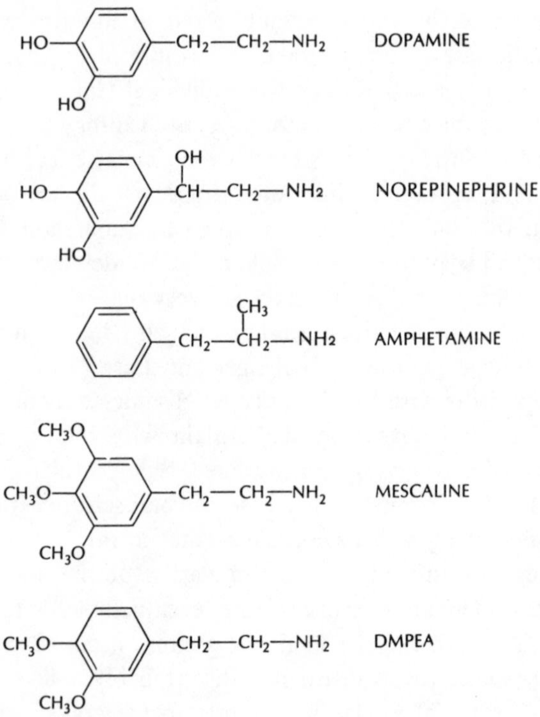

HO—⟨ring⟩—CH₂—CH₂—NH₂   DOPAMINE
(HO—)

$$HO-\text{(ring)}-CH_2-CH_2-NH_2 \quad \text{DOPAMINE}$$

$$HO-\text{(ring)}-\underset{\underset{OH}{|}}{CH}-CH_2-NH_2 \quad \text{NOREPINEPHRINE}$$

$$\text{(ring)}-CH_2-\underset{\underset{CH_3}{|}}{CH_2}-NH_2 \quad \text{AMPHETAMINE}$$

$$CH_3O-,\ CH_3O-,\ CH_3O-\text{(ring)}-CH_2-CH_2-NH_2 \quad \text{MESCALINE}$$

$$CH_3O-,\ CH_3O-\text{(ring)}-CH_2-CH_2-NH_2 \quad \text{DMPEA}$$

Fig. 5-2
STRUCTURE OF SOME
AMINES

For many years it has been known that mescaline and amphetamines can induce psychosis. The structural similarity between these methylated compounds and the catecholamines (Fig. 5-2) prompted the suggestion that abnormal methylation of catecholamines may lead to the formation of an amine with psychotogenic properties. The search for such an amine in schizophrenics has led us into many blind alleys. One of the most promising findings was the discovery by Friedhoff and Van Winkle (1962) of 3,4 dimethoxyphenylethylamine (DMPEA) in the urine of schizophrenic patients. This is a nonpsychotogenic dimethylated derivative of

Table 5-3
Neurotransmitters Affected by Antidepressant Drugs[a]

Antidepressant Drug	Affected Neurotransmitter			
	Serotonergic	Noradrenergic	Dopaminergic	Anticholinergic
"First Generation"				
Imipramine	+	++		++
Amitriptylene	++	+		+++
"Second Generation"				
Tricyclic				
Anoxapine	+	++	−	++
Tetracyclic				
Maprotiline		+++		+
Mianserin		+		○
Others				
Trazadone	++			○
Zimelidine	+++			
Fluoxetine	+++			○
Nomifensine		+++	+	○
Bupropion			+	○
Alprazolam[b]			−	○

[a] Almost all have similar clinical efficacy
[b] Affects primarily GABA system

dopamine, identical to mescaline except that it lacks one methoxy group. It was thought that DMPEA might be a metabolite of a psychotogenic precursor in schizophrenic patients. As it turned out, excretion of this compound is affected by both drugs and diet, especially those to which institutionalized psychiatric patients are exposed. It can also be found in the urine of some normal individuals.

Another approach to the possibility that an abnormally methylated amine could cause schizophrenia was the infusion of methyl donors (methionine and betaine) into schizophrenics, other psychiatric patients, and normal individuals (Kety, 1967). Though toxic to some degree to all groups, these compounds clearly increased the schizophrenic symptoms of schizophrenic patients. This rather frail reed is the only support for the theory that abnormally methylated compounds cause schizophrenia.

There is little direct evidence that, in schizophrenia, either an abnormal amine or an excess of normal amine exists. Bowers (1974) has assayed HVA and 5-HIAA levels in the spinal fluid of schizophrenics before and after treatment. He found that 5-HIAA levels were normal but that HVA levels were significantly reduced before treatment. These rose after phenothiazine therapy was initiated. Bowers drew an analogy between this and the administration of apomorphine, which lowers HVA levels in the spinal fluid. Apomorphine is thought to stimulate postsynaptic dopamine receptors directly and to suppress activity in dopaminergic cell bodies, presumably by means of a negative neural feedback loop that inhibits dopaminergic cells and consequently reduces dopamine turnover and HVA production. Phenothiazine, which block dopamine receptors, elicit more rapid firing of dopaminergic neurons, presumably by interrupting the negative feedback loop. This leads to increased dopamine turnover and HVA production. Bowers's findings thus provide indirect evidence that the excitability of dopamine receptors may be increased in schizophrenia.

There has been much recent work on the role of dopamine receptors in psychosis (Whitaker, 1981; Kleinman, 1982). Snyder (1981) noted that there are at least two dopamine receptors which show differential responses to various neuroleptics. Phenothiazines bind to both DA-1 and DA-2 receptors, thus blocking dopamine, whereas butyrophenones tend to affect primarily DA-2 receptors, and apomorphine seems selective for DA-1 receptors.

A discovery that may provide a basis for understanding the complications of therapy is that neuroleptic treatment *increases dopamine receptor binding and increases the total number of dopamine receptors,* possibly as a response to neuroleptic dopamine blockade (McKay, 1980; Staton and Brumback, 1980). These increases, particularly in the neostriatum and mesolimbic pathways, may underlie tardive dyskinesia as well as what has been called "supersensitivity psychosis" (Chouinard and Jones, 1980). Chouinard and Jones describe the latter condition as follows: (1) Psychotic symptoms appear when neuroleptics are stopped or the dosage decreased after at least a few weeks of treatment. (2) There are concomitant signs of tardive dyskinesia. (3) Patients have high prolactin levels. (4) Signs of tolerance are apparent, that is, neuroleptic doses must be continually increased to maintain effect. (5) As in tardive dyskinesia, the most effective treatment is the causative agent itself. Perhaps most disconcerting to theoretical formulations about the biochemical nature of psychosis is the fact that although the drugs used to treat psychosis affect the dopamine system, no consistent biochemical changes in groups of psychotics treated with these agents have yet been demonstrated. Linnoila and co-workers (1983) recently reported a series of patients (drug-free chronic schizophenics) whose spinal fluid was examined for norepinephrine, MHPG, HVA, and 5HIAA repeatedly. The main finding was considerable variability in the same individuals over time as well as between individuals.

Other indirect evidence of the role of amines in psychosis can be marshaled from clinical experience with drugs that affect amines and can induce, make worse, or alleviate schizophrenia or schizophrenialike psychoses. In discussing these drugs, we will limit ourselves to the agents already mentioned in the sections on movement and affective disorders.

The first effective antipsychotic drugs were the *Rauwolfia* alkaloids, of which reserpine was the most widely used. They have proven to be effective in reducing impulsivity, agitation, excitement, and chronic paranoid irritability. Such side-effects as hypotension, gastrointestinal bleeding, impotence, and depression, together with the long half-life of the compounds that makes control of side-effects by dosage adjustment difficult, have led most psychiatrists to prefer phenothiazines and related major tranquilizers for the treatment of psychosis. The phenothiazines are especially helpful in controlling the following symptoms of psychosis: psychomotor agitation, delusional and paranoid ideation, auditory hallucinations, blocking, inappropriate affect, and social withdrawal (Goldberg et al., 1965). The phenothiazines are as effective in treating drug-induced psychosis as they are in treating idiopathic schizophrenia. The antipsychotic effects of *Rauwolfia* alkaloids and phenothiazines could be understood if psychosis were shown to result from abnormal amines, an excess of normal catecholamines or indoleamines, or of receptor hypersensitivity, to normal amines.

The same hypothesis can be invoked to explain the effect of drugs known to worsen or induce psychosis; their mechanisms of action have already been discussed. The amphetamines, chronic use of which leads to a psychotic state virtually indistinguishable from paranoid schizophrenia, potentiate amine release. Amphetamines may also be active themselves at amine receptor sites. Anticholinergics and tricyclic mood elevators, which reduce amine uptake, may induce psychosis in some sensitive, nonpsychotic individuals and may cause a worsening of psychosis in schizophrenics. Amantadine, which can induce a drug psychosis, acts by enhancing amine release. The MAO inhibitors that prevent the degradative metabolism of both catechol- and indoleamines can induce or make worse psychosis in sensitive individuals. L-DOPA, which is a precursor of both dopamine and norepinephrine, causes confusion, paranoia, agitation, and excitement in roughly 5 percent of patients receiving it for Parkinsonism and tends to aggravate preexisting psychotic problems (Yaryura-Tobias et al., 1970).

One inconsistency in this scheme is that several antipsychotic drugs with potent dopamine receptor-blocking ability show a lower incidence of extrapyramidal side-effects than would be expected. These drugs were found to have antimuscarinic properties. It has been shown that the greater the antimuscarinic properties of the antipsychotic drugs, the less frequent the extrapyramidal side-effects (Snyder et al., 1974).

SLEEP

Before leaving the subject of biogenic amines and brain disorders, it seems appropriate to review some of the salient features of sleep disorders, especially narcolepsy. If we could understand this condition, we would have taken a great step in bridging the hiatus between psychosis and neurochemistry, since narcolepsy involves a sleep disturbance, motor alterations, hallucinations, EEG changes, and is remarkably affected by drugs that influence cerebral amines.

There are four cardinal symptoms in narcolepsy: sleep attacks, cataplexy, sleep paralysis, and hypnagogic hallucinations. In only 10 percent of the cases in which the diagnosis is made are all four symptoms present. In 70 percent of the cases, sleep attacks and cataplexy alone exist. There is often a family history of narcolepsy, which spans several generations. This has led to the proposal of a single, dominant mode of inheritance (Zarcone, 1973).

The SLEEP ATTACKS may be sudden, coming on without warning, or they may be preceded by an irresistible urge to sleep. The attacks vary in duration, lasting from several minutes to an hour or more. Some patients are normally alert between attacks, but others are constantly drowsy and become drowsier as they tire, especially toward the end of the working day. These patients often fall asleep under boring social circumstances conducive to sleep. This is often misunderstood, and the patients are considered lazy, impolite, neurotic, or worse. The most serious threat posed by the condition is accidental death, which results from a sleep attack or cataplectic attack. Automobile accidents are a much more frequent complication of narcolepsy than of epilepsy. Of a group of narcoleptics, 40 percent admitted that they had fallen asleep while driving (Bartels and Kuskacioglu, 1965).

CATAPLEXY can be defined as the sudden loss of muscle tone that causes a patient to slump or fall to the floor. It is unassociated with unconsciousness, and it is usually precipitated by such strong, sudden emotions as laughter, anger, or surprise. It is usually brief, lasting several seconds to several minutes.

The first two symptoms are the most incapacitating and are more likely to cause a patient to seek medical attention than the remaining two. SLEEP PARALYSIS is a state that occurs upon awakening and affects all skeletal muscles except those of respiration and the extraocular muscles (EOM). It typically lasts for a few seconds to a few minutes and is associated with alertness, a desire to get up, great fear, and, often, vivid visual and auditory nightmares that persist from the sleeping into the waking states; these are called *hypnagogic hallucinations*.

The entire narcolepsy syndrome was once considered to be purely "functional," since it was unassociated with any objective abnormality; the EEG in the waking state is normal. Sophisticated psychological explanations for the phenomena were provided by some on a post hoc basis. The condition thus serves to remind us that our classification of disease as functional is more often a reflection of our ignorance than our cleverness.

Sleep studies of the last decade have indicated that sleep can be divided into several stages, perhaps the most important being the REM and non-REM phases. The former is associated with a desynchronized EEG, loss of muscle tone in all skeletal muscles except the EOM and muscles of respiration, and dreaming. The non-REM phase is associated with high voltage, slow-wave electroencephalographic activity, and normal skeletal muscle tone. Dreaming does not occur in this phase. In normal controls, REM phases occur in intervals of ever-increasing duration beginning about 90 minutes after the onset of sleep and ultimately account for about

20 percent of the total sleeping time. Patients with narcolepsy, however, characteristically enter the REM phase immediately after falling asleep and spend more time in REM sleep than do controls (Dement et al., 1966).

Narcolepsy is now considered to be the result of overactivity of the REM system: sleep attacks are episodic REM sleep phases; cataplexy and sleep paralysis are the result of REM-associated loss of muscle tone, which spares only the EOM and respiratory muscles; hypnagogic hallucinations are persistent REM-associated dreams.

The ideal drug for the treatment of narcolepsy would have the effect of reducing REM attacks without increasing non-REM sleep or producing drowsiness. Virtually all sedatives reduce REM, but clearly they could not be used to treat narcolepsy. Amphetamines in large doses are the drugs of choice, though they only ameliorate sleep attacks and do not affect the other symptoms of narcolepsy. All the side-effects that attend their use in other conditions are encountered in narcolepsy, and amphetamines may well be the cause of the high incidence of "schizophrenia" in narcolepsy (Sours, 1963).

Other drugs that potentiate amine action and reduce REM may be effective in narcolepsy; MAO inhibitors relieve all four of the symptoms even in previously intractable cases (Wyatt et al., 1971), and imipramine is effective in relieving cataplexy (Hishikowa et al., 1966). Other drugs discussed in this chapter have not been systematically investigated in relation to narcolepsy.

Several observations suggest that brain serotonin is intimately involved in the biochemistry of sleep. Non-REM sleep is potentiated, and REM sleep suppressed, by parenteral injections of the serotonin precursor 5-hydroxytryptophan or by intraventricular injection of serotonin. Non-REM sleep is reduced when brain serotonin is reduced by blocking its synthesis with *p*-chlorophenylalanine. Reserpine also reduces non-REM sleep and triggers the EEG components of REM sleep (Jouvet, 1967).

REM sleep has also been thought to depend upon a cholinergic mechanism because it is suppressed by atropine. In view of the evidence that synthetic atropinelike drugs inhibit catecholamine

uptake (Coyle and Synder, 1969), it may be that atropine suppresses REM and potentiates non-REM sleep by this mechanism,
which is shared by the tricyclic antidepressants.

Hauri and Hawkins (1973) have described an abnormal phase
of non-REM sleep they all "alpha-delta" sleep. It is an electro-
encephalographically defined stage of sleep consisting of 5 to 20
percent delta waves mixed with large amplitude alpha waves. It
appears to replace delta-wave sleep in some patients who suffer
from chronic malaise and fatigue. Delta-wave sleep is a phase of
sleep in which delta waves (1 to 3 Hz) dominate the recorded
rhythms. The etiology is unknown.

Alpha-delta sleep has been observed in patients with a form of
psychosomatic illness that is often called the "chronic fibrositis
syndrome" (Moldofsky et al., 1975). This syndrome consists of
aching and stiffness of the paraspinal skeletal muscles that extend
over a period of more than three months, chronic fatigue and work
intolerance, a sleep disturbance, morning aching and stiffness, and
poor appetite. Damp weather provokes the aching pain, and heat
gives temporary relief. On examination, these patients reveal local
muscle tenderness but no muscle spasm, an unrestricted normal
range of musculoskeletal movement, and evidence of emotional
distress, including depression, anxiety, and irritability. X-rays of
the skeleton are normal, as are the sedimentation rate, serum glutamic oxaloacetic transaminase (SGOT), creatine phosphokinase,
latex fixation, and antinuclear factor. Electromyographic studies
have not demonstrated any physiological evidence of "involuntary
muscle spasm" (Kraft et al., 1968). Seven of the ten "fibrositic"
patients studied by Moldofsky et al. (1975) had the alpha-delta
sleep disturbance described by Hauri and Hawkins (1973). The
three patients without this sleep pattern showed a complete or almost complete absence of delta waves during sleep.

To determine whether sleep disturbance is primary or secondary to this syndrome, Moldofsky et al. extended their observations
to healthy volunteers. While EEG recordings were made, the
delta sleep pattern of these subjects was disturbed or temporarily
abolished by noises throughout the night that did not awaken

them or reduce their total sleeping time. Interestingly, these normal individuals experienced musculoskeletal symptoms and a mood disturbance comparable to the fibrositis syndrome, and there was a statistically significant remission of these symptoms after a night of undisturbed delta sleep. On the basis of these findings, the authors suggested that the fibrositis syndrome, generally regarded as a functional psychiatric disorder, is in fact the result of a slow-wave sleep disturbance.

Another sleep disorder related to EEG-defined stages of sleep, which is as yet incompletely understood, is the syndrome of somnambulism, night terror (pavor nocturnus), and enuresis. In contrast to narcolepsy, in which behavior usually associated with sleep occurs in the waking state, somnambulism and its closely related symptoms, consist of behavior that is typical of the alert state but occurs during sleep. Somnambulism, enuresis, and night terror arise during stage 3 or 4 sleep (delta-wave sleep) and not during REM. That these symptoms are in some way related is suggested by the fact that they coexist frequently and that there is a high family incidence of somnambulism among patients with enuresis (Broughton, 1968). They may, however, exist separately.

It has been suggested that this triad represents a disorder of arousal from sleep. Typically, a patient is in stage 3 or 4 sleep and suddenly gives evidence of arousal. There is body movement, intense autonomic activation, mental confusion and disorientation, automatic behavior, relative nonreactivity to external stimuli, poor response to efforts to provoke behavioral wakefulness, a retrograde amnesia for most of the intercurrent events, and a fragmentary recall or no recall of dreams. Though the subject is not asleep when the night terror is enacted, he is not in a fully alert, waking state either; the EEG may show an alpha rhythm. Other evidence suggesting that this triad represents a disorder of arousal is that it can be induced artificially by sounding a buzzer during stage 3 or 4 sleep, but it cannot be induced by thus awakening a patient from REM sleep (Fischer et al., I, 1973).

Night terror is associated with screaming or other vocalization and usually lasts for several minutes. The episode is associated with

Table 5-4
Biogenic Amines
Drugs, Movement, Mood, and Psychosis

Drugs	Parkinson's Disease	Depression	Mania	Psychosis	Chorea	Probable Major Amine Mechanism[a]
Anticholinergics	better	?better	?	worse	worse	Inhibits DA uptake
L-DOPA	better	?better	worse	worse	worse	↑ DA synthesis
Phenothiazines	worse	worse	better	better	better	Blocks postsynaptic receptors of DA and NE
MAO inhibitors	better	better	worse	worse	worse	↓ catabolism of DA, NE, and serotonin in presynaptic cell
Tricyclics	?better	better	worse	worse	worse	Inhibits NE and serotonin uptake
D-amphetamine	better	better	worse	worse	worse	Inhibits NE and DA uptake
L-amphetamine	better (animals)	no change	?	no change	?	Inhibits DA uptake
Lithium	?worse	?	better	?	?better	? ↓ NE release; ↑ NE uptake
Reserpine	worse	worse	better	better	better	Releases all stored biogenic amines
α Methylparatyrosine	worse	?	better	?better	better	Prevents DA and NE synthesis
Physostigmine	worse	?	better	?	better	Antiacetylcholinesterase (effect on amines not studied)

[a] DA, dopamine; NE, norepinephrine

marked hyperventilation, tachycardia, and a marked decrease in galvanic skin resistance. In the majority of cases, the subjects return to sleep within minutes. Many subjects become sleepy while being spoken to and may fall asleep in the middle of a sentence. The return to sleep so quickly after such intense manifestations of terror is striking and surprising. The next morning, typically, there is total amnesia for the events of the night and only a vague feeling that sleep had been disturbed.

Despite the marked similarity of this syndrome to complex partial seizure states, there is no EEG abnormality, even during the events of the episode, and anticonvulsants have no effect upon this syndrome. There is some evidence that night terror can be suppressed by diazepam and that with suppression there is a coincident decrease in the amount of stage 4 sleep (Fischer, II, 1973).

We are just beginning to understand the array of possible sleep disorders. Through studies of sleep, some disorders that were

Table 5-5
Drugs, Movement, Mood, and Psychosis

Mood	Parkinson's Disease	Chorea	Depression	Psychosis
Better				
Primary	belladonna L-DOPA amantadine	reserpine phenothiazines major tranquilizers	MAO inhibitors tricyclics	reserpine phenothiazines major tranquilizers
Secondary	amphetamine MAO inhibitors tricyclics		amphetamines ?L-DOPA ?belladonna	
Worse	reserpine phenothiazines major tranquilizers	L-DOPA amphetamines belladonna tricyclics	reserpine phenothiazines major tranquilizers amphetamine withdrawal	amphetamines belladonna amantadine L-DOPA MAO inhibitors tricyclics

thought to be functional have been placed in a physiological context. Incompletely explained are the clinical observations that sleep disorders are common concomitants of anxiety, affective disorders, and schizophrenia. Most movement disorders stop during sleep. Investigations concerning the role of neural transmitters and neural humors in producing the sleep disturbances seen in these psychiatric conditions and the relationship of neurological diseases to sleep have only just been started.

The effects of the drugs discussed in this chapter and their major mechanisms of action are summarized in Tables 5-4 and 5-5.

REFERENCES

Abraham, H. C., U. B. Kanter, I. Rosen, and J. L. Standen. A controlled clinical trial of imipramine (Tofranil) with outpatients. *Brit. J. Psychiat.* 109:286, 1963.

Ader, R. Developmental psychoneuroimmunology. *Dev. Psychobiol.* 16:251, 1983.

Akiskal, H. Dysthymic disorder. *Amer. J. Psychiat.* 140:11, 1983.

Altrocchi, P. H. and L. S. Forno. Spontaneous oral-facial dyskinesia: Neuropathology of a case. *Neurology* 33:802, 1983.

American College of Physicians. The dexamethasone suppression test for the detection, diagnosis, and management of depression. *Ann. Intern. Med.* 100:307, 1984.

Amsterdam, J., A. Winokur, S. Coroff, and J. Conn. The dexamethasone suppression test in outpatients with primary affective disorder and healthy control subjects. *Amer. J. Psychiat.* 139:287, 1982.

Angst, J., P. We's, P. C. Baastrup, and M. Schou. Lithium prophylaxis in recurrent affective disorders. *Brit. J. Psychiat.* 116:604, 1970.

Aquilonius, S. M. and R. Sjöström. Cholinergic and dopaminergic mechanisms in Huntington's chorea. *Life Sci.* 10:405, 1971.

Arnold, L. E., R. D. Huestis, D. J. Smeltzer, et al. Levoamphetamine vs. dextroamphetamine in minimal brain dysfunction. *Arch. Gen. Psychiat.* 33:292, 1976.

Asnis, G. and N. Ryan. The psychoneuroendocrinology of schizophrenia. In: *Schizophrenia and Affective Disorders*, T. Rifkin, J. Wright. PSG, Boston, 1983, p. 205.

Avery, D., G. Wildschiodtz and O. Rafaelsen. REM latency and temperature in affective disorder before and after treatment. *Biol. Psychiat.* 17:463, 1982.

Baastrup, P. C. and M. Schou. Lithium as a prophylactic agent against recurrent depressions and manic depressive psychosis. *Arch. Gen. Psychiat.* 16:162, 1967.

————, J. C. Poulsen, M. Schou, K. Thomsen, and A. Amdisen. Prophylactic lithium: Double-blind discontinuation in manic depressive and recurrent depressive disorders. *Lancet* 1:326, 1970.

Bacopoulos, N. Dopaminergic 3H-agonist receptors in rat brain: New evidence on localization and pharmacology. *Life Sci.* 34:307, 1984.

Ballenger, J. C. and R. M. Post. Carbamazepine in manic-depressive illness: a new treatment. *Amer. J. Psychiat.* 137:782, 1980.

Barbeau, A. Discussion. Association for Research in Nervous and Mental Disease. *Neurotransmitters* December, 1970.

Bartels, E. C. and O. Kuskacioglu. Narcolepsy: A possible cause of automobile accidents. *Lahey Clin. Found. Bull.* 14:21, 1965.

Beck, A. T., C. H. Ward, M. Mandelson, J. Mock, and J. K. Erbaugh. An inventory for measuring depression. *Arch. Gen. Psychiat.* 4:561, 1961.

Beigel, A. and D. L. Murphy. Unipolar and bipolar affective illnesses. *Arch. Gen. Psychiat.* 24:215, 1971.

Bernheimer, H. and O. Hornykiewicz. Brain amines in Huntington's chorea. In: *Advances in Neurology*, vol. 1, A. Barbeau, T. N. Chase, and G. W. Paulson, eds. Raven Press, New York, 1973, p. 525.

Bird, E. D. Biochemical studies on gamma amino butyric acid metabolism in Huntington's chorea. In: *Biochemistry and Neurology*, H. W. Bradford and C. D. Marsden, eds. Academic Press, London, 1976, p. 83.

Birkmayer, W. Der α methyl ρ tyrosine effekt bei extrapyramidalen erkrankungen. *Wien. Klin. Wochensch.* 81:10, 1969.

Blumenthal, M. P. Heterogeneity and research on depressive disorders. *Arch. Gen. Psychiat.* 24:524, 1971.

Boller, F., T. Mizutani, U. Roessmann, and P. Gambetti. Parkinson disease, dementia, and Alzheimer disease: Clinicopathological correlations. *Ann. Neurol.* 4:329, 1980.

Botney, M. and H. L. Fields. Amitriptyline potentiates morphine analgesia by a direct action on the cerebral nervous system. *Ann. Neurol.* 13:160, 1983.

Bowers, M. B. Cerebral dopamine turnover in schizophrenic syndromes. *Arch. Gen. Psychiat.* 31:50, 1974.

Broughton, R. J. Sleep disorders: Disorders of arousal? *Science* 159:1070, 1968.

Buchsbaum, M., F. Goodwin, D. Murphy, and G. Borge. AET in affective disorders. *Amer. J. Psychiat.* 128:19, 1971.

Bunney, W. E., Jr., H. K. H. Brodie, D. L. Murphy, and F. K. Goodwin. Studies of alpha methyl paratyrosine, L-DOPA and L-tryptophan in depression and mania. *Amer. J. Psychiat.* 127:7, 1971.

Calne, D. B., P. F. Teychenne, C. E. Clavaria, et al. Bromocriptine in Parkinsonism. *Brit. Med. J.* 4:442, 1974.

Calzetti, S., L. J. Findley, and M. A. Gresty. Effect of a single oral dose of propranolol on essential tremor: A double blind study. *Ann. Neurol.* 13: 165, 1983.

Carlsson, A., H. Corrodi, K. Fuxe, and T. Hökfelt. Effect of antidepressant drugs on the depletion of intraneuronal brain 5-hydroxytryptamine stores caused by 4 methyl α ethyl meta tyramine. *Europ. J. Pharmacol.* 5:357, 1969.

Carman, J. B. Anatomic basis of surgical treatment of Parkinson's disease. *New Eng. J. Med.* 279:919, 1968.

Carrea, R., M. E. and F. A. Mettler. Functions of the primate brachium conjunctivum and related structures. *J. Comp. Neurol.* 102:151, 1955.

Carroll, B., M. Feinberg, J. Greden, et al. A specific test for the diagnosis of melancholia: Standardization, validation, and clinical utility. *Arch. Gen. Psychiat.* 38:15, 1981.

Chase, T. N. and L. K. Y. Ng. Central monoamine metabolism in Parkinson's disease. *Arch. Neurol.* 27:486, 1972.

————. Biochemical and pharmacologic studies of monoamines in Huntington's chorea. In: *Advances in Neurology*, vol. 1, A. Barbeau, T. N. Chase, and G. W. Paulson, eds. Raven Press, New York, 1973, p. 533.

Chouinard, G. and B. D. Jones. Neuroleptic-induced supersensitivity psychosis: Clinical and pharmacologic characteristics. *Amer. J. Psychiat.* 137:16, 1980.

Clark, A. W., I. M. Parhad, S. E. Folstein, et al. The nucleus basalis in Huntington's disease. *Neurology* 33:1262, 1983.

Claveria, C. E., P. F. Teychenne, D. B. Calne, et al. Dopaminergic agonists in Parkinsonism. In: *Advances in Neurology*, vol. 9, D. B. Calne, T. N. Chase and A. Barbeau, eds. Raven Press, New York, 1975, p. 343.

Cochrane, R. and A. Robertson. The life events inventory: A measure of the relative severity of psychosocial stress. *J. Psychosom. Res.* 17:135, 1973.

Cooper, I. S. Involuntary Movement Disorders. Harper & Row, New York, 1968.

Cooper, J. R., F. E. Bloom, and R. H. Roth. *The Biochemical Basis of Neuropharmacology*. 4th ed. Oxford University Press, New York, 1982.

Coppen, A. The biochemistry of affective disorders. *Brit. J. Psychiat.* 113:1237, 1967.

Corrodi, J., K. Fuxe, and U. Ungerstedt. Evidence for a new type of dopamine receptor stimulating agent. *J. Pharm. Pharmacol.* 23:989, 1971.

Cotzias, G. C., P. S. Papavasiliou, and R. Gellene. Modification of Parkinsonism—chronic treatment with L-DOPA. *New Eng. J. Med.* 280:337, 1969.

Coyle, J. T. and S. H. Synder. Antiparkinsonian drugs: Inhibition of dopamine uptake in the corpus striatum as a possible mechanism of action. *Science* 166:899, 1969.

Crowe, R. R., K. K. Namhoodiri, H. B. Ashley, et al. Segregation and linkage analysis of a large kindred unipolar depression. *Neuropsychobiology* 7:20, 1981.

Curzon, G. Relationships between stress and brain 5-hydroxytryptamine and their possible significance in affective disorders. In: *Brain Chemistry and Mental Disease*, B. Y. Ho and W. M. McIsaac, eds. Plenum, New York, 1971, p. 163.

Dalos, N. P., P. V. Rubins, B. R. Brooks, et al. Disease activity and emotional state in multiple sclerosis. *Ann. Neurol.* 13:573, 1983.

Davies, R., G. J. Tucker, M. Harrow, and T. Detre. Confusional episodes and antidepressant medication. *Amer. J. Psychiat.* 128:95, 1971.

Davis, J. M. Antidepressant drugs. In: *Comprehensive Textbook of Psychiatry/IV*, H. Kaplan and B. Sadock, eds. Williams & Wilkins, Baltimore, 1985.

Davis, J. M., D. S. Janowsky, and M. K. El-Yousef. The use of lithium in clinical psychiatry. *Psychiat. Ann.* 3:78, 1973.

———— and W. E. Fann. Lithium. *Ann. Rev. Pharmacol.* 11:285, 1971.

Dement, W., A. Rechtschaffen, and G. Gulevich. The nature of the narcoleptic sleep attack. *Neurology* 16:18, 1966.

DeMuth, G. W. and S. H. Ackerman. A-methyldopa and depression: A clinical study and review of the literature. *Amer. J. Psychiat.* 140:534, 1983.

Detre, T., J. Himmelhoch, M. Swartzburg, C. M. Anderson, R. Byck, and D. J. Kupfer. Hypersomnia and manic depressive disease. *Amer. J. Psychiat.* 128:1303, 1972.

———— and H. Jarecki. *Modern Psychiatric Treatment*. J. P. Lippincott, Philadelphia, 1971.

Donnelly, E. F. and T. N. Chase. Intellectual and memory function in parkinsonism and non-parkinsonian patients treated with L-DOPA. *Dis. Nerv. System* 34:119, 1973.

Dunner, D. L., F. Stallone, and R. R. Fieve. Lithium carbonate and affective disorders V: A double-blind study of prophylaxis of depression in bipolar illness. *Arch. Gen. Psychiat.* 33:117, 1976.

English, O. S. and S. M. Finch. *Introduction to Psychiatry*. W. W. Norton, New York, 1954.

Fahr, S. Long-term treatment of tardive dyskinesia with presynaptically acting dopamine-depleting agents. *Adv. Neurol.* 37:267, 1983.

Fahr, S. Treatment of dystonia with high-dose anticholinergic medication. *Neurology* 29:605, 1979.

Farnebo, L. O., K. Fuxe, M. Goldstein, B. Hamberger, and U. Ungerstedt. Dopamine and noradrenaline release action of amantadine in the central and peripheral nervous system: A possible mode of action in Parkinson's disease. *Europ. J. Pharmacol.* 16:27, 1971.

Fieve, D. R., D. L. Dunner, T. Kambarachi, and F. Stallone. Lithium carbonate in affective disorders IV: A double-blind study of prophylaxis in unipolar recurrent depression. *Arch. Gen. Psychiat.* 32:1541, 1975.

Fischer, C. A., E. Kahne, A. Edwards, et al. I. A psychological study of nightmares and night terrors. *J. Nerv. Ment. Dis.* 157:75, 1973.

————. A psychophysiological study of nightmares and night terrors. II. The suppression of stage 4 nightmares with diazepam. *Arch. Gen. Psychiat.* 28:252, 1973.

Fogarty, S. J. and D. R. Hemsley. Depression and the accessibility of memories. *Brit. J. Psychiat.* 142:232, 1983.

Freeman, J. M., A. M. Aron, J. E. Collard, and M. C. MacKay. The emotional correlates of Sydenham's chorea. *Pediatrics* 35:42, 1965.

Friedhoff, A. J. and E. Van Winkle. Characteristics of amine found in urine of schizophrenic patients. *J. Nerv. Ment. Dis.* 135:550, 1962.

Garron, D. C., H. L. Klawans, and F. Narin. Intellectual functioning of persons with idiopathic parkinsonism. *J. Nerv. Ment. Dis.* 154:445, 1972.

Gershon, E. The genetics of affective disorder. In: *Psychiatry Update*, vol. II, L. Grinspoon, ed. American Psychiatric Press, Washington, 1983, p. 434.

Glaeser, V. S., W. H. Vogel, D. B. Oleweiler, and T. A. Hare. GABA levels in cerebrospinal fluid of patients with Huntington's chorea: A preliminary report. *Biochem. Med.* 12:380, 1975.

Gold, P., G. Chrousos, C. Kellner, et al. Psychiatric implications of basic and clinical studies with corticotropin-releasing factor. *Amer. J. Psychiat.* 141:619, 1984.

Goldberg, S. C., G. C. Klerman, and J. O. Cole. Changes in schizophrenic psychopathology and ward behavior as a function of phenothiazine treatment. *Brit. J. Psychiat.* 111:120, 1965.

Gollomps, S. M., S. Fahr, R. E. Burke, et al. Therapeutic trials in Meige's syndrome. *Adv. Neurol.* 37:207, 1983.

Gomez, M. R. and D. W. Klass. Epilepsies of infancy and childhood. *Ann. Neurol.* 13:113, 1983.

Goodman, L. S. and A. Gilman. *The Pharmacological Basis of Therapeutics.* 4th ed. Macmillan, London, 1970.

Granacher, R. P. Differential diagnosis of tardive dyskinesia: An overview. *Amer. J. Psychiat.* 138:1288, 1981.

Greenblatt, M., G. H. Grosser, and H. Wechsler. Differential response of hospitalized depressed patients to somatic therapy. *Amer. J. Psychiat.* 120:935, 1964.

Gumby, P. DNA probe offers possibility of genetic linkage testing for Huntington's disease. *Arch. Intern. Med.* 144:243, 1984.

Gusella, J., N. Wexler, P. M. Conneally, et al. A polymorphic DNA marker genetically linked to Huntington's disease. *Nature* 306:234, 1983.

Hamilton, M. Standardized assessment and recording of depressive symptoms. *Psychiat. Neurol. Neuroclin.* 72:201, 1969.

Hartmann, E. Longitudinal studies of sleep and dream patterns in manic-depressive patients. *Arch. Gen. Psychiat.* 19:311, 1968.

Hauri, P. and D. R. Hawkins. Alpha delta sleep. *Electroenceph. Clin. Neurophys.* 34:233, 1973.

Hawkins, D. R. and J. Mendels. Sleep disturbance in depressive syndromes. *Amer. J. Psychiat.* 123:682, 1966.

Heathfield, K. W. G. Huntington's chorea: Investigation into the prevalence of this disease in the area covered by the North East Metropolitan Regional Hospital Board. *Brain* 90:203, 1967.

Hill, D. Depression: Disease, reaction or posture. *Amer. J. Psychiat.* 125:445, 1968.

Himwich, H. E. and H. S. Alpers. Psychopharmacology. *Ann. Rev. Pharmacol.* 10:313, 1970.

Hishikawa, Y., H. Ida, K. Nakai, and Z. Kaneko. Treatment of narcolepsy with imipramine (Tofranil) and desmethylimipramine (Pertofran). *J. Neurol. Sci.* 453, 1966.

Hollister, L. E. Excretion of 3 methoxy-4 hydroxyphenylglycol in depressed and geriatric patients and normal persons. *Int. Pharmacopsychiat.* 16: 138, 1981.

Hornykiewicz, O. Dopamine (3 hydroxytyramine) and brain function. *Pharmacol. Rev.* 18:925, 1966.

———. Dopamine and extrapyramidal motor function and dysfunction. Presented at ARNMD meeting, New York, 1970.

———. Parkinson's disease: From brain homogerate to treatment. *Fed. Proc.* 2:183, 1973.

Insel, T. R., N. H. Kalin, L. B. Guttmacher, et al. The dexamethasone suppression test in patients with obsessive compulsive disorder. *Psychiat. Res.* 6:153, 1982.

Iversen, L. L., A. S. Horn, and R. J. Miller. Actions of dopaminergic agonists on cyclic AMP production in rat brain homogerates. In: *Advances in Neurology*, vol. 9, D. B. Calne, T. N. Chase, and A. Barbeau, eds. Raven Press, New York, 1975, p. 147.

Iversen, L. L., G. P. Reynolds, and S. H. Snyder. Pathophysiology of Schizophrenia—Causal role for dopamine or noradrenaline. *Nature* 305:577, 1983.

Jacobson, A. and W. T. Kinney. Affective disorders. In: *Treament of Mental Disorders*, J. Greist, J. Jefferson, and R. Spitzer, eds. Oxford University Press, New York, 1982, p. 184.

Jankovic, J. and J. Ford. Blepharospasm and orofacial-cervical dystonia: Clinical and pharmacological findings in 100 patients. *Ann. Neurol.* 13: 402, 1983.

Janowsky, D. S., M. K. El-Yousef, J. M. Davis, and J. Sekerke. Parasympathetic suppression of manic symptoms by physostigmine. *Arch. Gen. Psychiat.* 28:542, 1973.

———, ———, ———, ———, D. R. Morris, and B. Decker. Effects of amantadine on tardive dyskinesia and pseudo-Parkinsonism. *New Eng. J. Med.* 286:784, 1972.

Jouvet, M. Neurophysiology of the states of sleep. In: *The Neurosciences*, G. C. Quarton, T. Melnechuk, and F. O. Schmitt, eds. A Study Program. Rockefeller University Press, New York, 1967, p. 529.

Kaiko, F. M., K. M. Foley, P. Y. Oraiviski, et al. Central nervous system excitating effect of meperidine in cancer patients. *Ann. Neurol.* 13:180, 1983.

Kallman, F. J. The genetics of psychoses: An analysis of 1232 twin index families. *Int. Cong. Psychiat. Rapports* 6:1, 1950.

———. Genetics principles in manic-depressive psychosis. In: *Depression*, P. H. Hoch and J. Zubin, eds. Grune and Stratton, New York, 1954.

Kane, J. M. and J. M. Smith. Tardive dyskinesia. *Arch. Gen. Psychiat.* 39:473, 1982.

Kelwala, S., D. Jones, and N. Bitrom.   Monamine metabolites as predictors of antidepressant response. *Prog. Neuro-Psychopharmacol. Biol. Psychiat.* 7:229, 1983.

Kendall, R. E.   The Classification of Depressive Illness. Oxford University Press, London, 1968.

Kety, S. S.   Current biochemical approaches to schizophrenia. *New Eng. J. Med.* 276:325, 1967.

Kiloh, L. C. and R. F. Garside.   The independence of neurotic depression and endogenous depression. *Brit. J. Psychiat.* 109:451, 1963.

Klawans, H. L., Jr.   A pharmacologic analysis of Huntington's chorea. *Europ. Neurol.* 4:148, 1970.

————.   The pharmacology of tardive dyskinesias. *Amer. J. Psychiat.* 130: 82, 1973.

———— and R. Rubovits.   Central cholinergic-anticholinergic antagonism in Huntington's chorea. *Neurology* 22:107, 1972.

————, G. G. Paulsson, R. P. Ringel, and A. Barbeau.   Use of L-DOPA in the detection of presymptomatic Huntington's chorea. *New Eng. J. Med.* 286:1332, 1972.

———— and A. Barr.   Prevalence of spontaneous lingual-facial-buccal dyskinesia in the elderly. *Neurology* 32:558, 1982.

Klein, D. F. and J. M. Davis.   *Diagnosis and Drug Treatment of Psychiatric Disorders.* Williams & Wilkins, Baltimore, 1969.

Kleinman, J. E., D. R. Weinberger, A. D. Rogol, L. B. Bigelow, S. T. Klein, J. C. Gillin, and R. J. Wyatt.   Plasma prolactin concentrations and psychopathology in chronic schizophrenia. *Arch. Gen. Psychiat.* 39:655, 1982.

Koller, W. C.   Edentulous orodyskinesia. *Ann. Neurol.* 13:97, 1983.

Kraft, G. H., E. W. Johnson, and M. M. Laban.   The fibrositis syndrome. *Arch. Phys. Med. Rehab.* 49:156, 1968.

Kuhn, R.   The treatment of depressive states with G22 355 (imipramine hydrochloride). *Amer. J. Psychiat.* 115:459, 1958.

Kupfer, D. J. and M. E. Thase.   The use of the sleep laboratory in the diagnosis of affective disorder. *Pschiat. Clin. N. Amer.* 5:3, 1983.

————.   Validity of major depression: A psychobiological perspective. Presented at APA Conference on DSM-III, Washington, D.C., October, 1983.

Lewy, A. J., T. A. Wehr, F. K. Goodwin, et al.   Manic depressive patients may be sensitive to light. *Lancet* 1:383, 1981.

Linnoila, M., P. Ninon, M. Scheinin, et al.   Reliability of norepinephrine and major monoamine metabolite measurements in CSF of schizophrenic patients. *Arch. Gen. Psychiat.* 40:1290, 1983.

Loosen, P. T. and A. J. Prange.   Serum thyrotropin response to thyrotropin releasing hormone in psychiatric patients: A review. *Amer. J. Psychiat.* 139:405, 1982.

Loosen, P. T., K. Kistler, and A. J. Prange.   Use of TSH response to TRH as an independent variable. *Amer. J. Psychiat.* 140:700, 1983.

Maas, J. W.   Biogenic amines and depression: biochemical and pharmacological separation of two types of depression. *Arch. Gen. Psychiat.* 2: 1357, 1975.

Mayeux, R., Y. Stern, J. Rosen, and J. Leventhal. Depression, intellectual impairment, and Parkinson disease. *Neurology* 31:645, 1981.

McAllister, T. Pseudodementia. *Amer. J. Psychiat.* 140:528, 1983.

McKay, A. V. C., E. D. Bird, and E. G. Spokes. Dopamine receptors and schizophrenia. *Lancet* 2:915, 1980.

Mendels, J. and A. Frazer. Brain biogenic amine depletion and mood. *Arch. Gen. Psychiat.* 30:447, 1974.

Mindham, R. H. S. Psychiatric symptoms in Parkinsonism. *J. Neurol. Neurosurg. Psychiat.* 33:188, 1970.

Moldofsky, H., P. Scarisbrick, R. England, and H. Smythe. Musculoskeletal symptoms and non REM sleep disturbance in patients with "fibrositis" syndrome and healthy subjects. *Psychosom. Med.* 37:341, 1975.

Murphy, D. L., H. K. Brodie, and F. K. Goodwin. Regular induction of hypomania by L-DOPA in "bipolar" manic-depressive patients. *Nature* 229:135, 1971.

Nakaro, I. and A. Hitaro. Neuron loss in the nucleus basilis of Reynert in Parkinson-dementia complex of Guan. *Ann. Neurol.* 13:87, 1983.

Nauseida, P. A., L. A. Bieliauskas, L. D. Bacon, et al. Chronic dopaminergic sensitivity after Sydenham's chorea. *Neurology* 33:750, 1983.

Nemeroff, C. and Evans, D. Correlation between the dexamethasone suppression test in depressed patients and clinical response. *Amer. J. Psychiat.* 141:247, 1984.

Noll, K. and Davis, J. Biological theories in schizophrenia. In: *Schizophrenia and Affective Disorders*, A. Rifkin, J. Wright. PSG, Boston, 1983, p. 139.

Noyes, A. P. and L. C. Kolb. *Modern Clinical Psychiatry*. 6th ed. W. B. Saunders, Philadelphia, 1963.

Parkes, C. M. The first year of bereavement. *Psychiatry* 33:444, 1970.

Paykel, E. S. and A. Coppen. *Psychopharmacology of Affective Disorders*. Oxford University Press, Oxford, 1979.

Pollitt, J. D. Suggestions for a physiologic classification of depression. *Brit. J. Psychiat.* 111:489, 1965.

Post, R. M., E. K. Gordon, F. K. Goodwin, et al. Central norepinephrine metabolism in affective illness: MHPG in the CSF. *Science* 179:1002, 1973.

Post, R. M., T. W. Uhde, J. C. Bellenger, et al. Prophylactic efficacy of carbamazepine in manic-depressive illness. *Amer. J. Psychiat.* 140:1602, 1983.

Post, R. M., T. Uhde, F. Putnam, et al. Kindling and carbamazepine in affective illness. *J. Nerv. Ment. Dis.* 170:717, 1982.

Quitkin, F. M., A. Rifkin, and D. F. Klein. Prophylaxis of affective disorders: Current status of knowledge. *Arch. Gen. Psychiat.* 33:337, 1976.

Reynolds, G. P. Increased concentrations and lateral asymmetry of amygdala dopamine in schizophrenia. *Nature* 305:527, 1983.

Riklan, M. and E. Levita. *Subcortical Correlates of Human Behavior*. Williams & Wilkins, Baltimore, 1969.

Risch, S. C., L. Y. Huey, and D. S. Janowsky. Plasma levels of tricyclic antidepressants and clinical efficacy: Review of the literature—Part I. *J. Clin. Psychiat.* 40:4, 1979.

———. Plasma levels of tricyclic antidepressants and clinical efficacy: Review of the literature—Part II. *J. Clin. Psychiat.* 40:58, 1979.

Robins, E. and S. Guze. Classification of affective disorders. In: *Recent Advances in the Psychobiology of the Depressive Illnesses.* DHEW Publications No. 709053, 1972. U.S. Government Printing Office, Washington, D.C., p. 283.

Rogers, M. P., D. Dubey, and P. Reich. The influence of the psyche and the brain on immunity and disease susceptibility: A critical review. *Psychosom. Med.* 41:147, 1979.

Rosenthal, N., D. Sock, C. Gilleri, et al. Seasonal affective disorder. *Arch. Gen. Psychiat.* 41:72, 1984.

Rubin, R. and S. Morder. Biological markers in affective and schizophrenic disorders. In: *Affective and Schizophrenic Disorders*, M. Zales, ed. Brunner/Mazel, New York, 1983, p. 53.

Sachar, E. J. Corticosteroids in depressive illness. *Arch. Gen. Psychiat.* 17:544, 1967.

Schiffer, R. B., E. D. Caine, K. A. Bamford, and S. Levy. Depressive episodes in patients with multiple sclerosis. *Amer. J. Psychiat.* 140:1498, 1983.

Schildkraut, J. J. Neurochemical studies of the affective disorders. *Amer. J. Psychiat.* 127:358, 1970.

———. Norepinephrine metabolites as biochemical criteria for classifying depressive disorders and predicting responses to treatment. *Amer. J. Psychiat.* 130:695, 1973.

Schildkraut, J., P. Orsulak, A. Schatzberg, et al. Laboratory tests for discriminating subtypes of depressive disorders based on measurements of catecholamine metabolism. In: *Affective and Schizophrenic Disorders*, M. Zales, ed. Brunner/Mazel, New York, 1983, p. 103.

Schleifer, S. J., S. E. Keller, M. Camerino, J. C. Thornton, and M. Stein. Suppression of lymphocyte stimulation following bereavement. *JAMA* 250:374, 1983.

Schwab, R. S., H. D. Fabing, and J. S. Pritchard. Psychiatric symptoms and syndromes in Parkinson's disease. *Amer. J. Psychiat.* 107:901, 1951.

Shopsin, B., S. Wilk, S. Gershon, et al. Cerebrospinal fluid MHPG and assessment of norepinephrine metabolism in affective disorders. *Arch. Gen. Psychiat.* 28:230, 1973.

Slater, E. and V. Cowie. *The Genetics of Mental Disorders.* Oxford University Press, London, 1971.

Small, J. C., I. F. Small, and D. F. Moore. Experimental withdrawal of lithium in recovered manic-depressive patients. *Amer. J. Psychiat.* 127:131, 1971.

Snyder, S. H. Psychoactive drugs and central neurotransmitters. Presented at the Association for Research in Nervous and Mental Disease, New York City, 1970.

————. Catecholamines in the brain as mediators of amphetamine psychosis. *Arch. Gen. Psychiat.* 27:169, 1972.

————. Dopamine receptors, neuroleptics, and schizophrenia. *Amer. J. Psychiat.* 138:460, 1981.

————, D. Greenberg, and H. I. Yamamara. Antischizophrenic drugs and brain cholinergic receptors. *Arch. Gen. Psychiat.* 31:58, 1974.

————, H. Greenberg, and H. I. Yamamara. Antischizophrenic drugs: Affinity for muscarinic cholinergic receptor sites in the brain predicts extrapyramidal effects. *J. Psychiat. Res.* 11:91, 1974.

Sotaniemi, K. Valproic acid in the treatment of non-epileptic myoclonus. Report of three cases. *Arch. Neurol.* 39:448, 1982.

Sours, J. A. Narcolepsy and other disturbances of the sleep waking rhythm: a study of 115 cases with review of the literature. *J. Nerv. Ment. Dis.* 147:525, 1963.

Spars, J. E. and R. Grener. Does the dexamethasone suppression test distinguish dementia from depression? *Amer. J. Psychiat.* 139:238, 1982.

Sroka, H., T. S. Elizan, M. D. Yahr, A. Burger, and M. R. Mendoza. Organic mental syndrome and confusional states in Parkinson's disease. *Arch. Neurol.* 38:339, 1981.

Staton, D. D. and R. A. Brumback. Neuroleptic-induced reinnervation sprouting in the central nervous system. *J. Clin. Psychiat.* 41:427, 1980.

Stevens, J. R. Motor disorders in schizophrenia. *New Eng. J. Med.* 290:110, 1974.

Sulser, F. and E. Sanders-Bush. Effects of drugs on amines in the CNS. *Ann. Rev. Pharmacol.* 11:209, 1971.

Taylor, K. M. and S. H. Snyder. Amphetamine: differentiation by D and L isomers of behavior involving brain norepinephrine or dopamine. *Science* 168:1487, 1970.

———— and ————. Differential effects of D and L amphetamine on behavior and on catecholamine disposition in dopamine and norepinephrine-containing neurons of rat brain. *Brain Res.* 28:295, 1971.

Theodore, W. H. and Porter, R. J. Removal of sedative-hypnotic anti-epileptic drugs from the regimens of patients with intractable epilepsy. *Ann. Neurol.* 13:320, 1983.

Uhl, G. R., D. C. Hilt, J. C. Hedreen, et al. Pick's disease: Depletion of neurons in the nucleus basalis of Reynert. *Neurology* 33:1470, 1983.

Van Woert, M. H., L. M. Ambani, and M. B. Bowers, Jr. Levodopa and cholinergic hypersensitivity in Parkinson's disease. *Neurology* 22:86, 1972.

Walters, J. R., B. S. Burney, and R. H. Roth. Piridebil and apomorphine: Pre- and post-synaptic effects on dopamine synthesis and neuronal activity. In: *Advances in Neurology*, vol. 9, D. B. Calne, T. N. Chase and A. Barbeau, eds. Raven Press, New York, 1975, p. 273.

Wehr, T. and F. Goodwin. Biological rhythms and psychiatry. In: *American Handbook of Psychiatry*, vol. VII, S. Arieti, ed. Basic Books, New York, 1981.

Weintraub, M. I. and M. H. Van Woert. Reversal of cholinergic hypersensitivity in Parkinson's disease by levodopa. *New Eng. J. Med.* 284:412, 1971.

Weitkamp, W. R., H. C. Stancer, E. Persad, et al.   Depressive disorders and HLA. *New Eng. J. Med.* 305:1301, 1981.

Wettstein, A.   No effect from double-blind trial of physostigmine and lecithin in Alzheimer's disease. *Ann. Neurol.* 13:210, 1983.

Whatmore, G. B. and R. M. Ellis.   Further neurophysiologic aspects of depressed states. *Arch. Gen. Psychiat.* 6:243, 1962.

Whitaker, P. M., T. J. Crow, and I. N. Ferrier.   Tritiated LSD binding in frontal cortex in schizophrenia. *Arch. Gen. Psychiat.* 38:278, 1981.

Whitehouse, P. J., J. C. Hedreen, C. L. White III, et al.   Basal forebrain neurons in the dementia of Parkinson's disease. *Ann. Neurol.* 13:243, 1983.

Whitlock, F. A., and M. M. Siskund.   Depression as a major symptom of multiple sclerosis. *J. Neurol. Neurosurg. Psychiat.* 43:861, 1980.

Whittier, J., G. Haydu, and J. Crawford.   Effect of imipramine (Tofranil) on depression and hyperkinesia in Huntington's disease. *Amer. J. Psychiat.* 118:79, 1961.

Whybrow, P. C. and J. Mendels.   Towards a biology of depression: Some suggestions from neurophysiology. *Amer. J. Psychiat.* 125:1491, 1969.

—— and P. M. Silberfarb.   Neuroendocrine mediating mechanisms: from the symbolic stimulus to the physiological response. *Int. J. Psychiat. Med.* 5:531, 1974.

—— and T. C. Hurwitz.   Psychological disturbances associated with endocrine disease and hormone therapy. In: *Hormones, Behavior, and Psychopathology*, E. J. Sachar, ed. Raven Press, New York, 1976.

Winokur, G., R. Cadoret, J. Dorzab, and M. Baker.   Depressive disease: A genetic study. *Arch. Gen. Psychiat.* 24:135, 1971.

Wittenborn, J. R., M. Plante, F. Burgess, and H. Maurer.   A comparison of imipramine, electroconvulsive therapy and placebo in the treatment of depressions. *J. Nerv. Ment. Dis.* 135:131, 1962.

Wyatt, R. J., D. H. Fram, R. Buchbinder, and F. Snyder.   Treatment of intractable narcolepsy with a monoamine oxidase inhibitor. *New Eng. J. Med.* 285:987, 1971.

Yahr, M. D. and R. C. Duvoisin.   Drug therapy of Parkinsonism. *New Eng. J. Med* 287:20, 1972.

Yaryura-Tobias, J. A., B. Diamond, and S. Merlis.   The action of L-DOPA on schizophrenic patients (A preliminary report). *Curr. Ther. Res. Clin. Exp.* 12:528, 1970.

Yen, S. H., D. S. Haroupian, and R. D. Terry.   Immunocytochemical comparison of neurofibrillary tangles in senile dementia of Alzheimer type, progressive supranuclear palsy and postencephalitic Parkinsonism. *Ann. Neurol.* 13:172, 1983.

Zarcone, V.   Narcolepsy. *New Eng. J. Med.* 288:1156, 1973.

Zung, W. K. K.   A self-rating depression scale. *Arch. Gen. Psychiat.* 12:63, 1965.

Chapter 6

DISTINGUISHING NEUROLOGIC
FROM NEUROTIC DISORDERS

Hyperventilation syndrome, headache, hysteria, and hypochondriasis seem quite disparate, but they often coexist. Though commonly classified as symptoms of neurosis, they are often encountered in depression and also occur in personality disorders, and even in schizophrenia. In most individuals with the hyperventilation syndrome, other psychophysiological reactions, conversion hysteria, and hypochondriasis commonly appear. In other words, hyperventilation and other psychophysiological reactions, hysteria, hypochondriasis, and certain types of headache are psychosomatic conditions that together form a syndrome that occurs in a number of psychiatric disorders. The prognosis of this syndrome probably depends on the basic psychiatric conditions with which it is associated.

HYPERVENTILATION SYNDROME

Of all psychophysiological reactions, probably the most common one dealt with by physicians is the hyperventilation syndrome. Because its manifestations in different body systems can mimic other conditions, this syndrome is frequently unrecognized, and patients are often shunted from doctor to doctor undergoing numerous diagnostic tests, which are unnecessary and upsetting. Often the result of anxiety, hyperventilation produces changes in body functions that themselves become the focus of anxiety. Fear and confusion are compounded when a doctor tells his patient that his symptoms are factitious, "all in his nerves." The patient knows his symptoms are not imagined and supposes he has a life-threatening illness. The symptoms of the hyperventilation syndrome include faintness, visual disturbances, inability to concentrate, nausea, vertiginous instability, headache, fullness in the head and chest and epigastrium, breathlessness, palpitations, hot flushing, cold sweating, paresthesias, and occasionally vomiting. This panoply of symptoms results from physiological alterations that can be caused simply by overbreathing.

A study of the hyperventilation syndrome in neurological practice was undertaken by reviewing the charts of the 550 patients seen by one of us (JHP) over a five-year period at the Yale New Haven Hospital in the private outpatient neurology clinic.* All referred patients were suspected of having a neurological condition. Age, sex, past medical history, present symptoms, and past history of psychosomatic illnesses were noted. The diagnosis of the hyperventilation syndrome was made on the basis of the patient's response to overbreathing. Each patient who complained of any of the symptoms associated with this syndrome was asked to overbreathe by mouth for up to three minutes or until he became dizzy. If the symptoms of which he complained were thus reproduced in their entirety and if no other explanation for the symptoms could be adduced from physical examination, medical history or laboratory tests, the diagnosis was considered established.

Thirty patients met these criteria. They ranged in age from 15 to 60 years. In order to ascertain whether hyperventilation syndrome was more prevalent at certain ages and among women, a control group of 58 patients was randomly selected from the remaining 520 for detailed review, and these were fairly evenly distributed between the ages of several months to 75. Of the study group, 86 percent but only 24 percent of the control group, were between the ages of 15 and 30 ($p < 0.01$). Of the study group, 87 percent, but only 49 percent of the control group, were women ($p < 0.05$) (Table 6-1). Of all the women referred for neurologi-

---

* The data quoted were derived from the student thesis of Bruce B. Haak at the Yale University School of Medicine.

Table 6-1
Patients with Hyperventilation Syndrome
and Neurological Controls[a]
by Age and Sex

Age	0–15	15–30	30–45	45–60	60–75	Total
Syndrome						
(M)	0	2	1	1	0	4
(F)	0	16	5	5	0	26
						30
Control[a]						
(M)	7	8	3	5	7	30
(F)	5	6	6	6	5	28
						58

[a] Controls were drawn at random from the same private neurological outpatient clinic population of 550, from which the 30 patients with the syndrome had been drawn.

cal consultation between the ages of 15 and 30, 29 percent had the hyperventilation syndrome as the sole cause of their chief complaint. This was true of less than 5 percent of the men in the same age group.

A history of psychosomatic illness in the past was more common in the study group. This term encompasses complicated medical symptoms with negative evaluations, conversion reactions, psychophysiological reactions, and multiple visits to physicians for minor conditions (hypochondriasis). Of the patients with the hyperventilation syndrome, 77 percent had a history of psychosomatic illness in the past as compared with 28 percent in the control group ($p < 0.5$). Psychosomatic illness was twice as prevalent among women with the syndrome, between the ages of 15 and 45 as among control women of the same age ($p < 0.05$).

The chief complaints of the study group were usually multiple, involving at least two organ systems in 86 percent of the patients and three or more organ systems in over 30 percent. These included *neurological complaints* (lightheadedness, 80%; paresthesias, 50%; headache, 37%; weakness, 27%; inability to concentrate,

Table 6-2
Incidence of Psychosomatic Illness[a] in Patients with
Hyperventilation Syndrome and Neurological Controls
by Age and Sex

Age	0–15	15–30	30–45	45–60	60–75	Total
Syndrome						
(M)	0	1/2	1/1	1/1	0/0	3/4
(F)	0	13/16	5/5	2/5	0/0	20/26
Control						
(M)	1/7	1/8	1/3	0/5	1/7	4/30
(F)	0/5	2/6	3/6	5/6	1/5	11/28

[a] Psychosomatic illness was taken to mean a previous history of medical symptoms the investigation of which produced negative results or conversion reactions, and/or multiple visits to physicians for minor problems (hypochondriasis).

23%; loss of consciousness, 6%; and tetanus, 3%), *gastrointestinal complaints* (inability to swallow, 23%, and abdominal pains, 10%), and *cardiac complaints* (dyspnea, 23%; palpitations, 20%; and chest pain, 17%).

The symptom frequency noted above is obviously colored by the fact that these patients were referred for neurological evaluation. Studying the hyperventilation syndrome in a population of 500 consecutive patients seen by a gastroenterologist, McKell and Sullivan (1947) reported frequencies of 76, 60, and 55 percent for breathlessness, palpitations, and chest pain, respectively. All these patients had gastrointestinal complaints.

The mechanism by which hyperventilation causes such symptoms is the lowering of pCO_2. Two deep breaths produced by yawning or sighing are enough to alter pCO_2 significantly and produce symptoms. The lowered pCO_2 reduces cerebral blood flow, since there is a direct relation between pCO_2 and the caliber of the cerebral blood vessels. In 240 seconds of overbreathing, cerebral blood flow can be reduced by 40 percent (Plum and Posner, 1972). Thus, hyperventilation leads to cerebral hypoxia, and this is the cause of the EEG slowing so often seen with overbreathing (Gotoh et al., 1965). Prolonged hyperventilation can produce respiratory alkalosis, which in turn can induce tetany.

Hyperventilation is a routine part of electroencephalographic testing and may induce an epileptiform abnormality. Of course, it can also induce actual seizures. Hyperventilation in response to anxiety may, in fact, be a major mechanism by which emotional tension induces seizures in susceptible individuals (Mattson et al., 1970). The cerebral hypoxia caused by hyperventilation, when compounded by a mild degree of orthostatic hypotension and/or the Valsalva maneuver, may reduce cerebral blood flow to the degree that the patient faints or has a tonic convulsion. (Many young boys have learned to induce syncope by overbreathing and then performing the Valsalva maneuver for the amusement of their friends.)

Hyperventilation can also cause nonspecific ST- and T-wave changes in the electrocardiogram (EKG) (Christensen, 1946), and many hyperventilation syndrome patients showing such EKG changes have been admitted to coronary care units. Hyperventilation is often associated with air swallowing and this, in turn, can lead to epigastric distress and gastrointestinal symptoms.

Hyperventilation is a very common response to anxiety. One might almost call it a universal human reaction to anxiety, since it is part of the autonomic response to threatening situations. That it becomes a symptom that leads people to seek medical attention primarily when they are predisposed to conversion reaction, hypochondriasis, or psychosomatic illnesses is suggested by our finding a history of such problems in more than three-quarters of the hyperventilation syndrome patients. Young women aged 15 to 30 seem to be particularly susceptible. Preadolescents and patients at retirement age appear to be less so.

Seven of the 30 patients with the syndrome had organic diseases as well, including regional ileitis, arthritis, adrenal insufficiency, carpal tunnel syndrome, orthostatic hypotension, and endometriosis. Of these seven, five were over 30 years of age. For this reason, it would seem prudent, especially in patients over 30, to consider the possibility of associated medical illnesses even in the face of the hyperventilation syndrome.

HEADACHE

Determining the cause of headache is one of the most critical diagnoses a physician has to make. Headache can be a symptom of anxiety or depression, or it can be the first symptom of a brain tumor. It is not our purpose to provide a comprehensive discussion of headache. For this the reader is referred to two excellent books, Dalessio's edition of Wolff (1980) and Friedman and Merritt (1959). We will merely put forward the criteria from the patient's history that are helpful in distinguishing headaches of psychogenic origin from those of neurological origin.

In general, if the headache is "the worst" headache ever experienced by the patient, if it is a new headache, or if it is associated with neurological signs, the physician must assume that an acute or life-threatening situation may be present, and a full investigation should be promptly initiated. A CT scan should be the first test. If normal, lumbar puncture should follow. When this rule is followed, the diagnoses of subarachnoid hemorrhage, meningitis, encephalitis, or brain tumor will not often be missed. For teaching purposes, we advise medical students to fully investigate any headache that is "the worst, the first, or cursed (by neurologic abnormalities)." Conversely, any headache that has been present for more than a year, almost irrespective of its character, is rarely caused by a serious or progressive disorder.

Headaches that are dull, generalized, and constant for many days in a row usually have no neurological cause. Patients with such headaches often describe "a pressure feeling," which is what they mean by headache. These patients almost always have an impressive past history of psychosomatic illness and are depressed. The unremitting character of the headaches and the patient's complaints of their severity usually contrast with the fact that he is nonetheless able to work. Analgesics, tranquilizers, and sedatives are usually ineffective, but antidepressants often help. In general, headaches of sudden onset, headaches that awaken a patient from sleep, or unilateral headaches are not caused by purely emotional factors, even if they persist for days, weeks, or months.

Tension headaches are presumably caused by muscle tension. When the muscles in the posterior neck and temples are under the stress of continuous contraction, they begin to ache just as muscles anywhere in the body do when they have been overworked. The pain reflection is then generalized over the head. Such headaches are dull and steady, though occasionally, a sustained muscle contraction headache is followed by a typical vascular (throbbing) headache, and the two types of headache will coexist in an attack. Tension headaches can usually be attributed to emotional tension, but sometimes cervical pathology, such as osteoarthritis or cervical disc disease, will cause headache by cervical muscle contraction. Tension headaches characteristically occur in the morning on awakening or in the late afternoon. These headaches are worse during the working week and tend to be relieved on weekends and vacations. They are generally relieved by aspirin and sedatives. Tension headaches are often mistakenly attributed to essential hypertension or chronic sinusitis. With few exceptions, by the time a patient comes to a doctor for treatment of tension headaches, he will have had them for months or years. Surprisingly, this holds true for children too. Some patients who initially deny the long-standing nature of their headaches, when pressed will admit that they have had similar headaches in the past, though perhaps not so severe or so frequent. This point is important in distinguishing ordinary tension headaches from those caused by brain tumors.

Headaches are caused by brain tumors in two ways, by increased intracranial pressure and by traction of the mass on pain-sensitive structures within the skull. No single headache is characteristic of a brain tumor. Headaches caused by increased intracranial pressure are, if anything, remarkable for being nonspecific. They are mild, dull, aching, and very often bifrontal or bioccipital. They may be present in the morning on awakening, last a few hours, and get better as the day goes on. They may not occur every day. Thus, they may be quite similar to tension headaches. Headaches produced by increased intracranial pressure, however, are characteristically of recent onset, usually starting within a few weeks before the patient presents himself to the physician. We have found this to be the single most important feature in distinguishing tension headaches from those caused by increased intracranial pressure.

When brain tumors cause headaches by traction on pain-sensitive structures, headaches are often lateralized or localized to one spot. Intraventricular tumors can cause headaches that may be exacerbated or relieved by changes in position. Thus, when a patient complains of a headache that is brought on by putting his head in one position and relieved by changing the position, a mechanical factor must be considered and the possibility of a tumor investigated thoroughly. It is an ominous sign if headache is relieved by sitting up.

Headaches that follow the performance of a lumbar puncture are mechanical in origin, too, and the result of traction on pain-sensitive structures at the base of the brain after loss of spinal fluid that normally cushions these structures from the skull beneath. Reclining in a supine position promptly relieves such headaches. Contrary to common belief, emotional factors do not play an important role in producing these headaches.

Prostrating headaches that are throbbing and severe, lasting several hours, and associated with nausea, and/or vomiting are usually migrainous. This is so whether or not they are unilateral or preceded by typical ischemic symptoms such as flashing lights, scintillating scotomata, or sensory or motor symptoms. Migraine headaches begin with throbbing but as the blood vessels become maximally dilated and the pain reaches its zenith, the throbbing may stop. Usually the pain at this time is unbearable, prostrating, and associated with vomiting and photophobia. Curiously, at this point in the headache, many patients can fall asleep and if so, they awaken improved. The incidence of migraine is the same in men and women but, presumably because of hormonal factors, headaches are usually more severe and more frequent in women. Patients with such prostrating headaches usually have a positive family history of migraine, which suggests a hereditary basis. Migraine headaches occur primarily in the young, often begin in the first decade, and hardly ever develop for the first time after the age of 30 years. They may tend to occur more frequently on weekends and vacations and are seldom satisfactorily relieved by ordinary analgesics. Contrary to popular belief, emotional factors usually play a minor role in the etiology of migraine headaches and psychotherapy does not relieve them. Ergot-containing preparations are usually effective in stopping such headaches if they are taken in the early stages of the attack, especially during the prodromal period. Propranolol has become a useful therapeutic agent in reducing the frequency and severity of attacks. Antidepressants are also widely used with good effect but one wonders if tension headaches associated with depression have been labelled migraine in many patients who have experienced relief from antidepressants.

The syndrome of temporomandibular joint (TMJ) pain is characterized by a usually unilateral, deep-seated pain in the side of the face, which is brought on or exacerbated by movements of the lower jaw. The pain is related to spasm of the muscles that operate the jaw, mainly the temporalis and pterygoid, and rarely, the masseter. It is not usually associated with actual pathology of the temporomandibular joint so that the name is somewhat misleading. Radiographs of the joint are abnormal in only a small minority of cases. The syndrome is most common in young women. The characteristics of the pain are typical of muscle pain: it is steady (nonthrobbing) and severe. After several hours, throbbing can develop. The pain is exacerbated by quick stretches of the muscle, as in mouth opening, and by more prolonged use of the painful muscle, as in chewing. It may follow visits to the dentist when prolonged opening of the mouth and stretching of the muscles of mastication are necessary: bruxism, yawning, shouting, singing, fellatio, and direct trauma to the jaw are other contributing factors.

Since temporomandibular joint pain is usually experienced around or behind the eye and along the temple, palpation of the temporalis muscle and attempted lateral movement of the jaw against pressure usually produces pain. When the body of the pterygoid muscle is palpated from inside the mouth, there is great tenderness, and the muscle itself often feels tense and hypertrophied to the examiner. Direct pressure over the temporomandibular joint may also cause pain.

Many patients with this syndrome are depressed, do not sleep well, and awaken feeling tired. They often grind their teeth during sleep and yawn a great deal in the morning after awakening. Thus, bruxism and yawning seem to be the major contributing factors in many cases.

This syndrome is very commonly seen in neurological practice (Table 6-3). It is often misdiagnosed by neurologists as typical migraine, atypical facial pain, or a functional disorder. The steady, nonthrobbing nature of the pain at onset distinguishes it from migraine. Also, some headaches may last only a few minutes. The occasional very brief headache, lasting minutes, and the lack of throbbing at the onset are most helpful features in distinguishing the TMJ syndrome from migraine. The tenderness of affected muscles distinguishes it from atypical facial pain, and the unilaterality of the pain should distinguish it from functional or ordinary tension headache.

Table 6-3
Incidence of Temporomandibular Joint (TMJ) Syndrome among 365 Consecutive Private Neurological Outpatients[a]

	No. of Patients	Chief Complaint Headache	Tension Headache (Bilateral)	TMJ Syndrome[b]	Migraine[b]	Other Headache
Male	171	28	7	6	7	8
Female	194	48	16	14	8	10
Total	365	76	23	20	15	18

[a] All patients were referred; most of them by internists. All the headache patients had been unsuccessfully treated. In no instance had the temporomandibular joint syndrome been considered in the differential diagnosis by the referring physician.

[b] All patients had predominantly or exclusively unilateral headaches.

The syndrome is easier to diagnose than to treat. Conservative therapy consists of heat applied to the affected area, a diet of soft foods, limitation of mouth opening, and mild analgesics and muscle relaxants. Certain exercises may be helpful (Small, 1974), and antidepressants are appropriate in some cases in which depression has caused sleeplessness, bruxism, lassitude, and frequent yawning and these manifestations of depression have caused pain.

Another form of headache that is common but perhaps little known to psychiatrists often follows minor or major head trauma. This occurs in the posttraumatic syndrome, a form of traumatic encephalopathy that also involves giddiness, irritability, sensitivity to noise, and minor memory and concentration difficulties. Lishman (1968) noted that the symptoms were unrelated to either the extent or location of brain damage. Jacobsen (1969), however, noted that the symptoms were more likely to occur if the patient had been rendered unconscious at the time of impact. He observed that the headaches usually stopped within two months of the injury and that most patients were free of all symptoms within four years. This syndrome is not usually associated with radiographic or electroencephalographic changes and many have questioned its organic basis, suggesting that the symptoms resolve, "when the lawsuit arising from the injury is settled (two months to four years usually)." The distinctiveness of the syndrome argues against this psychosomatic view of its etiology, in our opinion, as does the fact that it may occur in individuals with no history of psychosomatic disease or pending lawsuits.

HYSTERIA

Hysteria is a much abused word. It can be used to refer to a *personality type* or to a *psychosomatic reaction* (conversion) or, in a pejorative way, to indicate a generalized *disorganized response to stress* (e.g., hysteria). In our discussion we will ignore the third use of the term.

The *hysterical personality* has been described as vain, egocentric, labile, excitable, dramatic, attention-seeking, overly conscious of sex, provocative but frigid, dependent, and demanding. Though this label is applied to both men and women, it is most often attached to attractive, overly madeup, underdressed, seductive, and exhibitionistic women. It is not an uncommon personality type.

The hysterical personality type is encountered only in a minority of those who manifest hysterical (conversion) symptoms (Ljungberg, 1957). Chodoff and Lyons (1958) found that of 17 patients they considered to have conversion hysteria, only three had hysterical personalities. Stephens and Kamp (1962) found only nine hysterical personalities among 100 patients with conversion hysteria. Conversion symptoms are probably more prevalent among people with hysterical personalities than in the general population, but this is by no means an obligatory association (Zeigler et al., 1960; Zeigler and Imboden, 1962). Hysterical psychosis is also seen in patients with hysterical personalities (see ch. 3).

Our discussion of hysteria will be limited mainly to those *conversion reactions* that can be confused with neurological illnesses. By conversion reactions we mean the loss or impairment of such normal neurological functions as seeing, moving, feeling, swallowing, and so on, which does not result from physiological abnormalities. The differentiation of conversion symptoms from neurological disease is a frequent problem in neurological, medical, and psychiatric practice.

Perley and Guze (1962) developed an elaborate and restrictive system for diagnosing hysteria (Briquet's syndrome). They assigned the diagnosis if patients had (1) a dramatic or complicated medical history before age 35, (2) a minimum of 15 symptoms of (45) distributed in at least nine of ten categories defined by the authors, and (3) no medical diagnosis that adequately explained their symptoms. For six to eight years, Perley and Guze studied a group of 39 patients in whom these criteria were met. Of these patients, 90 percent did not develop any other illness that might have explained their symptoms. The patients' tendency to develop further psychosomatic complaints continued over the years. Thus, the criteria put forth by Perley and Guze for diagnosing hysteria were fully validated. This study called attention to the importance of a thoroughly detailed history in establishing a correct diagnosis for patients suspected of hysterical conversion reaction.

On examining the criteria used by Perley and Guze, however, one finds that the hyperventilation syndrome could cause 18 of the symptoms distributed in seven of their ten categories. With only a few other complaints, the hyperventilation syndrome, a psychophysiological reaction, could thus satisfy their strict criteria. Most of our patients with hyperventilation syndrome (see p. 287) had seen gastroenterologists and/or cardiologists for their related symptoms and had excessive bodily concerns manifested by frequent visits to physicians for minor problems and menstrual and sexual difficulties. In other words, most of these patients with the hyperventilation syndrome had histories resembling those of hysterical patients.

Some physicians believe that hysteria, as defined by these criteria, can be differentiated from "isolated" conversion symptoms. In our experience, conversion symptoms rarely occur in isolation. When doctors label unexplained findings "conversion reaction" in patients lacking a history of hypochondriasis, psychophysiological reactions (chief among which is the hyperventilation syndrome), and/or other conversion reactions, the diagnosis is almost invariably wrong. We have found that two criteria are extremely important in making a positive diagnosis of conversion reaction. Unless both are present, the diagnosis should be held in doubt. These criteria are (1) that no medical diagnosis explains the patient's symptoms and (2) that there is, even in children, a past history of psychosomatic illness (conversion reaction, hypochondriasis, or psychophysiological reaction).

Table 6-4 shows how helpful the presence or absence of a past history of psychosomatic illness can be in establishing or ruling out a diagnosis of hysteria. Of 12 patients under the care of one of us (JHP) during the 1975-1976 year, for whom the diagnosis of hysteria was initially incorrectly made or incorrectly missed, seven had originally been considered hysterical by the primary physician but ultimately received another diagnosis. In five of these seven, there was no past history of psychosomatic illness. Of the five patients

Table 6-4

Occurrence of Psychosomatic Illnesses in Twelve Patients
Considered To Have Conversion Reactions[a]

Patient	Sex	Age	Chief Complaint	Initial Diagnosis[b]	Past History of Psychosomatic Symptoms	Final Diagnosis
1	F	34	generalized weakness	conversion reaction	−	Parkinson's disease
2	M	40	headache, amnesia	conversion reaction	+	meningitis
3	F	50	seizure	conversion reaction	+	epilepsy
4	F	50	generalized weakness, fatigue	neuresthenia, conversion reaction	−	cerebral metastases
5	F	35	blindness	conversion reaction	−	uveitis-meningitis
6	M	50	headache, ataxia	conversion reaction	−	cerebellar hemorrhage
7	M	32	vertigo, ataxia	hypochondriasis, conversion reaction	−	ependymoma
8	F	21	dyspnea	lactose intolerance, migraine, diaphragmatic flutter	+	conversion reaction
9	F	50	hemi-anesthesia and paresis	epilepsy, migraine, multiple sclerosis	+	conversion reaction
10	M	40	quadriparesis	multiple sclerosis	+	conversion reaction and multiple sclerosis
11	F	40	seizures, paraparesis, ataxia	epilepsy, multiple sclerosis	+	conversion reaction
12	F	36	ataxia, hemiparesis	brain tumor	+	conversion reaction

[a] All patients were examined by one of the authors (JHP) and were part of a total of 485 in- and out-patients seen between July 1, 1975 and July 30, 1976.
[b] Diagnosis of the refering (primary) physician.

referred for treatment of medical conditions in whom the diagnosis of hysteria was eventually established, all had a past history of psychosomatic illness. Conversion reaction was established by a negative, thorough investigation in these patients whose symptoms and course could not be otherwise explained.

Slater and Glithero (1965) made a retrospective study of 85 patients diagnosed as hysterical by various clinicians (presumably on the basis of various criteria) after 10 years had passed. Of the 85 patients with a chart diagnosis of hysteria, they found on follow-up that 22 had later been given a diagnosis of an organic disease that could have explained their initial symptoms. At the time they were diagnosed as hysterical, 19 of the patients had medical illnesses that could have explained their symptoms. Eight had died of their medical conditions. Well over half the total population of "hysterics" had medical problems that were mistaken as psychogenic or that had precipitated emotional reactions. Four patients had committed suicide. Roy (1979) reported that 14 of 22 patients with hysterical seizures had on one or more occasions attempted suicide and 19 of the 22 were clinically depressed at the time of their presentation. This suggests that depression may often occur in patients who manifest conversion symptoms. These studies emphasize the need for cautious and precise medical and psychiatric diagnosis, as the following case illustrates:

A 55-year-old factory worker had been involved in an industrial accident, which injured his back. He had worked for the same company for 15 years and had only rare absences for illness. There was no history of psychiatric or psychosomatic illness. There was a compensation suit pending. The patient was referred to the Department of Orthopedics for evaluation of his back. X-rays showed minor changes of the body of the 12th dorsal vertebra, which could have been related to old trauma, neoplasm, or infection, and it was decided to perform a punch biopsy of that vertebra. One hour after the performance of the biopsy, the patient announced blandly and calmly that he would never walk again. Examination revealed total paraplegia, depressed tendon reflexes in the lower extremities, and normal touch, pinprick, vibration, and position sensation.

His obvious indifference to his circumstances, the clear "secondary gain," and the inability of his physicians to explain how a lesion that destroyed all motor function below the first lumbar segments could fail to cause any sensory symptoms led to the diagnosis of "conversion reaction or malingering." Eight hours after the biopsy, he developed a sensory level of hypalgesia below L_1. A myelogram demonstrated a complete block, and shortly after the myelogram was done, he went into shock and died. At autopsy it was found that he had a metastatic carcinoma of the lung which had invaded his 12th dorsal vertebral body. The punch biopsy had caused extensive hemorrhage that compressed his cord.

Of key importance in this case was the absence of any previous tendency toward hypochondriasis or psychosomatic or conversion reaction. Because of the physicians' inexperience, *"la belle indifférence,"* "secondary gain," and neurological findings that "could not be explained" led them to make the erroneous diagnosis of hysteria. The two classical hallmarks of hysteria, *la belle indifférence* and secondary gain, have been, in our experience, more often misleading than helpful in establishing the diagnosis.

Apparent indifference is often a sign of stoicism, and stoical hospitalized patients are more often seriously ill than hysterical. Indifference to illness is also a common sign of brain damage. This is the basis of the "therapeutic" effect of frontal lobotomy. Many patients with progressive brain disease are "mercifully" indifferent to their desperate condition. Conversely, hysterical individuals may be excited and anxious when they develop conversion symptoms, though it is true that some do manifest *la belle indifférence*. Of the patients referred to (Table 6-4), only three manifested *la belle indifférence*. Two of these had neurological disorders (patients 1 and 7) and one had conversion hysteria (patient 11).

The secondary gain, which refers to the reward for the patient who develops a conversion reaction, is often difficult to identify. Sometimes it is no more than staying in the hospital and avoiding contact with the family, sometimes it may be a more subtle or even a fantasized gain. On the other hand, patients who have been injured in automobile or industrial accidents often have lawsuits or compensation claims pending, which are justified but could be mistaken as "secondary gain" by their physicians. No one has ever put forward criteria by which one can distinguish a "legitimate" from a "secondary" gain. The secondary gain may be quite clear after the diagnosis is established, but as a diagnostic aid, it is almost useless.

It has been our experience that most medical doctors consider a patient hysterical either when the physician cannot imagine an organic lesion that could explain his symptoms or when a patient with a well-known history of psychosomatic illnesses presents himself for examination. Mistakes are made because the physician's diagnostic acumen is naturally a function of his previous experience and his knowledge. No one can know everything, and peculiar facets of difficult cases of organic disease that even the most experienced clinician has not encountered before can appear. Also, the tendency toward psychosomatic illness does not confer immortality, and even hysterics can become sick and die.

Certain organic neurological diseases seem to predispose to conversion. Patients whose judgment is impaired by mental retardation, intoxications or other encephalopathies, encephalitis, brain tumor, or multiple sclerosis may elaborate symptoms and signs or exaggerate real symptoms. This may draw attention away from the real disease, sometimes with tragic results.

It may be worth while to consider some of the classic conversion symptoms that mimic neurological conditions. In doing so, we wish to demonstrate that symptoms that cannot be easily ascribed to an organic lesion constitute an inadequate basis for the diagnosis of hysteria. The diagnosis requires such symptoms *in addition to* a past history of psychosomatic illnesses. Both are necessary; neither is sufficient.

Inability to swallow or feeling a lump in the throat is typical of GLOBUS HYSTERICUS. Normal results on direct examination of the nasal and oral pharynx and on barium swallow studies are sufficient to rule out most lesions that could cause similar symptoms. On the other hand, both myasthenia gravis and polymyositis may begin with intermittent weakness of the swallowing mechanism. At the time of examination, the patient may be able to swallow normally and appear to be well. Similarly, pseudobulbar palsy, which interferes with swallowing, may wax and wane in severity. When unassociated with other signs of neurological disease, such symptoms have been mistakenly considered hysterical.

Hysterical HEMISENSORY LOSS usually involves half the entire body from head to feet and from the extremities to the midline. A pinprick felt normally on one side of the linea alba will not be felt on the other side. Sensory splitting at the exact midline and a shift of perception toward the side of normal sensation are considered by many to be hard-and-fast signs of hysteria; organic hemisensory deficits typically appear 1 or 2 cm toward the anesthetic side of the midline. This is because segmental sensory nerve fibers extend 1 or 2 cm across the midline from the "good" side into the anesthetic side. It is also said that the diagnosis of hysteria can be confirmed by testing vibratory sensation on the skull. A tuning fork placed on the skull or the sternum to one side of midline should be felt by neurological patients no matter which side the hemisensory loss is on because the oscillations of the tuning fork are transmitted throughout the entire bone. If the patient claims not to feel vibrations, he may be considered hysterical.

Unfortnuately, these sensory signs of hysteria are rather unreliable because some patients with neurological diseases report what they think their examiner wishes them to report, claiming that a change in sensation occurs at the midline when in fact this may not be so. In addition, it is conceivable that a minority of patients have a physiologically variant pattern of sensory function in which the anesthesia caused by a brain lesion does, in fact, change at the midline or to the "wrong" side of midline. Patients who report absent vibratory sensation on the anesthesia side of their skull or sternum may in fact feel the vibrations less on that side but report to the examiner that they feel nothing to be "consistent." Whatever the reason, it is an empirical fact that patients with lesions that are undeniably organic—strokes, tumors, demyelinating diseases—have reported sensory changes with characteristics that are considered to be typical of hysteria.

HYSTERICAL HEMIPLEGIA may be diagnosed in the following way: placing his hands underneath the patient's paralyzed heel while the patient is supine, the examiner asks the patient to raise his normal leg. The examiner can thereby determine whether or not the patient is able to move his paralyzed leg because the normal response while raising one leg is to push down with the other. If the patient pushes down with his "paralyzed" leg, the factitious nature of his paralysis should be clear. By reversing the process and asking the patient to raise the paralyzed leg, the examiner can determine whether or not the patient is actually trying to lift it. If the patient does not push down with the good leg, the examiner can conclude that he is not trying to raise the paralyzed leg. This test is only useful in complete hemiplegia, however, and will not help in distinguishing hysterical hemiparesis (which is more common than hysterical hemiplegia) from true hemiparesis. The presence of unilateral changes in deep tendon reflexes, spasticity, and Babinski's provides objective evidence indicating neurological disease. The absence of these alterations, however, cannot establish the diagnosis of hysteria.

PARALYSIS OF THE EXTRAOCULAR MUSCLES, those of the face and the tongue, does not occur in conversion syndromes. Paresis of the cervical muscles, with difficulty elevating the head from a pillow or with drooping of the head onto the chest, is extremely rare. Paralysis of the trunk muscles is also rare. Thus, hysterical paralysis or paresis usually involves one or more of the extremities. Weakness of the leg is more frequently encountered than weakness of the arm.

If the patient is ambulatory, the manner in which he moves, dresses, undresses, and mounts an examining table should be noted; for hysterical paralysis is mainly one of paralysis of movement as opposed to paralysis of individual muscles. The hysteric may complain that all movements at one joint are affected, but the object of the examination is to note the distribution of the paralysis as well as the muscles affected and to determine if the patient can still use the affected muscles to perform movements that he does not realize entail their use. Hysterical weakness implies simultaneous and equal contraction of agonistic and antagonistic muscles.

HYSTERICAL HEMIPARESIS is characteristically associated with "give-way" weakness. By this phrase is meant discontinuous resistance during direct muscle testing. Give-way weakness is absolutely diagnostic of factitious weakness, but occasionally a patient will exaggerate mild, real weakness in order to convince the examiner that he is, in fact, weak. In such cases, the patient may feel that the examiner is going to miss the diagnosis and so he "helps out." Reflex abnormalities, when present, can rule out hysteria, but the absence of such abnormalities will not establish the diagnosis.

Astasia-abasia, or hysterical gait, can sometimes be extremely difficult to differentiate from movement disorders. Physicians routinely place emphasis on the following indications that a disordered gait is hysterical. The patient walks well when unaware that he is being observed, never falls, and does not injure himself. The HYSTERICAL GAIT is usually recognized by its bizarre character and its dissimilarity from any disorder of gait produced by organic disease. In hemiplegia the affected leg is ostentatiously dragged along the ground and not circumducted as in organic hemiplegia. When severe, astasia–abasia will be manifested by the patient's attempting to fall as opposed to the organic patient who does his best to support himself. Some patients who walk with great difficulty, clinging to walls and furniture and to the examiners, manifest normal power and coordination while lying in bed. This kind of inconsistency suggests hysteria.

Since almost all movement disorders are worsened by anxiety, it is not wise to accept without reservation reports by nurses and other staff to the effect that the patient is able to walk nearly normally when unaware that he is being observed. If the patient is made nervous by an examiner or a large group of physicians on rounds, and his movement disorder worsens, this is only natural. Sometimes patients with hysterical gait problems do, in fact, fall and may accidentally hurt themselves so that a history of falls with occasional scrapes and bruises does not necessarily rule out hysteria.

Inconsistency of gait disturbance is common in gait apraxias caused by frontal or diffuse cerebral disease. Peculiarities of affect in such patients and an absence of the Babinski sign may lead to an incorrect diagnosis of hysteria. Formal mental status evaluation is helpful in identifying these patients.

In our experience, most MOVEMENT DISORDERS, whether organic

or hysterical, are likely to cause a certain amount of confusion among clinicians. It is not at all uncommon to find a minority of competent neurologists who will consider a given patient to be either organic or hysterical even in the face of an opposite majority view. Fortunately, there are relatively safe and fairly objective tests for hysteria in such cases: amytal infusion and hypnosis. Amytal is infused intravenously at a rate of 100 mg in 30 seconds until nystagmus develops. This usually requires 250 to 500 mg. As soon as nystagmus develops, the infusion is stopped and the patient is asked to perform the motor task that he previously found difficult. If there is a substantial improvement in his movement disorder, the diagnosis of hysteria is supported. If the gait deteriorates, the diagnosis of organicity is supported. This test is often extremely helpful but it can be misinterpreted. When anxiety is responsible for marked worsening of an organic movement disorder, amytal or hypnosis might occasionally improve the gait by relieving anxiety. When neither deterioration nor improvement is clear cut, no inference about the etiology of the gait disturbance can be made.

It is probably fair to say that hysterical dystonia and/or chorea virtually never occur. It is possible to be misled by certain inconsistencies. Some "inconsistencies" are virtually diagnostic. For example, in torticollis the examiner may not be able to straighten the patient's head even by exerting maximal effort, and yet the patient can often straighten his head considerably by merely touching his forehead with an index finger on the side toward which his head is tilted. This "inconsistency" is unexplained but characteristic of organic dystonia.

HYSTERICAL RIGIDITY increases in proportion to the effort made by the examiner to move the rigid extremity. This feature may also be present in the frontal lobe disorders that lead to "gegenhalten" or counterpull. Gegenhalten is a semivoluntary resistance the patient increasingly offers to passive movement of his limbs. When the examiner attempts to extend the patient's elbow, for example, the patient will resist, and his resistance will increase as the elbow is extended further. Forced grasping may be seen in response to tactile stimulation of the patient's palm by the examiner's fingers. When the examiner attempts to extend the patient's fingers while disengaging his own from the patient's grip, he may encounter counterpull in frontal lobe disorders.

VISUAL HYSTERICAL SYMPTOMS include monocular diplopia, triplopia, tunnel vision, and blindness. Though monocular diplopia is, in most cases, caused by hysteria, ocular pathology such as dislocated lenses, cataracts, and parietal lobe lesions can give rise to it (Kestenbaum, 1961). Triplopia, theoretically a physiological impossibility, was recently reported by a patient under our care who was recovering from well-documented disseminated leukoencephalitis.

A test for the hysterical etiology of tunnel vision depends upon the fact that the normal visual field expands in a cone of vision as the distance from the target to the patient is increased. If the patient's field is identical at 2 meters to what it is at 1 meter from his eye, the inconsistency suggests hysteria. Patients who are blind on the basis of neurological disease usually have no pupillary response to light. In disease of the parietal or occipital lobes, however, cortical blindness may be present and pupillary reflexes will remain normal. If a patient with blindness and normal pupillary responses is presented with a slowly rotating, vertically striped drum and develops involuntary tracking movements (optokinetic nystagmus) his blindness can be considered factitious.

There are two tests that can be useful in detecting unilateral hysterical blindness. The patient is asked to read a line of alternating black and red letters while a red glass is held over the "good" eye. In hysterical blindness the patient will be able to see the red letters with the "bad" eye and will read all the letters in the line. Also, a distorting prism can be placed over the "good" eye and the patient will still be able to perform tasks requiring intact vision. Convergence spasms and blepharospasm (the result of spasm of the orbicularis oculi) can be manifestations of hysterical disturbances of ocular movements. Defects in the lateral and vertical planes of gaze caused by hysteria may induce a kind of coarse nystagmus. However, blepharospasm can also be a sign of Meigs' syndrome, which is an organic involuntary movement disorder.

HYSTERICAL DEAFNESS can be easily demonstrated as the patient can be awakened from sleep by sound. A hysterical reduction of hearing (as opposed to deafness) is difficult to distinguish from organic disease of the ears. Variability of responses to audiological tests can reflect an organic brain syndrome as well as hysteria.

Hysterical amnesias, fugue states, and pseudodementia can also confound the diagnostician. In earlier chapters, particularly the one on epilepsy, we noted that transient fluctuations in consciousness can be associated with epileptic conditions and we suggested some guidelines for diagnosis (p. 23). Hysterical states may partially mimic epilepsy and can be confused with it. It is a rare psychiatrist or neurologist who has not been confronted with a patient who says he does not know who he is, or who he was at a particular time, or where he came from. Such hysterical states are most often seen in times of stress, for instance, among soldiers during war or in individuals indicted for crimes. Characteristics that help to distinguish those with psychogenic amnesia or dissociative states from neurological patients include the following: (1) In hysterical states the patients are able to carry out complex functions during the time of amnesia. (2) Memory loss and shift of identity to another person or personality are usually sudden. (3) The patient's behavior is fairly well integrated in that he usually has enough money to get where he is going and takes time to eat and drink. (4) Loss of memory usually affects a specific section of life or ability, that is, arithmetic or recognition of certain relatives. (5) The transition to a normal state is abrupt. (6) There is no history or physical evidence of neurological disease.

Berrington studied 37 cases of fugue state and noted that depression was a frequent concomitant. Interestingly, he noted that a high proportion of the patients had a history of head injury and he speculated that this may have precipitated the fugue state. He also observed that the patients were usually completely unaware of their identity and past life and acted as if they were in a dream. During the episodes, they could travel and seemed able to answer complex questions adequately. They had either partial or complete amnesia for the episodes.

Even if all the characteristics of amnesia indicate hysteria, unless the past history indicates a psychosomatic tendency the diagnosis should be held in doubt. Other conditions can cause dissociative states. For example, the clearly neurological syndrome of "transient global amnesia," described by Fisher and Adams (1958) and by Shuttleworth and Morris (1966) is marked by periods of confusion and disorientation to time and place that usually last a few hours. Patients in these two studies had no recollection of events and described themselves as feeling strange during the episodes of amnesia. In contrast to the above-mentioned syndromes of hysterical amnesia and fugue state, which usually affect individuals in the third or fourth decade, these patients were all middle-aged or elderly and had a history of hypertension or atherosclerosis. Although they did not lose their identity, they could not retain new information during these episodes. It was hypothesized that the episodes resulted from transient ischemia, specifically ischemia of the mamillary-hippocampal complex.

Complaints of pain are rarely hysterical. Patients who are considered to have HYSTERICAL PAIN syndromes complain of severe pain, but they exhibit none of the physical reactions that would be expected to be associated with pain of organic origin and thus present an appearance that belies their allegations of intense suffering. The diagnosis of hysterical pain may also be applied to patients who are unusually distressed and agitated by their pain. Some of the most common syndromes ascribed to hysteria are headaches, low back pain, abdominal pain, and atypical facial pain.

Many physicians regard low back pain as a common syndrome that can result from hysteria and are likely to consider diagnosis if there is no muscle spasm, if the neurological examination is normal, and if the work-up is completely normal (i.e., anterior-posterior and lateral x-rays of the spine and myelograms are normal). Unfortunately, a complete investigation might also include pelvic and rectal examinations and acid and alkaline phosphatase determinations. It might also include CT scans of the lumbar spine to rule out spinal stenosis, oblique films of the lumbar spine to rule out spondylolysis, and bone scans to rule out osteoid osteoma or inflammatory disease of the articular facets as well as other tests.

An incomplete and negative evaluation can erroneously seem to support the diagnosis of hysteria.

The most common physical cause of "atypical" facial pain is the temporomandibular joint (TMJ) syndrome (Table 6-3). Undiagnosable abdominal pain is very often the result of aerophagia. The statement of many physicians who attend pain clinics to the effect that two-thirds to three-quarters of their patients have solely psychosomatic pain (i.e., hysterical pain) are incorrect in our opinion. Though real pain is often exaggerated by patients, it is the responsibility of the physician to determine its underlying physical cause.

A variety of diagnostic myths that have been perpetuated with regard to pain: (1) *"Continuing pain in patients who have undergone multiple surgical procedures for pain without improvement means the pain is either psychogenic or an undesirable side-effect of surgery."* Often, all this may imply is that the original cause of the pain has not been diagnosed or treated. (2) *"A high intake of analgesics, or patient requests for analgesics more often than every four hours, indicate that the patient's problem is not pain but addiction."* In fact, some analgesics such as meperidine (Demerol hydrochloride) have a shorter duration of action than four hours (Goodman and Gilman, 1975). This drug, the most widely used narcotic analgesic in the United States, prescribed by 60 percent of physicians for acute painful conditions and by 22 percent for chronic conditions associated with pain, induced excitatory effects ranging from mild nervousness to seizures in 47 of 67 cancer patients receiving the drug acutely (Kaido et al., 1983). Mood changes such as apprehension, sadness, and restlessness occurred in some patients who were repeatedly given meperidine. These side-effects correlated with the buildup of the metabolite normeperidine. Therefore, patients with chronic pain who are being treated with increasing doses of meperidine and who manifest nervousness, depression, and tolerance may not be addicted but rather suffering from normeperidine toxicity. (3) *"A lawsuit combined with an undiagnosable pain problem is a sure sign of psychogenic origin. If the lawsuit is settled, the pain will disappear."* The data supporting this common assumption are lacking. Lawsuits are often justified and patients who settle them do not necessarily improve. (4) *"Negative findings on repeated tests and bizarre complaints with no physical findings indicate that pain is psychogenic."* Some of the most bizarre head pains we have seen were easily diagnosed as TMJ syndromes. True, repeated CT scans, EEG's, and standard neurological examinations revealed no abnormalities in these cases, but few physicians routinely palpate the head and face in headache patients. This is essential for the diagnosis of TMJ syndrome. Pain syndromes in other parts of the body may also be diagnosed when the correct test is done.

What we have tried to demonstrate with these examples is that the diagnosis of hysteria can be made in error, even when the conversion symptoms are "classical." It must be exceedingly rare for conversion reaction to be the first manifestation of a psychosomatic tendency. Conversion reactions are nearly always preceded, even in children, by other psychosomatic symptoms, many of which have not resulted in a visit to the physician. Stomachaches and headaches, with frequent school absences, sleep disturbances, and/or school phobia, precede conversion hysteria by many months or years in childhood. Unless there is a history of previous psychosomatic disorders, the diagnosis of conversion reaction should remain open to question. On the other hand, psychosomatic illness is so common, particularly in young women, that its presence should not blind the physician to the possibility of organic disease. Of patients referred for neurological examination, 25 to 40 percent have psychosomatic complaints (Tables 6–1 and 6–2).

Perhaps it is fitting that we have concluded this book with a chapter that deals in part with hysteria. The syndrome was first studied by a neurologist, Jean Martin Charcot (1825–1893), and it provided a springboard for modern psychiatry through the work of one of his most illustrious pupils, Sigmund Freud. It has been designated variously as a neurological syndrome, a psychiatric syndrome, and a disease of society (Vieth, 1965). To a degree it crystallized the dilemma we have had in writing this book: we have had to constantly check ourselves from referring to psychiatric illnesses as "functional," thereby implying a separateness from "organic" illness that does not exist. It should be apparent that almost every abnormal emotional state can be produced by one or more neurological syndromes. It is self-evident that all behavioral symptoms, whatever their etiology, are mediated by the central nervous system, a common pathway for many different pathological processes. Though most conversion syndromes exist in the absence of neurological disease, one wonders why one patient and not another develops hysteria in response to apparently similar life stresses. There is no clear answer to this problem yet. Genetic aspects have been incompletely explored, and we have not been able to identify causative environmental influences. Though our knowledge of hysterical conditions has increased considerably over the years (we no longer believe that the varied symptoms are related to a "wandering uterus," and we have been able to formulate criteria for their diagnosis), our skills are still exercised fundamentally at a descriptive level. This is still true of many neurological and psychiatric conditions. Though we look to basic medical research for the full understanding of these diseases, it behooves us meanwhile to polish our clinical skills and learn what we can from observation and description.

REFERENCES

Berrington, W. P., D. W. Liddell, and G. A. Foulds.   A re-evaluation of the fugue. *J. Ment. Sci.* 102:280, 1956.

Chodoff, P. and H. Lyons.   Hysteria, the hysterical personality and "hysterical" conversion. *Amer. J. Psychiat.* 114:734, 1958.

Christensen, B.   Studies on hyperventilation. II. Electrocardiographic changes in normal man during voluntary hyperventilation. *J. Clin. Invest.* 24:880, 1946.

Dalessio, D. J. (ed).   *Woeff's Headache and Other Head Pain*, 4th ed. Oxford University Press, 1980.

Fisher, C. M. and R. D. Adams.   Transient global amnesia. *Acta Neurol. Scand.* 40 (Suppl. 9):7, 1964.

Friedman, A. P. and H. H. Merritt.   *Headache: Diagnosis and Treatment.* F. A. Davis, Philadelphia, 1959.

Gelenberg, A. J.   The catatonia syndrome. *Lancet* 1:1339, 1976.

Goodman, L. S. and A. Gilman.   *The Pharmacological Basis of Therapeutics.* 5th ed. MacMillan, New York, 1975, p. 256.

Gotoh, F., J. S. Meyer, and Y. Takagi.   Cerebral effects of hyperventilation in man. *Arch. Neurol.* 12:410, 1965.

Jacobson, S. A.   Mechanisms of the sequellae of minor craniocervical trauma. In: *The Late Effects of Head Injury*, A. E. Walker, W. F. Caveness and M. Critchley, eds. C C Thomas, Springfield, Ill., 1969, p. 35.

Kaiko, R. F., K. M. Foley, P. Y. Grabinski, et al.   Central nervous system excitatory effects of meperidine in cancer patients. *Ann. Neurol.* 13:180, 1983.

Kestenbaum, A.   *Clinical Methods of Neuro-ophthalmologic Examination*, 2nd ed. Grune and Stratton, New York, 1961.

Lishman, W. A.   Brain damage in relation to psychiatric disability after head injury. *Brit. J. Psychiat.* 114:373, 1968.

Ljungberg, L.   Hysteria: a clinical, prognostic and genetic study. *Acta Psychiat. Scand. Suppl.* 112, 1957.

Mattson, R. H., G. R. Heninger, B. B. Gallagher, and G. H. Glaser.   Psychophysiological precipitants of seizures in epileptics. *Neurology* 20:406, 1970

McHugh, P. R. and M. F. Folstein.   Psychopathology of dementia: Implications for neuropathology. In: *Congenital and Acquired Cognitive Disorders*. eds. Robert Katzman Assoc. for Res. in Nerv. Ment. Dis. 57:17, 1979. Raven Press, New York.

McKell, T. E. and A. J. Sullivan.   The hyperventilation syndrome in gastroenterology. *Gastroenterology* 9:6, 1947.

Perley, M. J. and S. B. Guze.   Hysteria—the stability and usefulness of clinical criteria. A quantitative study based on a follow-up of six to eight years in 39 patients. *New Eng. J. Med.* 266:421, 1962.

Plum, F. and J. B. Posner.   *Diagnosis of Stupor and Coma*, 2nd ed. Contemporary Neurology Series. F. A. Davis, Philadelphia, 1972.

Roy, A.   Hysterical seizures. *Arch. Neurol.* 36:447, 1979.

Shuttleworth, E. C. and C. E. Morris.   The transient global amnesia syndrome. *Arch. Neurol.* 15:515, 1966.

Slater, E. and E. Glithero.   A follow-up of patients diagnosed as suffering from "hysteria." *J. Psychosom. Res.* 9:9, 1965.

Small, E. W.   Correlation of psychological findings and treatment results in temperomandibular joint pain-dysfunction syndrome. *J. Oral. Surg.* 32:589, 1974.

Stephens, J. H. and Kamp, M.   On some aspects of hysteria: a clinical study. *J. Nerv. Ment. Dis.* 134:305, 1962.

Theodor, W. H. and R. J. Porter.   *Ann. Neuro.* 13:243, 1983.

Veith, I.   *Hysteria*, University of Chicago Press, Chicago, 1965.

Ziegler, F. J. and J. B. Imboden.   Contemporary conversion reactions II: Conceptual model. *Arch. Gen. Psychiat.* 66:279, 1962.

———, ———, and E. Meyer.   Contemporary conversion reactions: clinical study. *Amer. J. Psychiat.* 116:909, 1960.

INDEX